KU-117-756

ICSSPE Perspectives
The Multi-disciplinary Series of Physical Education and Sport Science

By publishing Perspectives, ICSSPE aims to facilitate the application of sport science results to practical areas of sport by integrating the various sport science branches. In each volume of Perspectives, expert contributions from different disciplines address a specific physical education or sport science theme, which has been identified by a group of leading international experts.

ICSSPE editorial board members

Also available in this series:
Published by ICSSPE – www.icsspe.org
Published by Routledge – www.routledge.com/sport

Elite Sport and Sport-for-All
Bridging the Two Cultures?
Edited by Richard Bailey and Margaret Talbot

Sport, Education and Social Policy
The State of the Social Sciences of Sport
Edited by Gudrun Doll-Tepper, Katrin Koenen and Richard Bailey

Physical Activity and Educational Achievement
Insights from Exercise Neuroscience
Edited by Romain Meeusen, Sabine Schaefer, Phillip Tomporowski and Richard Bailey

Sport and Health
Exploring the Current State of Play
Edited by Daniel Parnell and Peter Krustrup

https://routledge.com/sport/series/ICSSPE

Sport and Health

It is a common assumption that sport is good for us and that participation in sport embodies public health benefits. With sport being increasingly used to deliver public health interventions worldwide, this book critically examines the rationale and evidence for sport as a public health policy tool. Featuring contributions from the United Kingdom, United States, Europe and Australia, it sheds new light on an emerging field of research which has significant implications for public health across the globe.

Each chapter looks at the effectiveness of sport interventions across the lifespan for biological, psychological and social benefits, including those that utilise a settings-based approach to health promotion such as schools and professional sport clubs. Drawing on cutting-edge research which examines policy and practice at community and elite levels, this book addresses key topics such as education, engaging children and young adults, mental health, sport sponsorship and volunteering.

Sport and Health: Exploring the Current State of Play is important reading for all students, scholars and policy makers with an interest in the sociology of sport, physical activity and public health.

Daniel Parnell is a Senior Lecturer in Business Management at Manchester Metropolitan University, United Kingdom. Dan is a collegiate scholar with a growing reputation for current, policy-relevant, empirically-rich research in areas that closely connect with sport business and management, who engages closely with the sport industry and can connect across multi-disciplinary areas and research programmes. Dan manages a number of research projects involving managing change and project evaluation using both quantitative and qualitative research methods regionally and internationally. He currently works with a number of professional sport clubs and national governing bodies in England and internationally. He has worked with the Premier League, Football League, Football Foundation (United Kingdom's largest sports charity) and the International Olympic Committee on research with policy makers, commissioners, chief executive officers, managers, coaches and participants. Currently, Dan leads the research on a unique

Masters in Sport Directorship executive education programme, coordinates a global platform for football researchers as a founder member ('The Football Collective') and is the Research Director for a platform to share community sport research with policy makers and practitioners ('Connect Sport').

Peter Krustrup is Professor of Sport and Health Sciences at the University of Southern Denmark, Odense, Denmark and an Honorary Visiting Professor at Exeter University, United Kingdom. Peter has authored 225 original research articles, with a total of 9,000 citations, achieving an H-index of 49. His three main research areas are muscle physiology, human performance and health effects of sport. Currently, Peter is continuing his pioneering work on the fitness and health effects of football and other team sports. His research includes investigations of the cardiovascular, metabolic and musculoskeletal effects of team sports compared with other types of physical activity (PA), and the potential of team sports for preventing and treating lifestyle diseases. He achieved the UEFA Pro Licence in 2017 and worked as assistant coach of the Danish Women's National Team that won a bronze medal at Euro 2013. He is an editor of the *European Journal of Applied Physiology* and the *British Journal of Sports Medicine* and has acted as guest editor of two Football for Health special issues of the *Scandinavian Journal of Medicine and Science in Sports*. He was chairman of the organising committee for the World Congress of Science in Football in 2015 (WCSF, 2015) and the Copenhagen Consensus Conference 2016 on Children, Youth and Physical Activity. He has received several research dissemination awards, including the Men's Health Award and the Faculty of Science Media Award.

Sport and Health

Exploring the Current State of Play

Edited by
Daniel Parnell and
Peter Krustrup

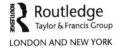

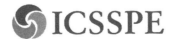

LONDON AND NEW YORK

First published 2018
by Routledge
2 Park Square, Milton Park, Abingdon, Oxon OX14 4RN

and by Routledge
711 Third Avenue, New York, NY 10017

Routledge is an imprint of the Taylor & Francis Group, an informa business

British Library Cataloguing-in-Publication Data
A catalogue record for this book is available from the British Library.

Library of Congress Cataloging-in-Publication Data
Names: Parnell, Daniel, editor. | Krustrup, Peter, editor.
Title: Sport and Health : Exploring the Current State of Play / Edited by Daniel Parnell and Peter Krustrup.
Description: Abingdon, Oxon ; New York, NY : Routledge, 2018. |
Series: ICSSPE Perspectives |
Includes bibliographical references and index.
Identifiers: LCCN 2017019508| ISBN 9781138290228 (hardback) |
ISBN 9781315266459 (ebook)
Subjects: LCSH: Sports—Sociological aspects. | Sports—Psychological aspects. | Sports—Health aspects. | Physical fitness—Health aspects. | Public health.
Classification: LCC GV481 .S663 2018 | DDC 306.4/83—dc23
LC record available at https://lccn.loc.gov/2017019508

ISBN: 978-1-138-29022-8 (hbk)
ISBN: 978-1-315-26645-9 (ebk)

Typeset in Sabon
by Florence Production Ltd, Stoodleigh, Devon, UK

Dedication

It has been a pleasure to collaborate on this work and hope it is the first of many. I would like to extend my gratitude to collaborators and chapter authors for their sterling work in creating excellent submissions and a quality addition to the sport and health literature. For me, this completes a number of years working in sport and health as a practitioner in the Sport and Physical Activity Alliance in the City of Liverpool (UK), through to managing an applied research unit within the Goodison Park, the Home of Everton Football Club – the Everton Active Family Centre. I am thankful to my ongoing network of support both colleagues and friends at the Business School at Manchester Metropolitan University, and the friendship and support of Kathryn Curran, Paul Widdop, Peter Millward, Ed Cope and Richard Bailey. Further, I would like to thank the International Council for Sport Science and Physical Education, both Katrin Koenen and Richard Bailey for their ongoing support. A special thank you to Cecily Davey and Simon Whitmore at Taylor and Francis (Routledge) for their patience, support and guidance. Finally, I would like to thank Sarah, Niamh, George and Betty for their ongoing love, care and belief.

Dan

From a personal point of view, this book is a milestone. My wife Birgitte, and I started out in 2003 with pioneering studies on the fitness and health effects of football for homeless men, for low-level seniors and for inactive computer-nerds (FC Zulu). Having worked with sport and health for 15 years, on descriptive studies, feasibility studies, small-scale randomised controlled trials and large-scale implementation projects, it is a great pleasure to see this book a reality. To illuminate the impact of sport on health and the potential of sport to drive improved health globally, it is of utmost importance to adopt a holistic research approach with contributions from multiple research fields. In order to understand the differential effects of various types of exercise on the risk of lifestyle diseases, we have to combine sports science approaches with methodologies, expertise and experience from sports medicine, and in order to understand the implementation potential of an exercise concept and its ability to make sustainable lifestyle changes, sports science and sports medicine research have to be combined with research in sports psychology, sociology and pedagogics. From that perspective, I have been privileged to work with many outstanding collaborators within each of these research fields, and I would like to thank them all for their valuable contributions. I am particularly thankful to my current and former research institutions – University of Southern Denmark, Exeter University and Copenhagen University – for supporting my sport and health work, and to numerous institutions around the world for supporting my colleagues in their work. I hope that many more will join in this work in the future. Furthermore, a special thanks to the Danish FA, the Danish Sports Confederation, FIFA, UEFA and IOC for their willingness to develop and implement evidence-based Sport for All concepts. This book, which brings together many years of research from many fields of expertise, provides a comprehensive up-to-date overview of the health effects of sport and how sport can be used as a vehicle for improving world health. On that basis, this book, the first on sport and health, may also be considered a milestone that can inspire sports organisations and policy-makers to get the full health benefit from sports. Thanks to Andrea, Sarah, Birgitte and my entire family. Finally, I would like to thank Dan for taking the initiative to produce this book and for working so hard to make it happen.

Peter

Contents

Figures

Tables

Contributors

Shawn M. Arent is currently an Associate Professor in the Department of Kinesiology and Health at Rutgers University. He is also the Director of the Rutgers Center for Health and Human Performance and Director of the Graduate Programme in Kinesiology and Applied Physiology. He is a Certified Strength and Conditioning Specialist with Distinction with the National Strength and Conditioning Association and a Fellow in the American College of Sports Medicine as well as the International Society of Sports Nutrition. His research focuses on the relationship between physical activity and stress and the implications for health and performance, with an emphasis on underlying biological and behavioral mechanisms. His recent work has focused on physiological responses to training-related stressors and their contribution to optimal performance and recovery. Dr. Arent also provides performance enhancement advice for youth, high school, collegiate and professional athletes in a number of sports, including soccer, hockey, football, wrestling, baseball, softball, gymnastics, rowing and cycling. He is currently the Sport Science Coordinator for the Texas Rangers (MLB), is on the national staff for the US Soccer Federation, and works closely with a number of teams at Rutgers University.

Richard Bailey PhD FRSA is Senior Researcher at the International Council of Sport Science and Physical Education, based in Berlin, Germany. Richard is a former University Professor, and he has carried out research in a wide range of topics connected with human development and sport. He was a leading contributor to the Designed to Move initiative (www.designedtomove. org), and numerous other international projects.

Søren Bennike is Post-Doctoral researcher at the 'Department of Nutrition, Exercise and Sports' and 'Copenhagen Centre for Team Sport and Health' at the University of Copenhagen. He completed a PhD degree in 2016 in the area of Humanities and Social Sport Sciences at the University of Copenhagen. His main research areas are rooted in policy and politics, institutions and organisations, implementation and innovation – all related to sport.

Ed Cope is Lecturer in Sports Coaching and Performance Science at the University of Hull. He is an established researcher in the field of sports coaching and youth sport. He has an expertise in qualitative research, particularly the use of visual research methodologies with young people and children. Ed has published this type of work in the leading journals in sport, health and exercise sciences, and has recently received an Advanced Research Grant from the International Olympic Committee, which investigated young children perceptions of the outcomes of their participation in sport and physical activity, and what these children valued about their participation, and a grant from Sport England focussed on the factors that explain children's attitudes and behaviours towards sport and physical activity. In addition to this, Ed researches, writes and publishes in the area of children's coaching pedagogy. Ed was also a senior researcher within a team of people who evaluated the Premier League's Physical Education and School Sport Programme. In addition to this, Ed is currently the Principal Researcher evaluating sport coach UK's online learning platform and its impact on coaches' beliefs, behaviour and practice. Central to this project is exploring how young people feel about the coaching they receive.

Tara Coppinger is a Lecturer and Researcher in the Department of Sport, Leisure and Childhood Studies at Cork Institute of Technology, Cork, Ireland. She has undertaken research in the United Kingdom, New Zealand and Ireland focusing on the promotion of physical activity and healthy eating in school children and is currently leading one such project in cork city and county (Project Spraoi) that has been delivered to over 3,000 children and more than 200 staff. She is a qualified netball coach and also a registered public health nutritionist.

Kathryn Curran is an Applied Researcher and Senior Lecturer in Physical Activity, Exercise and Health at Leeds Beckett University, United Kingdom. Kathryn's primary research interests and outputs centre on the design, implementation and evaluation of community physical activity and health interventions with hard-to-reach groups. Some of her work and research with hard-to-reach populations has been championed by the World Health Organization as an example of best practice.

Peter Elsborg is currently doing his PhD at the University of Copenhagen. His main research interests are motivation and self-regulation within the context of sport and exercise. His current research focuses on exercise specific volition and motivations influence on the task of weight loss maintenance following an intensive lifestyle intervention. Peter also has experience working as an applied sport psychology consultant with young elite athletes.

Emma George is a Lecturer in Health and Physical Education at Western Sydney University. With a background in physical activity and health promotion, her research aims to promote lifelong physical activity and improve health outcomes. Emma's research has involved working with middle-aged men, sport fans, older adults, emergency service volunteers, youth in organised sport and culturally diverse populations, and she has a particular interest in community engagement and health promotion initiatives delivered through sport.

Timothy J. Hall is a Senior Lecturer and Researcher within the School of Business at the University of Western Sydney who has a passion for the customer experience. Tim has worked with a number of commercial sporting organisations investigating the various elements which combine to create an overall fan experience, with a particular focus on the game day experience. This interest has seen Tim investigate aspects of the journey to and from game days as well as crucial elements within stadia such as hospitality offerings and stadium design.

Oscar Lederman is an Accredited Exercise Physiologist at the Prince of Wales Hospital, South Eastern Sydney Local Health District and a PhD Candidate at UNSW, Sydney, Australia. Oscar coordinates and supervises the Exercise Physiology programme at Eastern Suburbs Mental Health (incorporating inpatient units and community services). His research interests include: translational research, motivation for behaviour change and cardiometabolic risk factors among young people at risk of psychosis.

Keith Parry is a Lecturer with the School of Business at Western Sydney University. His research interests are based on the study of sport, with a focus on the sociology of sport, sports fandom and the spectator experience. His research has made use of innovative methodologies, such as Auto-ethnography, to provide a greater understanding of sports fans. He has collaborated with international colleagues to publish studies on international sports fandom and he has co-edited a book examining the relationship between football codes and community. He has recently published a series of interactive iBooks on the subject of Sport Entertainment while his knowledge and expertise have also been recognised with invitations to write for websites such as The Conversation and The Allrounder, allowing him to disseminate his knowledge to a wide audience.

Matthew Philpott is Executive Director of the European Healthy Stadia Network CIC, a social enterprise based in the United Kingdom working with sports clubs, stadium operators and governing bodies of sport to develop stadia as health promoting settings. With a MA and PhD in Social Sciences from the University of Warwick, Matthew now has over 12 years' experience of advocacy work and project management of public health and sports related projects in the private and NGO sectors.

Andy Pringle is Reader in Physical Activity and Public Health, he is 'Research Lead' for the Physical Activity and Health Subject and Chair of the Research

Ethics Review Group in the Institute of Sport, Physical Activity and Leisure at Leeds Beckett University, Leeds, United Kingdom. He is a Fellow of the Royal Society of Public Health and a Topic Expert (Physical Activity) on the Public Health Advisory Committee for the National Institute for Health and Care Excellence.

Laila Ottesen is Associated Professor at the Department of Exercise and Sport Sciences and Member of the steering committee at 'Copenhagen Centre for Team Sport and Health'. Both situated at the University of Copenhagen. She holds a PhD degree in European Ethnology from the University of Copenhagen. Her main research areas are rooted in sociology of sport and health summed up in the keywords: Voluntary Organisations, Implementation, Sport Policy, Health Promotion and Prevention.

Simon Rosenbaum is an NHMRC Early Career Fellow in the School of Psychiatry, UNSW Sydney, Australia, and an honorary fellow at the Black Dog Institute. He is a Director of Exercise and Sports Science Australia.

David Rowe, FAHA, FASSA is Professor of Cultural Research, Institute for Culture and Society, Western Sydney University and Honorary Professor, Faculty of Humanities and Social Sciences, University of Bath, UK. His books include *Sport, Culture and the Media: The Unruly Trinity* (McGraw-Hill, second edition, 2004), *Global Media Sport: Flows, Forms and Futures* (Bloomsbury, 2011), *Sport Beyond Television* (co-authored, Routledge, 2012), and *Sport, Public Broadcasting, and Cultural Citizenship: Signal Lost?* (co-edited, Routledge, 2014).

Morten Bredsgaard Randers is a Post Doc at the University of Southern Denmark, Odense, Denmark. He earned his PhD in 2011 from the University of Copenhagen with the thesis 'Physiological demands, fitness effects and cardiovascular health benefits of recreational football'. He has authored ~50 original research articles in the field of football – fitness and health effects for untrained and recreational players as well as testing and performance enhancement in elite football players. He has worked as a fitness coach in a Danish Premier League club and for the Danish elite referees.

Knud Ryom currently has a PhD. position with Copenhagen University and a part-time lecture position at Aarhus University. His main research interest is football, sports psychology and sport as integrative tool. His current research focus on social resilience, life-skills, social capital and active citizenship developed through a community psychological approach in a socially deprived area in Copenhagen, Denmark. Knud is also chairman of DIFO (the Danish sports psychological association).

Robert Snape is Reader in Leisure and Sport at the University of Bolton. He has published research on physical activity and health among British South Asian populations and has led funded evaluation projects in this field.

He is also Head of the Centre for Worktown Studies and has published on the history of leisure and sport in Bolton, the location of Mass Observation's Worktown study.

Brendon Stubbs is a clinical academic physiotherapist, with an interest in the mental-physical health interface, physical activity and healthy ageing based at Kings College London, United Kingdom and the South London and Maudsley NHS Foundation Trust. Brendon continues to provide clinical care for people in secure and acute mental health services and has published over 250 academic papers in the last 5 years on the aforementioned areas.

Lone Friis Thing is Associated Professor at the Department of Exercise and Sport Sciences, University of Copenhagen. She is head of the section 'Sport, Individual and Society' and head of three master programmes. She holds a PhD degree from Department of Sociology, University of Copenhagen. Her main research areas are rooted in health promotion and prevention in relation to sport and physical activity.

Davy Vancampfort is a Post-Doctoral Researcher at the KU Leuven Belgium. His research focuses on the importance of physical activity within the multi-disciplinary treatment of people with mental illness. He is chair of the International Organization of Physical Therapists in Mental Health research group on schizophrenia.

Alan Walker is currently a PhD candidate in the Kinesiology and Applied Physiology programme at Rutgers University, United States. He received his BS from Salisbury University ('12), his MS from Rutgers University ('14), and earned his CSCS in 2016. His current research focus is on the effects of training stressors on blood biomarkers, health, and performance in collegiate athletes, with his primary focus being on the female athlete. He has experience working with sports such as soccer, lacrosse, field hockey, swimming and diving, hockey, and boxing at both the collegiate and professional level.

Johan Wikman holds a position as Academic Officer at the Centre for Team Sports and Health, University of Copenhagen. His research interests are within the fields of talent development, sport psychological training, motivation and the psychological aspects of team games. Johan is also a board member of the Danish Sport Psychological Association and works as a sport psychology consultant for elite athletes.

Stephen Zwolinsky is a Research Officer within the Institute of Sport, Physical Activity and Leisure at Leeds Beckett University, Leeds, United Kingdom. He has extensive experience of undertaking applied research and consultancy projects for a range of organisations including the NHS, local government departments and commercial enterprises. He has published extensively within the field of physical activity and health in a range of different formats including project reports, blogs, books, letters and journal articles. He is currently funded by Leeds City Council to determine the prevalence and clustering of the proximal lifestyle risk factors that underpin non-communicable disease and their links to long-term conditions.

Introduction

In developing our idea and subsequently gathering the contributions to *Sport and Health: Exploring the Current State of Play*, we had a number of objectives. First, we wanted to offer an insight into an emerging field of research, with significant policy and practical implications. In doing so, we hoped to have a collection of articles that could stimulate politicians, policy makers, analysts, researchers and academics, sports developers, educationists and coaches, and the general public. Many of these stakeholders in sport and health who frequently assume that physical activity is good for us and that participation in sport can contribute to fight inactivity and are interested in knowing how sport can contribute to public health. Sport is being increasingly adopted as a vehicle to deliver public health intervention worldwide. On top of this, health issues in sport whether grassroots, amateur or elite contexts have become more common. In this respect, it appeared important to offer a collection that looked more closely at some of these issues. Alongside this, we have seen many professional sports evolve into hyper-commodified contexts. At the same time, the global economic downturn has changed state and regional investment in local sport and leisure. As such, it is hoped this book looks at some of the underpinning rationale supporting this approach across the lifespan, for biological, psychological and social benefits, in professional sporting contexts and through national and local perspectives.

Our second objective was that we wanted to attract a range of emerging and leading researchers in the field of sport and health. For us, the broad remit of sport and health is still an emerging field of unknowns. The intention of this is to allow researchers from across a multi-disciplinary background, involved in research across the lifespan in grassroots, community, amateur, elite and professional sport contexts to continue the academic discourse surrounding sport and health. It is hoped that this extension of the debate will help generate new understanding, new ideas, new collaborations and inspire emerging scholars to continue to build upon our current understanding in their respective discipline and research context. In places, offering a meaningful way forward in research and practice. Alongside exploring some of the more recent key research areas and applied practitioners and policy issues, to build on this existing research, and look to the future.

Finally, as the research continues to grow that builds the case for physical activity as a form of medicine that is good for us and our health, we now know there is a need to understand and critically explore what role sport can play. This book will critically describe the use of various types of sport to increase activity and to promote health aspects, where applicable, related to the type and intensity of sporting activity.

The book is divided into four themes. Richard Bailey provides a chapter to encapsulate theme one: *Sport participation and health: the evidence*. In his chapter, Richard is asking whether sport can play a role as part of the physical activity agenda. It focuses on the largest population of sports players, children and young people, and their most populous group, namely recreational players. It has been suggested that there has been a lack of critical discussion of the claims made on behalf of sport as a form of healthy physical activity, and these are considered. The empirical literature that relates to this question is reviewed and analysed, in order to achieve some sense of the potential of sport as a public health setting. Part of the difficulty with considerations of sport as physical activity is that the concepts of 'sport' and 'physical activity' are often ill-defined and misapplied, and the benefits identified for each are too-often conflated. It is hoped this chapter offers a degree of clarity on this topic for readers.

The second theme includes three-chapter contributions from Tara Coppinger, Ed Cope, and Andy Pringle and Stephen Zwolinsky. *Sport and health across the lifespan* is the primary focus of the second theme. Tara begins with examining sport, health and physical activity in children. As childhood obesity has grown significantly in recent years, a lack of physical activity physical activity linked, in part, to a fall in participation in sport, has been widely acknowledged as a key contributor. Similarly, the relationship between childhood physical activity and the impact this has on (i) child health, (ii) adult health and (iii) lifelong health behaviours, attracts widespread interest. Yet, the evidence to support these relationships remains relatively weak and much of the existing research focuses on adults. Children, with their unique behaviours and characteristics, require focused research and interventions that can improve long-term health outcomes. This chapter aims to discuss current evidence, address any misconceptions and enhance our understanding of the potential relationships between physical activity, sport and health. Key factors that influence children's participation at the macro, micro and individual level will also be discussed and identifying what sport and physical activity professionals can do to increase participation in both the physical activity and sporting domains are also addressed.

Ed Cope then offers a chapter that positions sport and physical activity in a child-friendly manner. Ed's chapter had two main purposes. First, the chapter discussed what constituted positive experiences, with a specific focus placed on what this looks like for children. Second, the available evidence was reflected upon and a judgement made of what is actually known about what children consider led to them experiencing physical activity and sports in a positive manner. The aim of the chapter is to offer a more critical take on the research evidence that has previously been afforded. This is particularly important for those involved in child-focused interventions whether at a policy, or practice level.

This theme has a clear focus on children and young people, and how sport and physical activity is delivered to these groups. Equally important is how physical activity and sport is delivered to older adults. The final chapter in this theme, by Andy Pringle and Stephen Zwolinsky discusses the literature on older adults, physical activity and public health. Older adults are a key physical activity and health priority. This chapter explores the definitions of older adults, the physical activity recommendations and levels of participation. The chapter makes the case for promoting physical activity with older adults including, the health consequences of physical inactivity, alongside the health benefits. For older adults, the adoption of physical activity is predicated by significant and wide-ranging determinants. In this respect and recognising the complex and specific needs that older adults have when adopting and maintaining physical activity, we share the key considerations for promoting and implementing physical activity interventions using case studies, including sport-based examples, that are also framed by theoretical frameworks and guidance.

Theme three focuses on the *political, social and psychological dimensions of sport and health* with four-chapter contributions. The first chapter considers health through state supported voluntary sport clubs, by Søren Bennike, Lone Friis Thing and Laila Ottesen. Søren *et al.* explore a very important part of the sport sector, not just in Europe, but globally. State supported, non-profit sport clubs play an important role in the sport sector, and make a number of contributions across society at a community, family and individual level. This chapter explores the role of voluntary sport clubs in delivering health outcomes, with a particular lens on Denmark. Understanding that this part of the sport sector links to and is affected by health outcomes is an important consideration for contemporary sport and health debates and this chapter offers key considerations for policy transfer. An element of voluntary sport club delivery is team sports. Team sports are assumed by many in policy and politic arenas to be a panacea to many social and health concerns. The next chapter in this theme, by Johan M. Wikman, Peter Elsborg and Knud Ryom, explores the psychological benefits of team sport. The chapter discusses if team sport offer psychological benefits above and beyond the benefits that can be acquired through individual physical activity. Psychological benefits of physical activity in general were compared to benefits of team sport. The chapter offers important considerations including that team sport holds an unused potential for psychological health improvement. This potential stems from the social qualities of team sport that both have a direct impact on psychological health and are indirectly important because it elicits higher motivation than individual physical activity. The chapter also provides considerations on the implications for practice and research.

Mental health is a key policy agenda across the globe. Indeed, more than one in five people will experience a mental disorder at some point throughout their lifetime. The third chapter in this theme, by Simon Rosenbaum, Davy Vancampfort, Oscar Lederman and Brendon Stubbs discusses mental health, physical activity and sport. Mental disorders are strongly associated with poor physical health including preventable conditions such as diabetes, heart disease and metabolic syndrome. Low participation in physical activity, including sport and exercise, and poor cardiorespiratory fitness are modifiable risk factors that can impact both physical and mental health. This chapter outlines the evidence for physical activity as an integrated component of both promoting mental wellbeing among the healthy population, and as a component of treatment among people experiencing mental illness. The final chapter of this theme is led by Robert Snape and Kathryn Curran, who discuss sport, physical activity and public health policy. The chapter, although Anglo centric discusses decades of government policy on sport which has assumed sport to be an effective means of increasing participation in physical activity. The chapter discusses how this impacts the funding for sport to increase participation and how physical activity has gained an increasingly prominent position in public health policy over the last 15 years in the United Kingdom. The chapter traces the historical development of policy in physical activity and sport to argue for a more holistic policy framework in which to address the need for increased rates of participation in physical activity for health.

The fourth theme of the book, which highlights *unique questions to the sport and health debate* consists of four-chapter contributions. Shawn M. Arent and Alan J. Walker offer an insight in the unique challenges of elite sport. The chapter highlights that participation in sport provides a number of benefits; however, elite sport presents a unique situation. The same positive outcomes that give the impression of a sort of 'superhuman' nature to these athletes may often be compromised in the pursuit of success. Despite enhanced performance, elite athletes are often willing to resort to performance-enhancing drugs, playing through injury and pain, permanent damage, addiction, and risk brain damage through concussion to win. This chapter will examine this conundrum and explore the positive and negative impacts of participation in elite sport on long-term health. Additionally, potential mechanisms for protecting athletes and helping them understand consequences are discussed.

Following this, Peter Krustrup and Morten Bredsgaard Randers examine the prevention and treatment of non-communicable diseases. Physical inactivity is the primary cause of most non-communicable diseases, which, according to the World Health Organization, are by far the leading cause of death in the world. The chapter highlights that high-intensity training seems superior to moderate- and low-intensity exercise for inducing cardiovascular and metabolic health benefits, and combination with strength training is recommended. While showing that small-sided recreational football offers an excellent combination of these types of training, with high heart rates and a high number of intense actions leading to broad-spectrum health-related improvements in cardiovascular, metabolic and musculoskeletal fitness. The chapter then discusses how small-sided recreational football, especially the Football Fitness concept, has been shown to be feasible for prevention and treatment for participants across the lifespan irrespective of gender, training status and technical skills, and can therefore serve as a model for large-scale health promotion through sports.

The third chapter of this final theme explores healthy sport consumption within professional sport stadia. In their chapter, Keith D. Parry, David Rowe, Emma S. George and Timothy J. Hall provide an analysis of the role of food and drink in the Australian sports fan experience. It contextualises the modern sporting experience and recent shifts towards a more mediated consumption of sport while recognising the influences of tradition and masculinity on consumption patterns. The cost, quality and healthiness of food and beverages are acknowledged as areas of dissatisfaction for fans. The potential for stadiums to play an important role in health promotion is discussed and the need for a holistic approach, incorporating measures such as a healthy eating policy, is highlighted. The sponsorship of venues by fast food and alcoholic beverage companies is identified as a key obstacle to stadium-based health promotion. The chapter concludes with a set of recommendations for venues to follow in order to promote healthy lifestyle choices.

The final chapter of the book extends upon the idea of a settings-based approach to health. Here Daniel Parnell, Kathryn Curran and Matthew Philpott offer a focused lens on the role of professional sports stadia and in amateur sport settings for health promotion. The chapter explores how these settings have been utilised to deliver health improvement interventions linked to the European Healthy Stadia Network (hereon Healthy Stadia). Healthy Stadia is a social enterprise based in the United Kingdom with over 300 members from a cross-section of European countries. Healthy Stadia endorses the concept of promoting public health through sports settings, and provides a platform to inform policy makers and promote good practice. This chapter aims to provide industry and research insights and considerations for promoting health at sport stadia settings through three case study examples, while offering some reflections for future interventions and research.

The collection of chapters provides a breadth of contributions that cover a range of disciplines on some of the major topics concerning sport and health. The individual chapters offer depth for those considering exploring specific topics, yet the full collection offers the reader whether involved in applied practice or scholarship and up-to-date and in depth insight into sport and health, and the current state of play.

Daniel Parnell
Peter Krustrup

Chapter 1

Is sport good for us?

Understanding youth sport as a public health setting

Richard Bailey

Introduction

It is widely accepted that regular physical activity can result in a range of positive outcomes (Bailey, Hillman, Arent, *et al.*, 2013). It is also acknowledged that large numbers of people around the world are not active enough to reap these benefits, often to the extent that they suffer life-threatening diseases (Kohl, Craig, Lambert, *et al.*, 2012). Consequently, governments and international agencies are investing considerable sums of money promoting physical activity in different settings. One setting that has received a great deal of attention has been sport (Commission of the European Communities, 2007; Centers for Disease Control and Prevention, 2000). However, discussions of the possible role sport might play in physical activity promotion have been highly contested. Some point to the fact that, by its nature, sport involves activity, and that it is often popular, especially among children and young people (Sport for Development and Peace International Working Group, 2008). Others claim that the competitive and potentially exclusionary character of sport is what makes it inappropriate in the context of health promotion (Waddington, 2000). The result of this contest has been conflicting messages: for example, many national governments produce enthusiastic statements celebrating sport's potential contribution to health, while at the same time, almost all of these same governments' policy documents for health either omit or marginalise sport (Michelini and Thiel, 2013).

This chapter addresses precisely this question: Can sport play a role as part of the physical activity agenda? It focuses on the largest population of sports players, children and young people, and their most populous group, namely recreational players. The empirical literature on the contribution that sport might be able to make to physical activity is reviewed, and analysed. The accusation that there has been a lack of critical discussion of the many claims on behalf of sport and exercise (Donnelly, 1996) is a fair one, and the hope is that this chapter will contribute to this much-needed discussion.

Defining terms

It is always useful to be clear about the terms we use, and lack of clarity can be the cause of unnecessary misunderstanding and confusion. This has not always been the case with the current topic with phrases like physical activity, sport, physical education and exercise sometimes employed by researchers with casual abandon. So, it is worthwhile spending a little time clarifying how some of the key terms will be used here.

Many governmental and sports agencies adopt the definition in the Council of Europe's European Sports Charter (CoE, 2001):

> Sport means all forms of physical activity which, through casual or organised participation, aim at expressing or improving physical fitness and mental wellbeing, forming relationships or obtaining results in competitions at all levels (Article 2).

This is an inclusive definition, which might explain its political employment. However, this is not how most people understand sport, and it would seem to allow numerous activities – jogging, gardening, folk dance, indoor exercise to a DVD – that would intuitively fall outside of the boundary of the concept of sport. Moreover, if such a broad conception of sport is used, what is the need for the concept of physical activity? If we follow the Council of Europe definition, both terms would mean the same thing. A stronger definition of sport comes from Coakley (2001), namely organised and competitive physical activities. Specifically, Coakley iden-tifies four attributes of sport that are characteristic of sport: physical activity, competition, institutionalisation and the desired outcome. The latter may be anything from enjoyment to health and other instrumental values. This reflects the ways in which the term is used in the literature (especially when drawing a distinction with other concepts), and it adds two important qualifications for some activity to count as sport: some sort of organisation, whether it is informal by the players themselves (such as in street games), or formal (such as at sports clubs). Sport encompasses a range of activities, including individual, partner and team forms, contact and non-contact, placing different emphases on strategy, chance and physical skills. People can play sport for a wide variety of reasons, and the inclusion of competition as a defining element does not at all mean that competition is the primary reason players play (Collins, Bailey, Ford, *et al.*, 2012).

Physical activity is understood here as any form of exercise where bodily movements are involved (World Health Organization, 2010). Physical activity is usually described in relation to intensity, duration, frequency and type, which together constitute the volume of activity (Corder, Ekelund, Steele, *et al.*, 2008). The World Health Organization (2010) recommends that school-aged children accumulate at least 60 minutes in moderate-to-vigorous physical activity (MVPA) every day. It also specifies that vigorous-intensity activities (VPA) should be incorporated, including those that strengthen muscle and bone, at least three times per week. This activity can take place in different contexts, such as travelling to and from school, leisure time activity, physical education classes, and sports participation. Health-enhancing physical activity (HEPA), as the name suggests, is any form of physical activity that benefits health and functional capacity without undue harm or risk (Foster, 2000). So, sport does not necessarily qualify as HEPA. Nor does it follow that people always engage in such activity primarily with health in mind, and a great deal of physical activity is incidental to other tasks. For example, people walk to work or the shops, cycle to school, run for a bus or train, and stretch, lift and carry as they do housework. Children participate in sport for a number of reasons, such as fun and enjoyment, the satisfaction of learning new skills, and the pleasure of being with family and friends. In many cases the enhancement of the health is not a significant motivating factor driving physical activity (Cope, Bailey and Pearce, 2013). Any health-related benefits of participation in sport are incidental to these other values.

Figure 1.1 suggests one way of thinking about the relationships between physical activity, sport and exercise.

The tendency towards treating sport as a relatively homogenous activity is evidenced in sociological writing on the relationship between sport and health, and consequently used to disqualify sport from discussions of health promotion. Waddington (2000), for example, discusses what he calls the 'sport-health ideology', framing sport as an inherently competitive activity which entails distinct social relations, and infused with aggressive masculinity

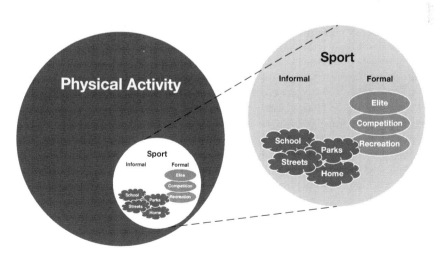

Figure 1.1 Relationships between physical activity and sport

and a relatively high tolerance of injury. He claims, 'The use of physical violence to a greater or lesser degree remains a central characteristic of modern sport . . . Many sports have, in present-day societies, become enclaves for the expression of physical violence' (Waddington, 2000, p. 27). He goes on to cite the patterns of commercial sponsorship as further evidence of the sport-health ideology, and implicitly, reason to doubt the role that sport can play in health promotion. Scambler (2005) extends this analysis by referring to the use of performance-enhancing drugs, and concludes that sport and health is one example of the way that contemporary public policies are 'designed as much to secure public legitimation as to be effective' (ibid., p. 92).

But treating sports as homogeneous, as these writers implicitly do, leads to claims that are simply not true. To extrapolate concerns with a context associated with a tiny minority of sports players to the whole is both misleading and unhelpful. Every sport has unique characteristics that appeal to different interests, abilities and expectations; their impact on players' health is enormously varied. Consider a list of the most popular sports in the world. All forms of sport and physical activity carry different levels of risk and health-related rewards, and are associated with different attitudes to violence and abuse. Moreover, there are vastly different levels of exertion and resultant health impacts from these activities.

1 Soccer
2 Cricket
3 Field Hockey
4 Tennis
5 Volleyball
6 Table Tennis
7 Baseball
8 Golf
9 Basketball
10 American Football
(Source: http://mostpopularsports.net (accessed 19/10/2016))

So, this discussion of definitions ends with two cautionary notes. First, it would be a mistake to assume that the benefits that have been found to be associated with physical activity in general necessarily accrue to sport. Second, it is an error to extrapolate concerns with an extreme and unrepresentative form of sport to all sport. In both of these cases, the veracity of claims are empirical matters, requiring empirical research.

Sport and the inactivity epidemic

The importance of regular physical activity is now well established, as are the harmful consequences of sedentary lifestyles (Kohl, Craig, Lambert, *et al.*, 2012). The trend towards sedentary lifestyles across most developed countries, and increasingly across developing countries is a source of considerable concern (Hallal, Andersen, Bull, *et al.*, 2012). The causes of this trend are complex, but there is little doubt that an important factor is the compound effects of industrial, automotive and information technology innovations, which have resulted in radical changes to the ways in which people carry out their daily tasks. Physical activity is being squeezed out of the Western, Educated, Industrialised, Rich and Democratic societies – WEIRD – societies (Henrich, Heine, and Norenzayan, 2010). The effects of some of these developments, such as cars and trains, have directly impacted on levels of physical activity, while others, such as televisions, computers and electronic entertainment are indirect and more ambiguous. The emergence and ready availability of new technologies has exaggerated these changes on physical labour and human energy expenditure (Hallal, Andersen, Bull, *et al.*, 2012).

The consequences of living in WEIRD societies can be considerable. A review of data from 105 countries found that four-fifths of adolescents did not reach recommended levels of physical activity (Hallal, Andersen, Bull, *et al.*, 2012). Children and adolescents spend more time after school in sedentary pursuits than free play, and fewer young people are commuting to school by foot or bicycle, further impacting avenues for daily physical activity in youth. These findings have serious health consequences because the lack of activity is one of the main risk factors of non-communicable diseases which are currently the leading causes of death worldwide (Lee, Shiroma, Lobelo, *et al.*, 2012). As a consequence, the promotion of physical activity is widely regarded as a global health priority, and the failure of large numbers of people, especially young people, to achieve even minimal levels of activity could justifiably be judged a health crisis. Led by initiatives from the World Health Organization, almost every country now has a physical activity strategy, supplemented by guidance for raising levels for differing age groups in different settings, and recommended daily targets.

What role can sport play in addressing this challenge? Surprisingly, perhaps, in almost all cases, top-level national and international guidance either omits or marginalises sport. The World Health Organization, in particular, has kept a cautious distance from sport in its guidance for physical activity. 'Settings' have long been at the centre of its approach (e.g. cities, workplaces, hospitals, schools), and while its goal remains the optimisation of individuals' health behaviours, the approach is premised on the view that this is best achieved within people's daily cultures and routines. No sporting or other leisure settings are mentioned in the list of appropriate settings for health promotion.

The omission of sport from public health discourse is a recent phenomenon as for centuries it was heralded as a useful way of making people fitter, stronger and more robust (Cachay and Thiel, 2000). Recently, though, the relationship has become more ambivalent, with many writers and policy makers questioning whether the nature of sport, the motivations to play and its dependence on volunteerism means that it is unsuited to substantially contribute to health objectives (Skille and Solbakken, 2014). Michelini (2015) aptly calls this recent tendency 'the disqualification of sport'. He argues that the source of the problem lies in a perceived incompatibility between the illness-orientated focus of health policies and the win/lose orientation of sport. According to this interpretation, sport becomes delegitimised as a potential type of healthy physical activity because it is performance- and not health-orientated. Michelini supports his claim by pointing to the language and omissions of policies from a range of countries, encompassing quite distinct political systems. According to Michelini's analysis, the United States stands as an outlier in international policies by its relative acceptance of sport within health discussions. Yet even here sport has been pushed to the margins. Berg *et al.*, describe sport as an 'afterthought in U.S. public health campaigns' (Berg, Warner, and Das, 2015, p. 20), as evidenced by the almost complete absence of the word from public health policy documentation designed to get people more physically active.

Many sport organisations have contributed to the absence of sport on the health agenda by focussing on elite performers, usually at the expense of grassroots players. As sport has become increasingly politicised there has been a significant shift in both policy rhetoric and funding from an emphasis on mass participation in physical activity towards elite sport (Collins, Bailey, Ford, *et al.*, 2012). Since the amount of resources available to sport or any other social activity has always been finite, the development of elite sport has usually occurred at the expense of mass participation. This is not inevitable, but there is a tendency because 'the scale of provision, the span of time needed and other favourable contextual policies to provoke major lifestyle and participation changes are huge, challenging and beyond the sport policy community, which is usually marginal' (Collins, 2008, p. 78). This situation is exacerbated by the prestige associated with elite sporting events, against which grassroots participation seems unable to compete.

Sport as a setting for health promotion

The settings approach to health promotion has become one of the dominant paradigms in the field, by shifting the focus from individual-based risk orientation and disease to social factors that support human health and wellbeing (Eriksson and Lindström, 2014). The application of the settings approach in schools has proved to be useful in terms of both impact and effectiveness with all age groups (Langford, Bonell, Jones, *et al.*, 2015). Advocates claim that sports participation can substantially increase energy expenditure and physical fitness for those who participate, as well as contributing to wide health outcomes (Samitz, Egger, and Zwahlen, 2011). Critics question these claims (Nielsen, Bugge and Andersen, 2016).

These discussions are part of a wider debate about the social impact of sport. Attempts to measure this impact have generally been context specific and for particular initiatives, or programmes in certain locations, and there have been a relatively limited number of studies that attempt to summarise and quantify the total impact of investment in sport. A recent analysis of the return on investment in sport in the UK reported that for every 1 pound invested in sport, the UK government gained a social return of 1.903 pounds (Davies, Taylor, and Ramchandani, 2016). Figures like these offer support for the case for investing in sport.

The case for the settings approach for sport as a feature of HEPA rests on a series of assumptions:

1   Large numbers of children and young people play sport regularly.
2   The physical activity dose from sport is sufficient to benefit the health of the player.
3   Participation in sport during childhood and youth tracks into physical activity later in life.

The justifications for these assumptions are examined below.

How many children and young people play sport?

Rates of participation in youth sport have been much less documented than general physical activity trends (Brettschneider and Naul, 2004), also a degree of caution needs to be maintained in discussions of this subject. Knight and Holt's (2014) estimation that 'somewhere between 50 and 70 per cent of young people participate in at least one sporting activity' (p. 11) is a plausible figure if it is taken to refer only to those in the developed world and participation is understood very liberally. For example, Australian research reported that 60 per cent of 5- to 14-year olds took part in organised sport within the previous year (Australian Bureau of Statistics, 2012). On average, children who participated spent 5 hours per fortnight playing and/or training in organised sport outside of school hours. Research from New Zealand data found that 60 per cent of boys and 50 per cent of girls participate in sports outside of school time (Adolescent Health Research Group, 2008). In England, data showed that in the 4 weeks prior to being interviewed, 81 per cent of 5- to 10-year olds took part in sport outside of school and 95 per cent of 11- to 15-year olds took part in sport in or outside of school. These results have remained stable since 2008-2009 (DCMS, 2013). In the United States, an estimated 4 million children and adolescents aged 6–18 years are engaged in organised sport, equating to 66 per cent of boys and 34 per cent of girls (NCYS, 2009). While figures like these paint a generally positive picture, their obvious limitation is that they use different timeframes and different levels of engagement (compare, for example, Australian and English criteria for participation).

Variation between national participation rates is predictable, and partly reflects differences between parental and cultural expectations, as well as the role of sport with educational systems. It also seems to reflect access to sport. In this respect, Germany is an interesting case study. Out of 91,000 existing sports clubs, 56,500 offer a range of activities in different types of sport from preschoolers, and 84,000 for school children and adolescents (Breuer and Wicker, 2009). This goes some way in explaining why 70 per cent of 7- to 10-year-old German children are regularly involved in sports clubs. In contrast to Anglo-American regions, sports clubs are available in most parts of Germany, even in rural areas (Baur and Burrmann, 2000). Membership in sports clubs is affordable for the majority of the German population, thus providing an opportunity for most Germans to be physically active. The proliferation of sports clubs in Germany goes back many years, but their potential to raise the general level of physical activity as part of nationwide health promotion interventions is shared by only a small number of other countries, such as Finland (Kokko, Kannas, and Villberg, 2009).

Gender inequality is a persistent and resistant concern, magnified by the relatively low levels of general physical activity among girls and women. The Australian study reported above found significant differences in rates of participation in organised sport between boys (67 per cent) and girls (54 per cent) (ABS, 2012), and where data are available similar patterns have been found elsewhere. For example, Bailey, Wellard and Dismore (2004) found consistently low levels of physical activity among women and girls, both relative to men and boys, and to physical activity recommendations. This and other studies report a clear trend of decreasing levels of activity as girls get older, and a widening disparity between girls' and boys' physical activity behaviours. For example, one study estimated that the decline in physical activity during secondary schooling is 7.4 per cent for girls, compared with 2.7 per cent for boys (Sallis, 1993). Another suggested that female adolescents were approximately 20 per cent less active than their male peers (Booth, 1997). The picture for sports participation is more positive in some (but not all) developed countries. In the United States, for example, there has been a significant increase in the number of girls and women participating in sports over recent decades (Cooky, 2009). However, even in the United States, there are still many girls who do not participate because of limited opportunities, structural barriers, and gender ideologies, and their participation do not match those of boys and men (Bailey, Wellard and Dismore, 2004).

Is the dose of the physical activity from sport sufficient?

It seems to be the case that any amount of physical activity in any domain (recreation, travel, housework and/or occupation) can contribute to health (Omorou, Erpelding, Escalon, *et al.*, 2013). Generally speaking, though, assessments are made with reference recognised criteria of frequency, intensity, duration and type of activity. By far the most common set of recommendations is from the World Health Organization (2010).

A large number of studies have examined the relationship between sports participation and physical activity levels, although there has been wide variation in methods used and outcomes measured. For example, several studies have reported participation in organised sport to be associated with increased levels of physical activity (e.g., Sacheck, Nelson, Ficker, *et al.*, 2011; Mota and Esculcas, 2002), but the confidence in their findings has been undermined by the use of research methods that might be inappropriate with children (such as self-report measures). Consequently, there has been tendency towards the use of objective measures of activity.

Some studies have used accelerometers to examine daily activity levels of engagement among sport participants. Wickel and Eisenmann (2007) investigated weekday levels of MVPA and VPA among 6- to 12-year-old American boys. They found average weekday MVPA and VPA to be 110 and 40 minutes per day, respectively, among Flag American Football, soccer and basketball players. They also reported levels of MVPA to be 30 minutes lower on a non-sports day compared to a sport day. Similar findings were reported by Machado-Rodrigues, Coelho-e-Silva, Mota, *et al.* (2012) in their study of MVPA of 13- to 16-year-old Portuguese boys. Sports players accrued 114 minutes per weekday of MVPA, and an average of 97 minutes per day across the week. The researchers calculated that this equated to between 11 to 13 per cent of total daily energy expenditure in organised sports which corresponds to 35 to 42 per cent of the MVPA of daily energy expenditure. Data from 9- to 15-year-old soccer players from France, Greece and England showed average daily MVPA to be 122 minutes per day, and daily VPA to be 25 minutes per day (Van Hoye, Fenton, Krommidas, *et al.*, 2013). These studies have also found the amounts of MVPA accrued during sport participation did not occur during non-playing days and was generally replaced with low-intensity and sedentary activities. This is consistent with other research indicating that children are unlikely to compensate for missed physical activity resulting from sports (Dale, Corbin and Dale, 2000), suggesting that sport might have the potential to increase levels of physical activity, and also be effective in reducing bouts of inactivity or sedentary behaviour (Kanters, McKenzie, Edwards, *et al.*, 2015).

Other studies have investigated levels of physical activity during sport time specifically to determine the extent to which participation contributes to meeting targets for MVPA and VPA. An Australian study of female netball, basketball and soccer participants (aged 11 to 17 years) found that for every hour of game play or practice time, participants accumulated approximately one-third of the recommended 60 minutes of MVPA per day (Guagliano, Rosenkranz and Kolt, 2013). A study from the United States found that both boys and girls (aged 7 to 14 years) engaged in approximately 45 minutes of MVPA, and 20 minutes of VPA during youth sport practice (Leek, Carlson, Cain, *et al.*, 2011). The findings also showed that 23 per cent of players met the recommended 60 minutes of MVPA per day during youth sport time. Comparatively lower levels of MVPA were reported by Wickel and Eisenmann (2007) in their study of 6- to 12-year-old boys, although their findings are similar to those from the studies reported above in terms of the proportion of time active (49 per cent).

More negatively, many of these studies also recorded large amounts of either sedentary or light intensity activity. Some studies show that children spend up to 70 per cent of their time playing sport engaged in activity either inactive or minimally active (e.g., Leek, Carlson, Cain, *et al.*, 2011; Wickel and Eisenmann, 2007). It needs to be remembered, of course that there is considerable variation within the youth population. Obese children and adolescents tend to be less active than their normal-weight peers during sport (Sacheck, Nelson, Ficker, *et al.*, 2011), and female players engage in higher levels of MVPA during training sessions compared to competition (Guagliano, Rosenkranz, and Kolt, 2013). Psychological factors probably also affect physical activity engagement, and numerous studies have highlighted the influence of perceptions of competence, autonomy, self-efficacy and enjoyment within activity settings (Harwood, Keegan, Smith, *et al.*, 2015). Also, coaches/teachers often base lessons on skill development and competition preparation, which are usually at sub-MVPA levels (Sasaki, Howe, John, *et al.*, 2016).

As has been discussed earlier, the efficacy of physical activity is usually described in relation to intensity, duration, frequency and type, and it seems clear that different sports offer difference levels of exercise for different players. For example, Leek *et al.*'s (2011) study (see earlier) reported levels of MVPA (and the proportion of session time engaged in MVPA) to be higher in soccer participants, compared to softball/baseball. Likewise, Katzmarzyk, Walker and Malina (2001), who studied the amount and quality of physical activity through direct notational observation of 11- to 14-year-old boys' and girls' recreational sports, found outdoor soccer to be the most robust activity opportunity, providing less sitting time than in-line hockey and ice hockey. Indoor soccer provided less sitting time than basketball, in-line hockey, and ice hockey. Outdoor soccer also had the greatest time spent jogging and sprinting. Leek *et al.* (2011) also found that 7- to 10-year-olds were more active than 11- to 14-year-olds, and boys were more active than girls. Other studies have found that younger participants engage in higher levels of MVPA than older participants (Wickel and Eisenmann, 2007); overweight and obese participants engage in lower levels of MVPA and VPA, and are inactive for more time, than their normal weight peers (Sacheck, Nelson, Ficker, *et al.*, 2011); those with access to designated sports facilities (Mandic, Bengoechea, Stevens, *et al.*, 2012), and that MVPA was higher during practice sessions than competitions (Guagliano, Rosenkranz, and Kolt, 2013).

Table 1.1 shows the results of a brief review of studies examining the relationship between children's sports participation and physical activity levels, using only studies published during the 2013 to 2016 period.

These recently published studies paint a generally positive picture about the potential role of sports participation as a contribution to children's daily physical activity. However, caution is needed in interpreting these findings for two reasons. First, while sports-playing children are generally more active, have greater energy expenditure and spend more time in MVPA than their non-participant peers, data are still limited about how their physical activity varies with types and levels of sports participation, and how these relationships contribute to other parameters of health, such as obesity (Silva, Andersen, Aires, *et al.*, 2013). Second, it has been reported that light intensity physical activity can be misclassified as MVPA in children aged 10 years and younger (Kim, Beets, and Welk, 2012). Consequently, levels of physical activity during youth sport may have been overestimated in studies involving younger participants (Leek, Carlson, Cain, *et al.*, 2011). In addition, as has been seen above, sport is not played regularly by all children. So, while existing studies indicate that participation in youth sport offers children and adolescents the opportunity to accrue substantial amount of MVPA and VPA, it seems to be the case that physical activity accrued during youth sport alone is not sufficient to meet recommended levels of MVPA.

Does participation in sport during childhood and youth track into physical activity later in life?

A large part of the rationale for policy attention on children's physical activity is the widely held belief that the early years of life provide the foundation of later activity (Bailey, Cope and Parnell, 2015). This presumption is given added support by the finding that past exercise behaviour is a reliable predictor of current activity status (Smith, Gardner, Aggio, *et al.*, 2015), and urgency by the fact that physical activity tends to decrease as individuals move into adulthood (Kwan, Cairney, Faulkner, and Pullenayegum, 2012). There are clear benefits of participating in sport during high school, from increased psychomotor competence and improved physical health to team works skills and new friendships (Bailey, Hillman, Arent, *et al.*, 2013), but the potential long-term benefits related to continued engagement in physical activity as an adult could be the most rewarding benefit of all, at least from

Table 1.1 The relationship between children's sports participation and physical activity levels, studies published 2013 to 2016

Study	Sample	Methods	Findings
Bocarro, Kanters, Edwards et al. (2014)	6,735 middle school students.	Percentage of children observed in sedentary and MVPA assessed by SOPLAY measures. Energy expenditure and physical activity intensity were also estimated by using MET values.	Within-school sports had higher MET values than between-schools sports, and Intermural sports ranked in four of the top five sports in terms of average MET values. Regression models found a significant interaction between school sport delivery model and gender, with boys significantly less physically active in IS programmes than boys in IM programmes.
De Meester, Aelterman, Cardon et al. (2014)	1,049 Belgian 11-year-olds.	Flemish Physical Activity Questionnaire.	Extracurricular school-based sports participants were significantly more physically active than children not participating in extracurricular school-based sports.
Fenton, Duda, Barrett, et al. (2015)	109 grassroots soccer players; mean age = 11.98.	Physical activity assessed via accelerometer for 7 days.	Youth football contributed 60.27 per cent and 70.68 per cent towards daily weekend MVPA and VPA, respectively. Overall, 36.70 per cent of participants accumulated >60 min MVPA and 69.70 per cent accrued > 20 min of VPA. For participants aged 13 to 16 years, MVPA and VPA were significantly higher during football sessions, and contributed a greater amount towards daily weekend MVPA and VPA than for participants aged 9 to 12 years.
Hebert, Møller, Andersen, et al. (2015)	1,124 Primary school students.	Organised leisure-time sport participation was reported via text messaging; physical activity was objectively measured over seven days with accelerometry.	Boys were more active than girls, and physical activity levels and guideline concordance decreased with age. Soccer participation at any frequency was associated with greater overall MVPA, equating to between 5 and 20 minutes more MVPA on the average day and 3- to 15-fold increased odds of achieving recommended levels of health-related physical activity. Similar associations were identified among children playing handball at least twice per week. Relationships with other sports (gymnastics, basketball, volleyball) were inconsistent.

Study	Sample	Method	Findings
Jekauc, Reimers, Wagner, et al. (2013)	4,529 German girls (49.5 per cent) and boys, aged between 4 and 17 years.	MoMo Physical Activity Questionnaire.	52 per cent of girls and 63.1 per cent of boys were members of sports clubs who exercised on average for 4 h per week with MVPA to VPA. The amount of MVPA was only significantly predicted by age, gender and residential area.
Marques, Ekelund and Sardinha (2016)	973 UK children and adolescents, aged 10–18 years.	Organised sport was self-reported. Physical activity and time spent in MVPA and sedentary time was assessed with accelerometers.	More boys than girls reported to be involved in organised sports participation. Those engaged in were more likely to achieve physical activity guidelines, spent more time in MPA, VPA and MVPA than those who did not participate in organised sports.
Nielsen, Bugge and Andersen (2016)	518 Danish children aged 9–10.	Accelerometry during 4 days, included 1–2 weekend days.	Children playing club football had higher total daily amounts of physical activity than both children taking part in other club-sports and children not taking part in club-sports at all. About half of the difference in total physical activity could be explained by higher activity levels during school recess. On a more general level, the results indicate that the influence leisure-time club sport participation has on physical activity may differ due to how well the sport can be transferred to and played in other daily contexts for children's self-organised physical activity, such as school recess.
Peralta, O'Connor, Cotton, et al. (2014)	34 indigenous Australian adolescents, mean age = 13.7 ± 1.16.	SOFIT observation system.	Students were engaged in MVPA for 58 per cent of lesson time.
Pharr and Lough (2014)	49,832 students in Southwestern United States	Cross-sectional, secondary analysis of survey data.	Black girls participated less and White girls participated more while White and Asian boys participated less than expected. Reported sport participation was high compared to national data when analysed by gender and ethnic group. Sport participation was higher in low SES schools compared to high SES schools.

continued

Table 1.1 continued

Study	Sample	Methods	Findings
Silva, Andersen, Aires, et al. (2013)	310 Danish youth (183 girls and 127 boys) aged 11–18 years.	Sports participation assessed by questionnaire; habitual physical activity measured objectively with accelerometers.	Participation in competitive sports at club levels increased the chances of being fit independently of MVPA levels. There were positive and significant trends in CRF and objectively measured physical activity across the levels of engagement in competitive sports.
Telford, Telford, Cochrane, et al. (2012)	289 8- to 16-year-olds.	Longitudinal-study using pedometers and accelerometers, and club sport participation by questionnaire.	Sports club participants were more physically active at all age groups than non-participants. Boys took an extra 1,800 steps and girls 590 steps per day. Boys engaged in an extra 9 minutes and girls 6 minutes more MVPA per day.
Van Hoye, Fenton, Krommidas, et al. (2013)	331 10–14 year-olds from England, France and Greece.	3-day valid accelerometer data and self-report measure of physical activity.	Players accumulated 122.33 minutes of MVPA and 488.19 minutes of sedentary time per day.
Vella, Cliff, Okely, et al. (2013)	12,188 adolescents from 238 secondary schools aged between 12 and 17 years.	Participation in organised sports, compliance with national physical activity guidelines, and other health-related factors were self-reported.	Organised sports participation was higher among males and those residing in rural/remote areas. Underweight adolescents reported the lowest levels of participation. Higher levels of participation were associated with an increased likelihood of complying with national physical activity guidelines.

the perspective of public health. In light of the high costs on inactivity and sedentary behaviours, childhood physical activity promotion offers a promise of a relatively cheap preventive strategy for a range of non-communicable diseases (Matheson, Klügl, Engebretsen, et al., 2013).

Tracking studies, which are longitudinal studies examining the tendency of individuals to maintain behaviours over time (Malina, 1996), have an obvious appeal within the context of physical activity research. These studies are relatively rare as they generally require a large financial investment and a long-term commitment of both participants and researchers. In addition to the emergence of new measurement methods and changing conceptions of physical activity, a host of confounding factors can occur in repeated measures (Hirvensalo, and Lintunen, 2011). Physical activity during childhood seems to predict physically active lifestyles in adolescence and adulthood (Anderssen, Wold, and Torsheim, 2005; Kjønniksen, Torsheim, and Wold, 2008). However, the tracking from sports participation to adult physical activity is less understood (Kjønniksen, Anderssen, and Wold, 2009). Also, the tracking of physical activity during transitions from childhood to adolescence and adulthood has been shown to be quite low, while the tracking of physical activity during adult life is relatively high (Telama, Yang, Leskinen, et al., 2013). This is hardly surprising, perhaps, as education, occupation, local environment, family status and other factors have been found to influence later activity (Tammelin, Näyhä, Hills, et al., 2003; Cleland, Ball, Magnussen, et al., 2009).

Dennison, Straus, Mellits, et al. (1988) carried out a precursor of tracking studies, although their focus was on childhood determinants of adult physical activity patterns. In a non-concurrent prospective study, the physical activity levels of 453 young men, aged from 23 to 25 years, were compared with their physical fitness test scores as children and adolescents (10- to 11-year-olds and 15- to 18-year-olds). The researchers found that physically active adults had significantly better childhood physical fitness test scores than did inactive adults, and that physical inactivity in young adulthood was linearly related to the number of low scores on run and sit-ups tests as children. Another early investigation, by Kuh and Cooper (1992), was more explicitly a tracking study: they examined the influence of childhood activity on adult activity patterns in a national sample of more than 3,300 36-year-old men and women in the United Kingdom, using a birth cohort database. Kuh and Cooper reported that adults who were most active in sport had been of above average ability at sports in school (and were also more outgoing socially in adolescence, had fewer health problems in childhood, were better educated, and had more mothers with a secondary education) than those who were less active. Studies examining the relationship between sports participation and later physical activity appeared a little later. For example, Finnish researchers reported that participation in sports competitions and sports club membership at 16-year-olds predicted physical activity 2 years later (Aarnio,

Winter, Peitonen, *et al.*, 2002), and a follow-up study with a large sample of 14- to 31-year-olds found that participation in sports twice a week or more after school hours, being a member of a sports club, and a high grade in school sports at age 14 years were associated with a high level of physical activity at age 31 years (Tammelin, Näyha, Hills, *et al.*, 2003).

The Amsterdam Longitudinal Growth and Health Study (Wijnstok, Hoekstra, van Mechelen, *et al.*, 2013) is an important contribution because, unlike most studies to that point, it has not relied on retrospective recall or cohort data. Measures have been taken from 13-year-olds who were followed-up until they were 43-year-old. These data suggest that organised youth sports made relatively important contributions to both weekly physical activity and energy expenditure in both males and females.

A more recent study found that participation in high school sports was the best predictor of physical activity after age 70 (Dohle and Wansink, 2013). In addition, Smith, Gardner, Aggio, and Hamer (2015) found that participation in sport at age 10 was highly associated with participation in physical activity at age 42. However, Mäkinen, Borodulin, Tammelin, *et al.* (2010a) have argued that physically active individuals are more likely to stay physically active from adolescence to adulthood, especially among those who participate in several different sports after school hours. This claim has been offered support by a number of longitudinal studies (Aarnio, Winter, Peltonen, *et al.*, 2002; Tammelin, Näyhä, Hills, *et al.*, 2003; Telama, Yang, Leskinen, *et al.*, 2013).

Table 1.2 summarises recent studies that have examined the tracking of physical activity from childhood sport.

It is clear from the literature that sports participation and associated experiences are not the only or even main determinants of physical activity during childhood and later in life (Hirvensalo and Lintunen, 2011; Cleland, Ball, Magnussen, *et al.*, 2009). For example, children's socioeconomic conditions can have a potent effect on leisure-time physical activity (Mäkinen, Kestilä, Borodulin, *et al.*, 2010b), including participation in different sports (Tammelin, Näyhä, Hills, *et al.*, 2003). Researchers have also found associations between participation in some sports with high grades in school sports and membership of a sports club that carried over into adult years (Tammelin, Näyhä, Hills, *et al.*, 2003). Australian researchers reported upward social mobility – reaching a higher level of educational attainment than one's parents – to be associated with a greater likelihood of high physical activity in adulthood and a greater likelihood of a high fitness level (Cleland, Ball, Magnussen, *et al.*, 2009). Psychosocial factors have also been found to mediate physical activity, and these seem to be especially marked for girls and women (Bailey, Wellard and Dismore, 2004). Qualitative research has highlighted the effect of body shape and weight management on girls' participation (Allender, Cowburn and Foster, 2006). Differences in the experiences and perceptions of boys and girls of early sport and physical

Table 1.2 The relationship between children's sports participation and physical activity levels in adolescence and adulthood, studies published 2013 to 2016

Study	Sample	Methods	Findings
Ball, Bice and Parry (2016)	516 university employees, university students and members of a state health organisation (28.6 per cent males; 71.2 per cent females)	International Physical Activity Questionnaire and Retrospective Evaluation	Participants who competed in individual sports while in high school reported to partake in significantly more days of VPA as an adult. There were more days of VPA with individuals who participated in individual sports, rather than team sports.
Basterfield, Reilly, Pearce, et al. (2015)	609 UK children at ages 7, 9 and 12 years	Cohort study data	Sports club participation was significantly associated with overall accelerometer-measured physical activity at 12 years, but not 9 years. An inverse relationship between fat mass and sport club participation, and between fat mass and accelerometer-measured physical activity was observed at 12 years, but not 9 years. Sports club participation at 9 years was highly predictive of participation at 12 years.
Bélanger, Sabiston, Barnett, et al. (2015)	673 Canadian adolescents, aged 12–13 years	Cohort study data	There was a positive linear relationship between number of years participating in sports (and running) in adolescence and physical activity level at age 24 years.
Dohle and Wansink (2013)	712 US males	Males who passed a rigorous physical examination in 1940s were surveyed 50 years later	The single strongest predictor of later-life physical activity was whether he played a varsity sport in high school.
Hardie Murphy, Rowe and Woods (2016)	5,397 Irish youth aged, 10–18 years	Self-report surveys 5 years apart	Participation frequency in club sport extracurricular sport significantly predicted physical activity 5 years later, adjusted for age, sex and urban/rural classification.

continued

Table 1.2 continued

Study	Sample	Methods	Findings
Schlechter, Rosenkranz, Milliken, et al. (2016)	111 US boys, aged 5–11 years	Physical activity was assessed using Accelerometry. physical activity was assessed from scheduled practice start time until practice completion	The proportion of practice time spent in sedentary ($13 \pm 1\%$), MVPA ($34 \pm 2\%$) and VPA ($12 \pm 1\%$). Practice contributed less half. Although sport provides a setting for youth to accrue MVPA, two-third of practice was spent sedentarily or in light activity. Neither greater experience nor participation in a coach training programme was not associated with higher MVPA.
Smith, Gardner, Aggio, et al. (2015)	6,458 UK children, aged 10 years	Cohort study data	Participants who often participated in sports at age 10 were significantly more likely to participate in sport/physical activity at age 42.
Sun, Vamos, Flory, et al. (2016)	5,381 US women	Longitudinal cohort data	Physical activity levels during adolescence significantly predicted physical activity adherence. Additionally, having 5 days of PE a week was a significant predictor.
Telford, Cunningham, Telford, et al. (2012)	289 Australian youth, aged 8–16 years	Pedometry and accelerometry, fitness by the 20 m shuttle-run, and club sport participation by questionnaire	Sports club participants were more physically active at all age groups than non-participants, especially boys. Fitness was higher among sports participants, and sport participant girls had 2.9 per cent less body fat. Higher fitness scores were maintained over time by sports participants but their greater physical activity diminished during adolescence, especially among girls.

activity is a persistent theme in the literature (e.g., Bailey, Wellard and Dismore, 2004; Cooky, 2009), and there seems to be little doubt that girls have traditionally been disadvantaged by the sports provision made available to them. Traditionally, more boys than girls are involved in organised youth sports in childhood (Prusak and Darst, 2002; Hovden, and Pfister, 2006), although the Lunn's analysis (2010) suggests that differences are greatest in team sports, and that opportunities are more equal in individual sports.

The quality of early experience is also an important factor, and it seems to impact on both genders. Unfortunately, not all trajectories or experiences are positive, and some studies have shown that participation in organised sport is associated with both short-term and long-term risks (Dworkin, and Larson, 2006; Linver, Roth, and Brooks-Gunn, 2009). Despite the self-evident value in understanding the harmful consequences of negative experiences of sport, the topic is under-researched (exceptions include Bean, Fortier, Post, *et al.*, 2014; Cardinal, Yan, and Cardinal, 2013).

Why, exactly, some sporting experiences are positive and others negative is not well-understood. However, some empirical studies have identified some clues. The review by Allender *et al.* (2006) reported that those who participated from youth to adulthood tended to recall the importance of positive influences at school in becoming and staying physically active (teachers, friends), while overly competitive classes, a lack of teacher support, negative experiences at school, and peer pressure and identity conflict were major barriers to physical activity. McPherson, Atkins, Cameron, *et al.*'s (2015) retrospective study of children's experience of sport found that while their adult participants reported the lasting developmental benefits of participation in organised sport as children, more than 50 per cent also reported negative experiences, including emotional and physical harm and sexual harassment.

Abuse and bullying aside, differences in children's engagement in certain sporting activities could be a matter of fit between the characteristics of the person and the characteristics of this particular physical activity. And the resultant outcomes may create a virtuous cycle whereby a child who has a positive experience of his or her engagement in a movement activity may be more likely to participate in the activity in the future, and is, therefore, more likely to have further positive experiences (whereas a person who experiences negative movement experiences is likely to drop out or have restricted future participation in movement contexts) (Agans, Säfvenbom, Davis, *et al.*, 2013). If this is the case, the phenomenon of negative experiences of sport is a very serious matter. Despite the common view that sport is inherently inclined towards benefitting players, this is not the case (Bailey, 2006; Coakley, 2011). Many (perhaps most) of benefits claimed for sport can be matched by empirically supported negative pairs. For example, while there is evidence that sport can build resilience and positive attitudes to physical activity in children and adolescence (Bailey, 2016; Makkai, Morris, Sallybanks, *et al.*,

2003), there is also evidence that certain types of sports experiences may lead to increased levels of stress (Scanlan, Babkes, and Scanlan, 2005), reduced motivation (Dworkin, and Larson, 2005), and risky behaviour (Habel, Dittus, De Rosa, *et al.*, 2010). Each of these negative outcomes increases the likelihood of disengagement from physical activities, which can, in turn, increase stress, de-motivation and unwise behaviour (Carr, 2006; Dworkin and Larson, 2006; Agans, Säfvenbom, Davis, *et al.*, 2013).

If sports participation follows parallel virtuous and vicious cycles, then negative experiences of sport during childhood might not just be a missed opportunity, but result in outcomes that could harm players' health, well-being and likelihood of sports participation for years in the future.

Conclusion

Sport as defined in this chapter – organised and competitive physical activities – may have become marginalised or 'disqualified' within health policy in recent years, but there are reasons to challenge this position. More young people in the developed world than ever before are participating in organised youth sports programmes (Bauman, Reis, Sallis, *et al.*, 2012). The simple facts that sport represents one of the main developmental contexts for children and youth, next to family and school (Rutten, Stams, Biesta, *et al.*, 2007), and that millions of children participate in sport across the globe (de Knop, 1996), mean that, in principle, youth sport represents an important and globally relevant domain for interventions seeking to promote physical activity, during childhood, adolescence and adulthood.

Sport has certain characteristics that suggest it can play a valuable role in the promotion of physical activity, during childhood, adolescence and adulthood. The findings from the studies reported in this chapter demonstrate that sport can make a useful, if not sufficient role in helping young people reach recommended physical activity levels. The effect this has on later physical activity is more ambiguous, as mediating factors seem to play more of a role. However, a plausible case can be made for a generally positive influence of childhood sporting experiences on the development of lifelong physical activity in a number of ways. First, sports participation seems to provide of the experiences and attitudes that underpin later capabilities to engage in physical activities. Indeed, some have suggested that the first 10 years or so help children overcome a 'proficiency barrier' of skills that would otherwise exclude large groups of activities for lack of basic confidence and competence (Bailey and Collins, 2013; Stodden, True, Langendorfer, *et al.*, 2010). Second, sport may provide opportunities for children to acquire the psychological skills and confidence that will facilitate participation in physical activities later in life (Bailey, Collins, Ford, *et al.*, 2010). Third, positive sports experiences and positive outcomes during childhood and adolescence may support the development of intrinsic motivation

(Larson, 2000), which may, in turn, lead to increased motivation to be physically active later in life (Kilpatrick, Hebert, and Bartholomew, 2005). At the moment, these are plausible hypotheses, but no more. Further research will be needed to properly understand the mechanisms why sport does and does not affect physical activity engagement during childhood and in later life.

One thing does seem clear: sports participation does not automatically result in long-lasting benefits. Simply put, participation is unlikely to be enough. It is possible to disagree with critics like Coalter (2007), who have questioned the empirical base of the various physical, physiological psychological and sociological outcomes claimed for sport, while accepting that there remains 'a widespread lack of even more valuable evidence relating to sufficient conditions: the type of sports and the conditions under which the potential to achieve the desired outcomes are maximised' (p. 23). As Svoboda (1994) stated some time ago, the presumed positive outcomes of sport are 'only a possibility', and a direct linear affect between simple participation and effect cannot be assumed. This is with good reason as there is ample evidence to suggest that participation in sport and physical activity can result negative as well as positive outcomes (Bailey, Cope and Parnell, 2015). This is not a danger specific to sport and physical activity, but all contexts with which children engage. So, although participation in sporting contexts can potentially promote positive, healthy development, 'it is best not to take the relationship as a "given"; it can be difficult to achieve; and can only be realised in association with a series of conducive "change mechanisms"' (Whitelaw, Teuton, Swift, *et al.*, 2010, p. 65). What are these mechanisms? The evidence base here is much less well-developed than that of outcomes, however, it seems clear that these outcomes are mediated by a host contextual factors, including the ways in which sport is presented, managed and valued. If sport is going to be recruited for wider policy concerns, then it is likely that there is intentionality in the design of the programmes so that programmes are deliberately structured and implemented to achieve the desired outcomes.

Acknowledgements

The research informing this chapter was made possible thanks to the generous support of Deutsche Gesellschaft für Internationale Zusammenarbeit(GIZ) 'Strategic Alliance with Nike Ltd. Designed to Move School: Enhancing Youth Social and Economic Development through Positive Physical Experience'. Thanks are due to Christiane Frische (GIZ), Will Norman (Nike), and Detlef Dumon (ICSSPE) for valuable insights and commentary. Thanks, too, to Jennifer Leigh (University of Kent), Rich Kite (British Weight Lifting), and Katrin Koenen (ICSSPE) for comments on earlier drafts of this chapter.

References

Aarnio, M., Winter, T., Peltonen, J., Kujala, U. M., and Kaprio, J. (2002). Stability of leisure-time physical activity during adolescence – A longitudinal study among 16-, 17- and 18-year-old Finnish youth. *Scandinavian Journal of Medicine & Science in Sports*, 12(3), 179–185.

Adolescent Health Research Group (2008). *Youth '07: The Health and Wellbeing of Secondary School Students in New Zealand*. Auckland: University of Auckland.

Agans, J. P., Säfvenbom, R., Davis, J. L., Bowers, E. P., and Lerner, R. M. (2013). Positive Movement Experiences. *Advances in Child Development and Behavior*, 45, 261–286.

Allender, S., Cowburn, G., and Foster, C. (2006). Understanding participation in sport and physical activity among children and adults: a review of qualitative studies. *Health Education Research*, 21, 826–835.

Anderssen, N., Wold, B., and Torsheim, T. (2005). Tracking of physical activity in adolescence. *Research Quarterly for Exercise and Sport*, 76(2), 119–129.

Australian Bureau of Statistics (2012). Children's Participation in Cultural and Leisure Activities, Australia, Apr 2012. Accessed on 1/8/16. http://abs.gov.au/AUSSTATS/abs@.nsf/Lookup/4901.0Main+Features1Apr%202012?OpenDocument

Bailey, R. P., Wellard, I., and Dismore, H. (2004). *Girls' Participation in Physical Activities & Sports: Benefits, Patterns, Influences & Ways Forward*. Geneva: World Health Organisation.

Bailey, R. P. (2006). Physical education and sport in schools: a review of benefits and outcomes. *Journal of School Health*, 76(8), 397–401.

Bailey, R. P., Collins, D., Ford, P., MacNamara, A., Toms, M., and Pearce, G. (2010). *Participant Development in Sport: An Academic Review*. Leeds: Sports Coach UK.

Bailey, R. P., Hillman, C., Arent, S., and Petitpas, A. (2013). Physical activity: an underestimated investment in human capital? *Journal of Physical Activity and Health*, 10, 289–308.

Bailey, R. P., Cope, E., and Parnell, D. (2015). Realising the benefits of sports and physical activity: the human capital model. *Retos: nuevas tendencias en educación física, deporte y recreación*, 28, 147–154.

Bailey, R. P. (2016). Sport, physical activity and educational achievement–towards an explanatory model. *Sport in Society*, doi.org/10.1080/17430437.2016.1207756

Ball, J. W., Bice, M. R., and Parry, T. (2016). Retrospective evaluation of high school sport participant and adult BMI status, physical activity levels, and motivation to exercise. *American Journal of Health Studies*, 31, 105–111.

Basterfield, L., Reilly, J. K., Pearce, M. S., Parkinson, K. N., Adamson, A. J., Reilly, J. J., and Vella, S. A. (2015). Longitudinal associations between sports participation, body composition and physical activity from childhood to adolescence. *Journal of Science and Medicine in Sport*, 18(2), 178–182.

Bauman, A. E., Reis, R. S., Sallis, J. F., Wells, J. C., Loos, R. J., Martin, B. W., and Lancet Physical Activity Series Working Group. (2012). Correlates of physical activity: why are some people physically active & others not? *The Lancet*, 380(9838), 258–271.

Baur, J. and Burrmann, U. (2000). *Unerforschtes Land: Jugendsport in ländlichen Regionen*. Aachen: Meyer & Meyer.

Bean, C. N., Fortier, M., Post, C., and Chima, K. (2014). Understanding how organized youth sport may be harming individual players within the family unit: a literature review. *International Journal of Environmental Research and Public Health*, 11(10), 10226–10268.

Bélanger, M., Sabiston, C. M., Barnett, T. A., O'Loughlin, E., Ward, S., Contreras, G., and O'Loughlin, J. (2015). Number of years of participation in some, but not all, types of physical activity during adolescence predicts level of physical activity in adulthood: results from a 13-year study. *International Journal of Behavioral Nutrition and Physical Activity*, 12(1), 1.

Berg, B., Warner, S., and Das, B. (2015). What about sport? A public health perspective on leisure-time physical activity. *Sport Management Review*, 18, 20–31.

Bocarro, J. N., Kanters, M. A., Edwards, M. B., Casper, J. M., and McKenzie, T. L. (2014). Prioritizing school intramural and interscholastic programmes based on observed physical activity. *American Journal of Health Promotion*, 28(sp3), S65–S71.

Booth, M. (1997). The NSW schools fitness & physical activity survey, 1997. *New South Wales Public Health Bulletin*, 8(5), 35–36.

Brettschneider, W. D., Naul, R., Armstrong, N., Diniz, J., Froberg, K., and Laakso, L. (2004). Study on young people's lifestyle and sedentariness and the role of sport in the context of education and as a means of restoring the balance. Final report. Paderborn: EC, Directorate General for Education and Culture, Unit Sport.

Breuer, C. and Wicker, P. (2009). *Die Situation der Sportvereine in Deutschland: ein Überblick*. Sportverlag Strauß, Köln.

Cachay, K. and Thiel, A. (2000). *Soziologie des Sports: Zur Ausdifferenzierung und Entwicklungsdynamik des Sports der modernen Gesellschaft*. Weinheim: Juventa-Verlag.

Cardinal, B., Yan, Z., and Cardinal, M. (2013). Negative experiences in physical education and sport: how much do? *Journal of Physical Education, Recreation & Dance*, 84(3), 49–53.

Carr, S. (2006). An examination of multiple goals in children's physical education: motivational effects of goal profiles and the role of perceived climate in multiple goal development. *Journal of Sports Sciences*, 24(3), 281–297.

Centers for Disease Control and Prevention. (2000). *Promoting better health for young people through physical activity and sports*. Atlanta, GA: Centers for Disease Control and Prevention.

Cleland, V. J., Ball, K., Magnussen, C., Dwyer, T., and Venn, A. (2009). Socioeconomic position and the tracking of physical activity and cardiorespiratory fitness from childhood to adulthood. *American Journal of Epidemiology*, 170, 1069–1077.

Coakley, J. (2001). *Sport in Society: Issues and controversies*, 7th edn. New York: McGraw-Hill.

Coakley, J. (2011). Youth sports: what counts as 'positive development?' *Journal of Sport & Social Issues*, 35(3), 306–324.

Coalter, F. (2007). *A Wider Social Role for Sport: Who's Keeping the Score?* London: Routledge.

CoE (Council of Europe)(2001). *European Sports Charter*. Strasbourg: CoE.

Collins, D., Bailey, R., Ford, P. A., MacNamara, Á., Toms, M., and Pearce, G. (2012). Three worlds: new directions in participant development in sport and physical activity. *Sport, Education and Society*, 17(2), 225–243.

Collins, M. (2008). Public policies on sports development can mass and elite sport hold together? In V. Girginov (ed.), *Management of Sports Development* (pp. 59–88). Oxford: Butterworth-Heinemann.

Commission of the European Communities (2007). White Paper on Sport. Retrieved from: http://europa.eu/documentation/official-docs/white-papers/index-en.htm

Cooky, C. (2009). 'Girls just aren't interested': the social construction of interest in girls' sport. *Sociological Perspectives*, 52(2), 259–283.

Cope, E., Bailey, R. P., and Pearce, G. (2013). Why do children take part in, and remain involved in sport? A literature review and discussion of implications for sports coaches. *International Journal of Coaching Science*, 7(1), 56–75.

Corder, K., Ekelund, U., Steele, R., Wareham, N., and Brage, S. (2008). Assessment of physical activity in youth. *Journal of Applied Physiology*, 105(3), 977–987.

Dale, D., Corbin, C. B., and Dale, K. S. (2000). Restricting opportunities to be active during school time: do children compensate by increasing physical activity levels after school? *Research Quarterly for Exercise and Sport*, 71(3), 240–248.

Davies, L., Taylor, P., Ramchandani, G., and Christy, E. (2016). *Social Return on Investment in Sport: A Participation-Wide Model for England Summary Report*. Sheffield: Sheffield Hallam University.

DCMS (Department of Culture, Media)(2013). Taking Part 2012/13 Annual Child Report. London: DCMS.

De Knop, P. (ed.). (1996). *Worldwide Trends in Youth Sport*. Champaign, IL: Human Kinetics.

De Meester, A., Aelterman, N., Cardon, G., De Bourdeaudhuij, I., and Haerens, L. (2014). Extracurricular school-based sports as a motivating vehicle for sports participation in youth: a cross-sectional study. *International Journal of Behavioral Nutrition and Physical Activity*, 11(1), 1.

Dennison, B. A., Straus, J. H., Mellits, E. D., and Charney, E. (1988). Childhood physical fitness tests: predictor of adult physical activity levels? *Pediatrics*, 82, 324–30.

Dohle, S. and Wansink, B. (2013). Fit in 50 years: participation in high school sports best predicts one's physical activity after age 70. *BioMed Central Public Health*, 13, 1100.

Donnelly, P. (1996). Approaches to social inequality in the sociology of sport. *Quest*, 48(2), 221–242.

Dworkin, J. and Larson, R. (2006). Adolescents' negative experiences in organized youth activities. *Journal of Youth Development*, 1(3), 1–19.

Eriksson, M. and Lindström, B. (2014). The salutogenic framework for well-being: implications for public policy. In J. H. Timo and J. Michaelson (eds), *Well-Being and Beyond: Broadening the Public and Policy Discourse* (pp. 68–97). Cheltenham: Edward Elgar Publishing.

Fenton, S. A., Duda, J. L., and Barrett, T. (2015). The contribution of youth sport football to weekend physical activity for males aged 9-to 16-years: variability related to age and playing position. *Pediatric exercise science*, 27(2), 208–218.

Foster, C. (2000). Guidelines for health-enhancing physical activity promotion programmes. Tampere, Finland: The European Network for the Promotion of Health-Enhancing Physical Activity.

Guagliano, J. M., Rosenkranz, R. R., and Kolt, G. S. (2013). Girls' physical activity levels during organized sports in Australia. *Medicine & Science in Sports & Exercise*, 45(1), 116–122.

Habel, M. A., Dittus, P. J., De Rosa, C. J., Chung, E. Q., and Kerndt, P. R. (2010). Daily participation in sports and students' sexual activity. *Perspectives on Sexual and Reproductive Health*, 42(4), 244–250.

Hallal, P. C., Andersen, L. B., Bull, F. C., Guthold, R., Haskell, W., and Ekelund, U. (2012). Global physical activity levels: surveillance progress, pitfalls, & prospects. *The Lancet*, 380(9838), 247–257.

Hardie Murphy, M., Rowe, D. A., and Woods, C. B. (2016). Impact of physical activity domains on subsequent physical activity in youth: a 5-year longitudinal study. *Journal of Sports Sciences*, doi.org/10.1080/02640414.2016.1161219

Harwood, C. G., Keegan, R. J., Smith, J. M., and Raine, A. S. (2015). A systematic review of the intrapersonal correlates of motivational climate perceptions in sport and physical activity. *Psychology of Sport and Exercise*,18, 9–25.

Hebert, J., Møller, N., Andersen, L., and Wedderkopp, N. (2015). Organized sport participation is associated with higher levels of overall health-related physical activity in children (CHAMPS Study-DK). *PLOS One*, 10(8), e134621.

Henrich, J., Heine, S. J., and Norenzayan, A. (2010). The weirdest people in the world? *Behavioral and Brain Sciences*, 33(2–3), 61–83.

Hirvensalo, M. and Lintunen, T. (2011). Life-course perspective for physical activity and sports participation. *European Review of Aging and Physical Activity*, 8, 13–22.

Hovden, J. and Pfister, G. (2006). Gender, power and sports. *Nordic Journal of Women's Studies*, 14(1), 4–11.

Jekauc, D., Reimers, A. K., Wagner, M. O., and Woll, A. (2013). Physical activity in sports clubs of children and adolescents in Germany: results from a nationwide representative survey. *Journal of Public Health*, 21(6), 505–513.

Kanters, M., McKenzie, T., Edwards, M., Bocarro, J., Bahar, M., Martel, K., and Hodge, C. (2015). Youth sport practice model gets more kids active with more time practicing skills. *Retos*, 28, 173–177.

Katzmarzyk, P., Walker, P., and Malina, R. (2001). A time-motion study of organized youth sports. *Journal of Human Movement Studies*, 40(5), 325–334.

Keung, A. (2016). Children's time and space. In J. Bradshaw (ed.), *The Well-being of Children in the UK*, 4th edn (pp. 149–178). Bristol: Polity Press.

Kilpatrick, M., Hebert, E., and Bartholomew, J. (2005). College students' motivation for physical activity: differentiating men's and women's motives for sport participation and exercise. *Journal of American College Health*, 54(2), 87–94.

Kim, Y., Beets, M. W., and Welk, G. J. (2012). Everything you wanted to know about selecting the 'right' Actigraph accelerometer cut-points for youth, but . . .: a systematic review. *Journal of Science and Medicine in Sport*, 15(4), 311–321.

Kjønniksen, L., Anderssen, N., and Wold, B. (2009). Organized youth sport as a predictor of physical activity in adulthood. *Scandinavian Journal of Medicine & Science in Sports*, 19(5), 646–654.

Kjønniksen, L., Torsheim, T., and Wold, B. (2008). Tracking of leisure time physical activity during adolescence and young adulthood: a 10-year longitudinal study. *International Journal of Behavioral Nutrition and Physical Activity*, 5(69), 1.

Knight, C. J. and Holt, N. L. (2014). Parenting in youth tennis: understanding and enhancing children's experiences. *Psychology of Sport and Exercise*, 15, 155–164.

Kohl, H. W., Craig, C. L., Lambert, E. V., Inoue, S., Alkandari, J. R., Leetongin, G., Kahlmeier, S., and Lancet Physical Activity Series Working Group. (2012). The pandemic of physical inactivity: global action for public health. *The Lancet*, 380(9838), 294–305.

Kokko, S., Kannas, L., and Villberg, J. (2009). Health promotion profile of youth sports clubs in Finland: club officials' and coaches' perceptions. *Health Promotion International*, 24(1), 26–35.

Kuh, D. J. and Cooper, C. (1992). Physical activity at 36 years: patterns and childhood predictors in a longitudinal study. *Journal of Epidemiology and Community Health*, 46(2), 114–119.

Kwan, M., Cairney, J., Faulkner, G., and Pullenayegum, E. (2012). Physical activity and other health-risk behaviors during the transition into early adulthood: a longitudinal cohort study. *American Journal of Preventive Medicine*, 42(1), 14–20.

Langford, R., Bonell, C., Jones, H., and Campbell, R. (2015). Obesity Prevention and the Health Promoting Schools Framework: essential components and barriers to success. *International Journal of Behavioral Nutrition and Physical Activity*, 12(1), 15.

Larson, R. W. (2000). Toward a psychology of positive youth development. *The American Psychologist*, 55(1), 170–183.

Lee, I. M., Shiroma, E. J., Lobelo, F., Puska, P., Blair, S. N., Katzmarzyk, P. T., and Lancet Physical Activity Series Working Group. (2012). Effect of physical inactivity on major non-communicable diseases worldwide: an analysis of burden of disease & life expectancy. *The Lancet*, 380(9838), 219–229.

Leek, D., Carlson, J. A., Cain, K. L., Henrichon, S., Rosenberg, D., Patrick, K., Sallis, J. F. (2011). Physical activity during youth sports practices. *Archives of Pediatric and Adolescent Medicine*, 165(4), 294–299.

Linver, M. R., Roth, J. L., and Brooks-Gunn, J. (2009). Patterns of adolescents' participation in organized activities: are sports best when combined with other activities? *Developmental Psychology*, 45, 354–367.

Lunn, P. D. (2010). The sports and exercise life-course: a survival analysis of recall data from Ireland. *Social Science & Medicine*, 70(5), 711–719.

Machado-Rodrigues, A. M., Coelho-e-Silva, M. J., Mota, J., Santos, R. M., Cumming, S., and Malina, R. M. (2012). Physical activity and energy expenditure in adolescent male sport participants and non-participants aged 13–16 years. *Journal of Physical Activity and Health*, 9(5), 626–633.

Mäkinen, T. E., Borodulin, K., Tammelin, T. H., Rahkonen, O., Laatikainen, T., and Prättälä, R. (2010a). The effects of adolescence sports and exercise on adulthood leisure-time physical activity in educational groups. *International Journal of Behavioral Nutrition and Physical Activity*, 7(1), 1.

Mäkinen, T., Kestilä, L., Borodulin, K., Martelin, T., Rahkonen, O., and Prättälä, R. (2010b). Effects of childhood socioeconomic conditions on educational differences in leisure-time physical activity. *The European Journal of Public Health*, 20(3), 346–353.

Makkai, T., Morris, L., Sallybanks, J., and Willis, K. (2003). *Sport, Physical Activity And Antisocial Behaviour In Youth*. Canberra: Australian Institute of Criminology.

Malina, R. M. (1996). Tracking of physical activity and physical fitness across the lifespan. *Research Quarterly for Exercise and Sport*, 67(suppl.), S1-S10.

Mandic, S., Bengoechea, E., Stevens, E., de la Barra, S., and Skidmore, P. (2012). Getting kids active by participating in sport and doing it more often: focusing on what matters. *International Journal of Behavioral Nutrition and Physical Activity*, 9(1), 86.

Marques, A., Ekelund, U., and Sardinha, L. B. (2016). Associations between organized sports participation and objectively measured physical activity, sedentary time and weight status in youth. *Journal of Science and Medicine in Sport*, 19(2), 154–157.

Matheson, G., Klügl, M., Engebretsen, L., Bendiksen, F., Blair, S. N., Börjesson, M., Budgett, R., Derman, W., Erdener, U., Ioannidis, J.P., and Ljungqvist, A. (2013). Prevention and management of non- communicable disease: the IOC consensus statement, Lausanne 2013. *British Journal of Sports Medicine*, 47, 1003–1011.

McPherson, L., Atkins, P., Cameron, N., Long, M., Nicholson, M., and Morris, M. E. (2015). Children's experience of sport: what do we really know? *Australian Social Work*, 1–12.

Michelini, E. (2015). Disqualification of sport in health-related promotion of physical activity: a global social phenomenon? *European Journal for Sport and Society*, 12(3), 257–280.

Michelini, E. and Thiel, A. (2013). The acceptance of 'sport' in the communication of the health system. A sociological analysis. *European Journal for Sport and Society*, 10(4), 325–344.

Mota, J. and Esculcas, C. (2002). Leisure-time physical activity behavior: structured and unstructured choices according to sex, age, and level of physical activity. *International Journal of Behavioral Medicine*, 9(2), 111–121.

NCYS (National Council on Youth Sports)(2009). NCYS report on trends and participation in organized youth sports. Stuart, FL: NCYS.

Nielsen, G., Bugge, A., and Andersen, L. B. (2016). The influence of club football on children's daily physical activity. *Soccer & Society*, 17(2), 246–258.

Omorou, Y. A., Erpelding, M. L., Escalon, H., and Vuillemin, A. (2013). Contribution of taking part in sport to the association between physical activity and quality of life. *Quality of Life Research*, 22(8), 2021–2029.

Peralta, L. R., O'Connor, D., Cotton, W. G., and Bennie, A. (2014). The effects of a community and school sport-based program on urban indigenous adolescents' life skills and physical activity levels: the SCP case study. *Health*, 6(18), 2469.

Pharr, J. and Lough, N. L. (2014). Considering sport participation as a source for physical activity among adolescents. *Journal of Physical Activity & Health*, 11(5), 930–941.

Prusak, K. A. and Darst, P. W. (2002). Effects of types of walking activities on actual choices by adolescent female physical education students. *Journal of Teaching in Physical Education*, 21(3), 230–241.

Rutten, E. A., Stams, G. J. J., Biesta, G. J., Schuengel, C., Dirks, E., and Hoeksma, J. B. (2007). The contribution of organized youth sport to antisocial and prosocial behavior in adolescent athletes. *Journal of Youth and Adolescence*, 36(3), 255–264.

Sacheck, J. M., Nelson, T., Ficker, L., Kafka, T., Kuder, J., and Economos, C. D. (2011). Physical activity during soccer and its contribution to physical activity recommendations in normal weight and overweight children. *Pediatric Exercise Science*, 23(2), 281–292.

Sallis, J. F. (1993). Epidemiology of physical activity and fitness in children and adolescents. *Critical Reviews in Food Science and Nutrition*, 33, 403–408.

Samitz, G., Egger, M., and Zwahlen, M. (2011). Domains of physical activity and all-cause mortality: systematic review and dose-response meta-analysis of cohort studies. *International Journal Epidemiology*, 40(5), 1382–1400.

Sasaki, J. E., Howe, C. A., John, D., Hickey, A., Steeves, J., Conger, S., Lyden, K., Kozey-Keadle, S., Burkart, S., Alhassan, S., and Bassett Jr, D. (2016). Energy expenditure for 70 activities in children and adolescents. *Journal of Physical Activity and Health*, 13(6 Suppl 1), S24–S28.

Scambler, G. (2005). *Sport and Society: History, Power and Culture*. Maidenhead, UK: Open University Press.

Scanlan, T., Babkes, M., and Scanlan, L. (2005). Participation in sport: a developmental glimpse at emotion. In J. Mahoney, J. Eccles, and R. Larson (eds), *Organized Activities as Contexts of Development* (pp. 275–309). Mahwah, NJ: Erlbaum.

Schlechter, C. R., Rosenkranz, R. R., Milliken, G. A., and Dzewaltowski, D. A. (2016). Physical activity levels during youth sport practice: does coach training or experience have an influence? *Journal of Sports Sciences*, doi:10.1080/02640414.2016.1154593

Silva, G., Andersen, L. B., Aires, L., Mota, J., Oliveira, J., and Ribeiro, J. C. (2013). Associations between sports participation, levels of moderate to vigorous physical activity and cardiorespiratory fitness in children and adolescents. *Journal of Sports Sciences*, 31(12), 1359–1367.

Skille, E. Å. and Solbakken, T. (2014). The relationship between adolescent sport participation and lifelong participation in physical activity in Norway. A Critical Analysis. *Scandinavian Sport Studies Forum*, 5, 25–45.

Smith, L., Gardner, B., Aggio, D., and Hamer, M. (2015). Association between participation in outdoor play and sport at 10 years old with physical activity in adulthood. *Preventive Medicine*, 74, 31–35.

Sport for Development and Peace International Working Group (2008). *Harnessing the Power of Sport for Development and Peace*. Toronto, ON: Right to Play.

Stodden, D. F., True, L. K., Langendorfer, S. J., and Gao, Z. (2013). Associations among selected motor skills and health-related fitness: indirect evidence for Seefeldt's proficiency barrier in young adults? *Research Quarterly for Exercise and Sport*, 84(3), 397–403.

Sun, H., Vamos, C. A., Flory, S. S., DeBate, R., Thompson, E. L., and Bleck, J. (2016). Correlates of long-term physical activity adherence in women. *Journal of Sport and Health Science*. Corrected Proof.

Svoboda, B. (1994). *Sport and Physical Activity as a Socialisation Environment: Scientific Review Part 1*. Strasbourg: Council of Europe.

Tammelin, T., Näyhä, S., Hills, A. P., and Järvelin, M. R. (2003). Adolescent participation in sports and adult physical activity. *American Journal of Preventive Medicine*, 24(1), 22–28.

Telama, R., Yang, X., Leskinen, E., Kankaanpää, A., Hirvensalo, M., Tammelin, T., Viikari, J. S. and Raitakari, O. T. (2013). Tracking of physical activity from early childhood through youth into adulthood. *Medicine and Science in Sports and Exercise*, 46(5), 955–962.

Telford, R. D., Cunningham, R. B., Telford, R. M., Kerrigan, J., Hickman, P. E., Potter, J. M., and Abhayaratna, W. P. (2012). Effects of changes in adiposity and physical activity on preadolescent insulin resistance: the Australian LOOK longitudinal study. *PloS One*, 7(10), e47438–e47438.

Van Hoye, A. l., Fenton, S., Krommidas, C., Heuzé, J.-P., Quested, E., Papaioannou, A., and Duda, J. L. (2013). Physical activity and sedentary behaviours among grassroots football players: a comparison across three European countries. *International Journal of Sport and Exercise Psychology*, 11(4), 341–350.

Vella, S. A., Cliff, D. P., Okely, A. D., Scully, M. L., and Morley, B. C. (2013). Associations between sports participation, adiposity and obesity-related health behaviors in Australian adolescents. *International Journal of Behavioral Nutrition and Physical Activity*, 10(1), 1.

Waddington, I. (2000). Sport and health: a sociological perspective. In J. Coakley and E. Dunning (eds), *Handbook of Sports Studies* (pp. 408–421). London: Sage.

Whitelaw, S., Teuton, J., Swift, J., and Scobie, G. (2010). The physical activity – mental wellbeing association in young people: a case study in dealing with a complex public health topic using a 'realistic evaluation' framework. *Mental Health and Physical Activity*, 3, 61–66.

Wickel, E. and Eisenmann, J. (2007). Contribution of youth sport to total daily physical activity among 6- to 12-yr-old boys. *Medicine and Science in Sports and Exercise*, 39(9), 1493–1500.

Wijnstok, N. J., Hoekstra, T., van Mechelen, W., Kemper, H. C., and Twisk, J. W. (2013). Cohort profile: the Amsterdam growth and health longitudinal study. *International Journal of Epidemiology*, 42(2), 422–429.

World Health Organization (2010). *Global Recommendations on Physical Activity for Health*. Geneva: World Health Organization.

Chapter 2

Sport, health and physical activity in children

Tara Coppinger

Introduction

As childhood obesity has grown significantly in recent years, a lack of physical activity (PA) linked, in part, to a fall in participation in sport, has been widely acknowledged as a key contributor. Similarly, the relationship between childhood PA and the impact this has on (i) child health (ii) adult health and (iii) lifelong health behaviours, attracts widespread interest. Yet, the evidence to support these relationships remains relatively weak and much of the existing research focuses on adults. Children, with their unique behaviours and characteristics, require focused research and interventions that can improve long-term health outcomes. This chapter aims to discuss current evidence, address any misconceptions and enhance our understanding of the potential relationships between PA, sport and health. Key factors that influence children's participation at the macro, micro and individual level will also be discussed and identifying what sport and PA professionals can do to increase participation in both the PA and sporting domains will also be addressed.

During this chapter we refer to childhood as the period between birth and adulthood (0–17 years) but if there is reference made to a specific age e.g. adolescence (the period from the beginning of puberty until adulthood) or younger children (the period before puberty), this will be made clear.

What classifies as physical activity during childhood?

PA is defined as any bodily movement produced by skeletal muscles that results in energy expenditure above resting level (Caspersen *et al.*, 1985). The World Health Organization (2004) classifies PA for individuals aged 5–17 years, to include a broad range of activities; including games, play, sport, transportation, chores, recreation, physical education (PE) or planned exercise. Each of these activities often takes place in the context of family, school or community. Health enhancing PA, when added to baseline activity, is any type of activity that leads to health benefits. Examples include, but are not limited to, walking briskly, jumping rope/skipping, dancing, playing tennis or soccer, lifting weights, climbing trees and playing on playground equipment at recess/break-time.

Benefits of physical activity for children

Figure 2.1 displays a broad range of health benefits that have been reported by Public Health England in relation to PA participation during childhood (Chalkey *et al.*, 2015). Research has demonstrated a strong positive relationship between PA and a number of health-related parameters such as cardiometabolic health, muscular strength, bone health, cardiorespiratory fitness (CRF), self-esteem, anxiety/stress, academic achievement, cognitive functioning, confidence and peer acceptance (Chalkey *et al.*, 2015). A systematic review

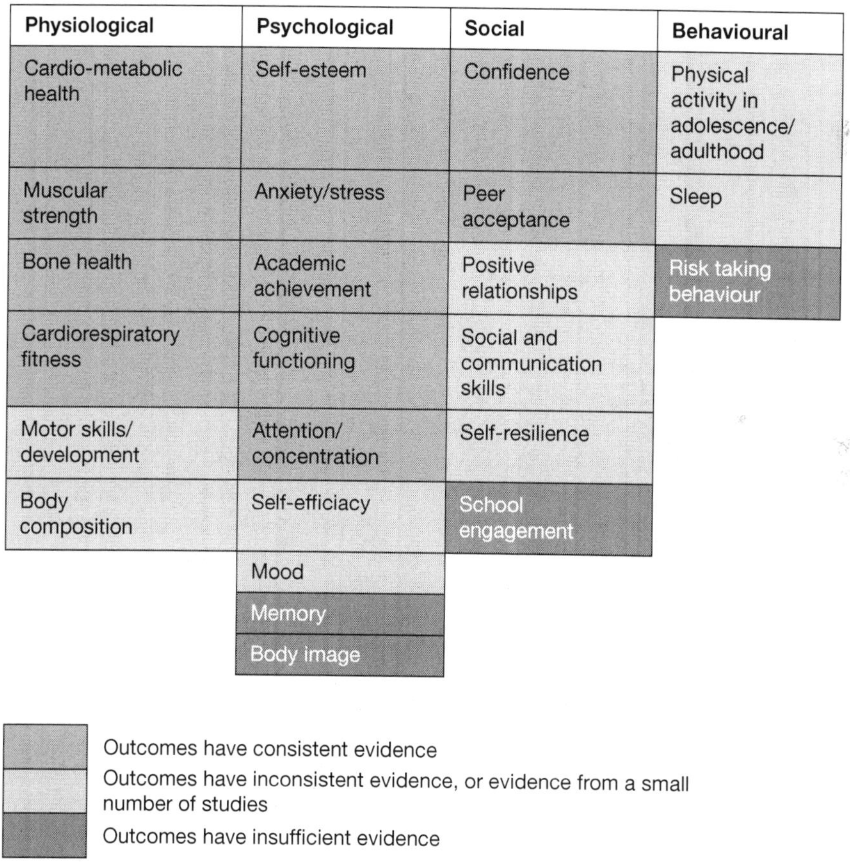

Physiological	Psychological	Social	Behavioural
Cardio-metabolic health	Self-esteem	Confidence	Physical activity in adolescence/ adulthood
Muscular strength	Anxiety/stress	Peer acceptance	Sleep
Bone health	Academic achievement	Positive relationships	Risk taking behaviour
Cardiorespiratory fitness	Cognitive functioning	Social and communication skills	
Motor skills/ development	Attention/ concentration	Self-resilience	
Body composition	Self-efficacy	School engagement	
	Mood		
	Memory		
	Body image		

Outcomes have consistent evidence

Outcomes have inconsistent evidence, or evidence from a small number of studies

Outcomes have insufficient evidence

Figure 2.1 Summary of the strength association between physical activity and each health outcome

Adapted from Chalkley et al., 2015

(Janssen and LeBlanc, 2010) found that the intensity of activity needs to be at least moderate to provide advantageous benefits; with the more PA undertaken, the greater the health benefits earned. Aerobic-based activities show the largest benefits to health, but the review also reported even small amounts of PA to benefit those youngsters deemed high-risk (e.g. obese) (Janssen and LeBlanc, 2010).

The majority of studies that have examined PA during childhood are observational in nature; in that subjects are merely observed, not assigned randomly to 'treatment' and 'control' groups like in traditional randomised control trials (RCTs). There are an increasing number of intervention studies but few of these are reported as RCT's. As diseases such as cardiovascular diease (CVD) and Type 2 diabetes are also rare in childhood, most research focuses on any associations between PA and markers for health such as adiposity or blood pressure. Consequently, research has been linked to over two dozen different parameters (Janssen and LeBlanc, 2010), depending on the measure of interest. For measures of adiposity alone, studies may have included some or all of the following: body weight, body mass index (BMI), numerous skinfold and circumference measures, total body fat, and several specific body fat depots. As a result, the markers for health reported in this chapter have aimed to offer a broad insight in to the area and do not try to cover every individual health parameter.

Risk factors for CVD

As CVD has been traditionally recognised as a disease of adulthood, the majority of research investigating potential relationships between PA and CVD during childhood relate to its risk factors; including blood pressure and blood lipids (Hardman et al., 2009; Twisk et al., 2000). Numerous cross-sectional studies have reported relationships between low levels of PA and/ or physical fitness and a heightened chance of risk factors for CVD (Rocha et al., 2014; Hardman et al., 2009); with overweight and obese children particularly at risk (L'Allemand-Jander, 2010). The authors of the European Youth Heart Study, which investigated systolic blood pressure, triglyceride, high density lipoprotein cholesterol, insulin resistance, skinfolds, aerobic fitness and PA in 1,732 9- and 15-year olds across Europe therefore conclude that we need to get children to undertake greater than 1 hour of moderate to vigorous physical activity (MVPA) per day, in order to avoid a clustering of risk factors for CVD (Andersen et al. 2006).

Evidence is mounting, however, to show that CVD is in fact commencing in childhood (Imhof et al., 2015; McGill et al., 2000). As high blood pressure (HBP) is one of the most important risk factors for CVD disease and the incidence of pre-HBP and HBP is already high in European children (de Moraes et al., 2015), Cesa et al. (2014) believes that we need to take action now by designing school-age prevention programmes for CVD that have PA as a core component.

Overweight and obesity

The global prevalence of obesity has increased substantially in children and adolescents in both developed and developing countries. Yet, no long-term success stories have been reported in the past three decades that prove to reduce these rates (Ngo et al., 2014). In a recent study that included 6,025 children aged 9–11 years, from 12 different countries, lifestyle behaviours (particularly low MVPA, short sleep duration, and high TV viewing) were all found to be important correlates of obesity among youth (Katzmarzyk et al., 2015). When examining PA alone, previous research has found small but suggestive associations on the effects of PA for both obese and non-obese children (Bar-Or and Baranowski, 1994; Riddoch, 1998) and one of the key recommendations from the WHO's (2016) Report of the Commission on Enduring Childhood Obesity was the promotion of physical activity (World Health Organization, 2016). Two reviews (Hills et al., 2011; Chalkley et al., 2015) lend to strengthen these findings and conclude that PA is an important determinant in the prevention of both overweight and obesity in youth, with it being associated with reductions in overall adiposity and visceral adiposity in children who are already overweight/obese. Yet, some inconsistencies in this relationship still remain (Physical Activity Advisory Committee, 2008 cited in Chalkey et al., 2015) and the dose-response relationship continues to be unclear.

Although Hills et al. (2011) state that PA on its own will not reduce obesity rates, they believe that it should hold the highest public health priority in order to tackle the condition in childhood. This is supported by a large-scale study undertaken by Must et al. (1992) that found overweight in adolescence to be linked to a broad range of negative health consequences in adulthood; each of which were independent of adult weight. Strategies need to be well resourced, comprehensive and population based with some suggesting the school setting as the most appropriate. A systematic review of 32 studies, with over 52,000 participants (Sobol-Goldberg et al., 2013) reported that school-based interventions demonstrated more convincing evidence of their effectiveness in reducing body mass scores because they tended to be longer, more comprehensive and included parental support. The greatest effects were seen in the interventions with a duration of greater than 1 year and included a wide range of multiple-level efforts; including PA (Sobol-Goldberg et al., 2013).

Musculoskeletal health

Boreham and Riddoch (2001) highlight the importance of PA for bone structure in relation to increasing peak bone mass in youth; and go as far as to say that there is a difference in bone mineral density of between 5 and 15 per cent among children who are low fit compared to high fit. This review supports work previously undertaken by Kemper et al. (2000), who found site-specific bone mineral density to be higher in youth that undertook weight bearing and high impact strength training programmes. It is still not clear though, how much PA is required to accrue these benefits. More specific research is therefore warranted, that quantifies the dosage of PA required to specifically improve bone health (Chalkley *et al.*, 2015).

Strength training leads to improvements in muscle strength among children in the majority of research undertaken in the field (Chalkley *et al.*, 2015; Riddoch, 1998). A review by Malina (2006) showed that resistance training improved muscle strength in both boys and girls, while at the same time, not impacting growth or maturation. Yet, caution is still advised, as not much is known about the optimal mode, intensity, volume and duration of this type of strength training among youth (Chalkley *et al.*, 2015; Blimkie and Bar-Or, 1996) and the risks from innappropriate/over training should, therefore, not be ignored.

Physical activity and psychological health

Depending on the psychological outcome of choice, the evidence to support PA for the promotion of psychological health in youth, is in part, mostly positive. The greatest amount of research has been undertaken investigating the relationship between PA and (i) self-esteem (ii) anxiety/stress (iii) academic achievement (iv) cognitive functioning (v) attention/concentration (vi) self-efficacy (vii) mood (viii) memory and (ix) body image; with only memory and body image proving to have insufficient evidence to report any such association (Chalkley *et al.*, 2015). Tortolero *et al.* (2000) undertook a review of 48 studies and reported either moderate or strong relationships between PA and fitness in youth and numerous positive mental health variables; including lower rates of stress and depression and higher scores on self-efficacy, physical competence, self-concept and self-esteem. In a review of reviews by Biddle and Asare (2011), however, although an association between PA and mental health in young people was evident, they noted that research designs were often weak and the effects found were only small to moderate.

How much physical activity should children undertake?

In contrast to PA requirements for adults, children need to be physically active for longer periods of time to improve cardiorespiratory and muscular fitness, bone health and cardiovascular and metabolic health markers. Hence, the World Health Organization (2010) recommend:

1   Children aged 5–17 years to accumulate at least 60 minutes of MVPA daily.
2   Children should engage in more than 60 minutes of PA to provide additional health benefits.

3   Children should mostly take part in aerobic, vigorous intensity physical activities, including those that strengthen muscle and bone, at least three times a week. Bone loading activities can be performed as part of playing games, running, turning or jumping.

The accumulation of shorter bouts, such as 10 minutes at a time is welcomed, as is the encouragement of any activity for youth that are currently inactive. Small amounts of PA that are gradually increased in duration, frequency and intensity over time are best for the most inactive but it's important to stress that any PA is better than none.

These recommendations are encouraged for all healthy children aged 5–17 years, regardless of race, gender, ethnicity or income level but should be interpreted with consideration for individual physical and mental capabilities. Age appropriate activities should be encouraged. For example, younger children do not need to undertake structured weight muscle strengthening programmes. Partaking in activities such as climbing (trees, climbing frames), playing on playground equipment or gymnastics are appropriate. During adolescence, however, they may choose to start to take part in structured weight strengthening activities that are commonly embedded into sports such as football and basketball (Centers for Disease Control, 2015).

Physical activity recommendations for early childhood (under 5s)

Prior to 2011, pre-school children (under 5s), did not have any specific PA recommendations. Some countries like the United Kingdom, United States, Australia, and New Zealand, however, felt that not addressing the needs of this particular age group meant that caregivers/parents/guardians were unsure as to what amount of activity was suitable for their pre-school child. Babies, toddlers and pre-schoolers have distinct physiological differences and capabilities compared to school-age children and, therefore, require their own specific PA guidelines. As a result, expert panels from the aforementioned countries put together recommendations for this age group, which were subsequently introduced by the United Kingdom's Department of Health in July 2011. There is still not, however, a global consensus.

Physical Activity Guidelines for early years (under 5s not yet walking)

- 'PA should be encouraged from birth, particularly through floor-based play and water-based activities in safe environments.'
- 'All under 5s should minimise the amount of time spent sedentary (being restrained or sitting) for extended periods (except time spent sleeping).'

Physical Activity Guidelines for early years (under 5s capable of walking)

- 'Children of pre-school age who are capable of walking unaided should be physically active daily for at least 180 minutes (3 hours), spread throughout the day.'
- 'All under 5s should minimise the amount of time spent sedentary (being restrained or sitting) for extended periods (except time spent sleeping).'

(Department of Health, 2011)

Levels of physical activity in children

Advancements in the objective measurement of PA of children have been welcomed in recent years, with accelerometers, doubly labelled water and GPS devices providing more accurate insights in to their levels of PA. Yet, few countries have collected this data consistently, particularly in relation to long-term trends (Hardman *et al.*, 2009), making it difficult for international comparisons to be made.

In 2014, the cooperation of 15 countries from across the world (Australia, Canada, Columbia, England, Finland, Ghana, Ireland, Kenya, Mexico, Mozambique, New Zealand, Nigeria, Scotland, South Africa, United States) saw, for the first time, the development of Report Cards on PA for children and youth (Tremblay *et al.*, 2014). These Report Cards, in the respective countries, utilised the best available evidence and followed harmonised procedures (Colley *et al.*, 2012), which has enabled researchers and policy makers to view the global PA situation among youth, highlighting international differences and disparities (Tremblay, 2014). In November 2016, the second global matrix on Physical Activity for Children and Youth was launched at the International Congress on Physical Activity and Public Health in Bangkok, Thailand, and included 38 countries, from 6 continents. It is the aim to expand the countries involved each year, in order to establish a global 'Active Healthy Kids' network that can work collaboratively to promote healthy childhood PA behaviours (Tremblay, 2014).

Results from these Report Cards have confirmed existing findings that globally, children's PA levels are inadequate (Tremblay *et al.*, 2014) and continue to decline. Boys, in general, are more active than girls (Hallal *et al.*, 2012) and levels decline further as these children move into adolescence (Metcalf *et al.*, 2015; Nader *et al.*, 2008). In a study produced for the *Lancet* on global PA levels of adolescents, Hallal *et al.* (2012) report the proportion of 13–15-year-olds doing fewer than 60 min of MVPA per day as 80 per cent. As physical inactivity shows strong links to inactivity in adulthood (Raitakari *et al.*, 1994), something urgently needs to be done to try and prevent a legacy of inactivity and associated ill-health in the future years for our young people (Bailey *et al.*, 2013). If we can get young people to be active, they stand more of a chance of being active as they age. Sport participation may be a viable option, as data from the 1970 longitudinal observational British Cohort Study, which followed 6,458 participants from the age 10 years to age 42 years, found those who took part in sport at age 10 were significantly more likely to participate in sport/PA at age 42 (Smith *et al.*, 2015).

Physical activity, fitness and future health

Physical fitness is defined as the ability to carry out tasks without undue fatigue and includes both skill and health-related components, of which CRF and muscular fitness are important elements (Cohen *et al.*, 2014). Research to support the importance of CRF in childhood and its impact on adult health is becoming increasingly persuasive (Dwyer *et al.*, 2009; Ruiz *et al.*, 2009). Yet, when discussing the evidence in relation to childhood PA and adult health, differing findings exist (Fernandes and Zanesco, 2010; Yang *et al.*, 2006; Malina 2001; Seefeldt *et al.*, 2002; Van Mechelen and Kemper, 1995). Ultimately, there remains limited evidence to suggest such a relationship, particularly in relation to the quantification of PA using objective measures.

Reasons behind such weak relationships are due, in part, to the difficulties in measuring children over long periods of time. Genetic predisposition also plays a part and as Fox and Riddoch (2000) state, 'you can't make a healthy child healthier', which makes statistically significant associations harder to find (Cale and Harris, 2005). The fact that mortality statistics, which are traditionally used in adult health epidemiological studies, are not applicable to children, makes it even more difficult (Fox and Riddoch, 2000). This gives rise to the majority of research into PA in childhood and its relationship with adult health, focusing on risk factors for adult onset diseases (Hardman *et al.*, 2009).

Researchers in the field, however, argue that although the data may be inconclusive, the positive relationships (Cale and Harris, 2005; Riddoch, 1998) that do exist should not be ignored and due to the rise in childhood cardiovascular health problems and obesity, it may be important to stress the importance of even small associations to promote lifelong health (Cale and Harris, 2005; Cavill *et al.*, 2001).

It cannot be ignored that PA remains the least expensive and most effective preventative means for combating the increasing worldwide problem of obesity. With its associated physical fitness outcomes, it may also represent the most effective strategy to prevent chronic disease (Bonow *et al.*, 2002; Bailey *et al.*, 2013). CRF and health in adults has shown positive associations in relation to its protection against disease (Hardman *et al.*, 2009), with low CRF linked to reduced metabolic health and an increased risk of early death (Artero *et al.*, 2011). Furthermore, as a change in habitual PA almost certainly leads to appreciable changes in fitness (Warburton *et al.*, 2006), it has been recommended that we consider changing the focus of all our attention on PA and obesity, and instead focus more of our efforts on examining the CRF levels of children (Hurtig-Wennlof *et al.*, 2007; Hardman *et al.*, 2009).

Globally, children's fitness levels have been declining in recent decades (Cohen and Sandercock 2014). In a study from the United Kingdom (Sandercock *et al.*, 2015) that tracked BMI and CRF in 157 boys and 150 girls, both boys (d=0.68) and girls' (d=0.47) fitness levels were significantly lower in 2014 than in 2008; and these declines were independent of any changes in BMI. Such findings warrant attention, as this study indicates childhood fitness is declining at a rate of 0.95 per cent per year, which is double the global average of 0.43 per cent. This may be having an even greater knock on effect on the health of these children than when the relationship between PA and health is measured in isolation, as such low fitness scores are below the health-related threshold (Sandercock *et al.*, 2015), which puts individuals at a threefold increased risk of chronic diseases, such as heart disease or diabetes, in adulthood. In response to these findings, Lady Grey-Thompson, chair of 'ukactive,' the not-for-profit health body for the PA sector, has called for the UK government to introduce fitness testing alongside the current height and weight measurement that is taking place in UK schools (ukactive, 2015).

Physical activity, sedentary behaviour and health

Sedentary behaviour is defined as 'any waking behaviour characterised by an energy expenditure of ≤1.5 METs, while in a sitting, reclining or lying posture' (Network SBR, 2012) and it is a common misconception that sedentary behaviour is the ultimate cause of low PA levels. In fact, sedentariness often has little association with MVPA (Biddle *et al.*, 2004; Ekelund *et al.*, 2006) and even among children who do meet PA recommendations, it is possible for these individuals to accumulate large amounts of sedentary time across a day (Healy *et al.*, 2008; Katzmarzyk *et al.*, 2009; Owen *et al.*, 2009; Tremblay *et al.*, 2010; Wong and Leatherdale, 2008). Evidence continues to find children choosing to engage in sedentary activities like watching television or playing video games during their discretionary time (Matthews *et al.*, 2008; Treuth *et al.*, 2009) and that these activities continue as they get older (Treuth *et al.*, 2005; Janz *et al.*, 2005).

The rise in sedentary activities is associated with increased risk of cardio-metabolic disease, all-cause mortality, and a variety of physiological and psychological problems (de Rezende *et al.*, 2014; Katzmarzyk *et al.*, 2009; Owen *et al.*, 2009). One study found TV viewing alone to be unfavourably linked to inflammation and endothelial dysfunction in children (Gabel *et al.*, 2015). Tremblay *et al.* (2011) undertook a large systematic review that examined sedentary behaviour and health indicators in school-aged children and found strong evidence from all study designs that reducing sedentary time was linked to reduced health risk in children aged 5–17 years. Specific evidence suggested that >2 hours of daily TV was associated with reduced physical and psychosocial health, and that lowering sedentary time lead to reductions in BMI. Yet, a more recent U.S. nationally representative longitudinal study of 14,645 kindergarten to first graders (Peck *et al.*, 2015) suggests that as little as 1–<2 h of television a day leaves children more likely to become overweight and obese over time.

Due to the fact that research on sedentary behaviour is a relatively new field of study (Tremblay *et al.*, 2017), there are a limited number of studies that have investigated the relationship between total sedentary time (SED) and screen time (ST) in the same population. A recently published study that investigated correlates of SED and ST from 5,844 children (45.6 per cent boys, mean age = 10.4 years) from across the globe, found children to average 8.6 hours of daily SED, with a further 54 per cent of children failing to meet ST guidelines. (LeBlanc *et al.*, 2015). Across all countries involved, boys had higher amounts of ST, were less likely to meet ST guidelines, and had higher BMI z-scores than girls. Yet, out of 9 of the 12 countries involved in the research, girls engaged in significantly more SED than boys, highlighting that both genders need to be targeted in any intervention trying to reduce sedentary behaviours in youth. Across all participants, frequent correlates of higher SED and ST included poor weight status, not meeting PA guidelines, and having a TV or a computer in the bedroom (LeBlanc *et al.*, 2015). These findings show that children from across the world adopt similar behaviours in relation to SED and ST and equal attention needs to be made to reduce both sedentary time and increase PA in youth.

Sport, physical activity and health

Sport has been defined as 'all forms of PA which, through casual or organised participation, aim at expressing or improving physical fitness and mental wellbeing, forming social relationships or obtaining results in competition at all levels' (Council of Europe, 2001). Participating in sport can therefore be one approach for being physically active and the sports movement has a great influence on the level of health-enhancing PA in the general population (WHO, 2011).

Sport, in the context of PA, can be viewed as an attractive and motivating form of exercise, which Bailey *et al.* (2013) believes can be very effective at empowering individuals, communities, and countries to take action to improve their health. Organised sport is important for healthy development, growth and wellbeing (Vella *et al.*, 2015); can be a useful tool for mobilising health-promoting resources (Ewing *et al.*, 2002) and can also help to enhance both the cultural and social lives of individuals and society as a whole (WHO, 2011).

One study from the United States analysed data from the Centers for Disease Control and Prevention's Youth Risk Behavior Surveys from 1999 through 2007 to examine any relationships by year between sport participation and numerous health risk behaviours among high school students (Taliaferro, 2010). Although there were some negative health behaviours found in certain subgroups, overall, the study found that the advantages of participating in sports during adolescence included: weight control, problem-solving skills, positive self-esteem, social competence and academic achievement. Taking part in sports was also found to result in a reduced incidence of juvenile arrests, teen pregnancies and school dropout (Taliaferro, 2010).

Research examining the relationship between child sport's participation and PA, however, has shown conflicting findings. Wickel and Eisenmann (2007) found youngsters who were involved in sport had higher levels of MVPA, estimated daily energy expenditure, and energy expenditure in PA. Participation in structured activity programmes during childhood was also found to track positively into adulthood in other studies (Clark and Metcalfe, 2002; Stodden et al., 2009). Yet, a recent longitudinal study found no such continuation of participation levels into adolescence (Telford et al., 2015) and only girls who participated in sports were more physically active, fit and had lower levels of body fat than those who did not take part in sports.

These variations may be influenced by a number of factors including the type of sport being undertaken, the number of coaches/teachers and the amount of individuals participating. Sedentariness is not uncommon in some sports and the skill of the coach/teacher may also impact on how much sustained activity is undertaken during a session (Nelson et al., 2011). The fact that most youngsters who partook in sport in the Telford et al. (2015) longitudinal study did not meet recommended levels of PA is also worth noting. Interestingly, when looking specifically at adolescents, taking part in organised PA seems to have a more positive affect on sustained PA levels into adulthood, compared to other indicators of activity (Malina, 2001), which could be linked to learned sports skills being readily transferable to other skills that support an active lifestyle (Bailey et al., 2013; Malina, 2012).

Sporting activity during childhood also has other notable benefits; particularly in relation to skill mastery, with evidence showing interrelationships between fundamental motor skills, physical fitness, PA and knowledge (Lloyd et al., 2010). Some researchers believe that it is through the mastery of fundamental skills that lifelong adherence to sport and PA is enabled, as through the learning of a wide range of movement skills in childhood, we have the physical competence to participate in a broader range of activities and sports (Bailey et al., 2013; Seefeldt and Haubenstricker, 1982; Clark, 2005). In fact, some theorists acknowledge the period of childhood as so important for movement skill learning that if they aren't given the opportunity to develop a broad foundation of skills during childhood, they never will (Balyi, 1998).

Although participation in sport alone is not enough to ensure that children can accrue the health benefits associated with being physically active, initiatives should be developed that facilitate better access for all children to sport. This would improve current levels of sport participation and prevent dropout (Vella *et al.*, 2015); particularly as there are limited other resources available to promote positive health behaviours (Taliaferro, 2010). Future research and surveillance methodologies should also be developed that standardised metrics to capture more detailed data regarding organised sport participation (Vella *et al.*, 2015).

What factors influence participation in sport and physical activity at the macro/micro/individual level?

A complex range of factors, ranging from individual, micro and macro factors, exist to explain why some individuals, groups or communities may be more physically active than others (Cavill *et al.*, 2006). These can also be viewed more broadly as personal (biological and psychological), social (family, friends) and environmental (availability of PA settings) factors (Pate *et al.*, 1995; Sallis *et al.*, 2008). At the individual level, belief in ability, personal attitudes towards PA and awareness of physically active opportunities closeby can all play a role (Sallis and Owen, 1999). At the micro level, the conduciveness of living surroundings to encouraging PA, the support of local communities and the social norms of the local society towards PA can be a factor. Whereas on the macro scale, environmental, cultural and socioeconomic conditions can all act as leading causes as to why somebody may or may not be physically active (Cavill *et al.*, 2006).

Macro factors

Socioeconomic status

Although for the majority of activities, being physically active does not involve a direct cost, socioeconomic factors have been found to be directly related to participation in PA (Cavill *et al.*, 2006). Less socioeconomically advantaged youth tend to participate in reduced amounts of leisure time PA compared to their higher socioeconomic status peers (Stalsberg and Pedersen, 2010), and these low participation rates continue to track into adulthood (Elhakeem *et al.*, 2015). Reasons put forward as to why these differences exist include: poorer children having less free time, living in environments that are not conducive to PA or having limited access to leisure facilities (Gordon-Larsen *et al.*, 2006). Children from lower social classes can also be more exposed to the dangers of urban living, which could also play a role. In the United Kingdom, for example, youth from lower social classes are more likely to live in busy, urban areas that have high rates of fast traffic and poorer road safety networks; contributing to them being five times more likely to be killed on the road than those from higher socioeconomic groups (Institute of Public Policy Research, 2002).

The physical environment

There has been a growing amount of evidence to support the notion that the built environment plays an important role in encouraging physically active behaviour in adults (Cavill *et al.*, 2006) but similar conclusive evidence is not currently available for youth. Of the available evidence, some ambiguous findings are present (Sallis *et al.*, 2000; Davison and Lawson, 2006). For example, a recent longitudinal study among 321 children and their parents examined changes in the perceived neighbourhood environment in relation to changes in PA from childhood to adolescence and found the neighbourhood physical environment to not be related to overall MVPA. The perceived neighbourhood environment was only related to PA that actually took place in the neighbourhood (in the streets, on sidewalks) (D'Haese *et al.*, 2015). This indicates that making changes to a child's neighbourhood to try and promote PA may not, in fact, impact on health enhancing PA levels among this population. It may be that other factors play a more important role when trying to understand children's overall MVPA. Another study that undertook a systematic semi-quantitative review of 150 studies on environmental correlates of youth PA (Ferreira *et al.*, 2007) found low crime incidence (in adolescents) to be a characteristic of the neighbourhood environment, which led to higher participation rates in PA. Yet, solid evidence to show that other environmental factors influenced PA was not found.

More research in this field is particularly important for young people, as due to them having less power over their behavioural choices, environmental influences can be especially relevant (Nutbeam *et al.*, 1989; Ferreira *et al.*, 2007). Finding out the factors in the physical environment that are associated with young people's PA; particularly their location-specific PA, would enable more effective intervention strategies to be designed (Sallis *et al.*, 1998; Haug *et al.*, 2010), while also allowing researchers to identify ways to increase children's PA in specific locations e.g. recreation facilities (D'Haese *et al.*, 2015).

Active transport

Most studies that have looked at the relationship between PA and active commuting in children have found positive outcomes (Cooper *et al.*, 2003; Tudor-Locke *et al.*, 2001; Larouche *et al.*, 2014) in that young people who actively travel to school engage in more PA than those who use cars or other forms of motorised transport. Yet, few studies to date have examined this relationship longitudinally and even less have examined the relationship between active commuting to school, PA and other health indicators such as body mass. Due to inconsistency in studies, one previous review (Lee *et al.*, 2008) suggested that there might actually be no association between active commuting and reduced weight or BMI in school children.

Despite the lack of available longitudinal data, it is believed that promoting active transport could reap great benefits for increasing children's overall PA levels (Hardman *et al.*, 2009; Hills *et al.*, 2007), as approximately 20 per cent of all UK car journeys undertaken during morning rush hour have been found to be made up of parents dropping children to school. As safety, social interactions, and the presence of facilities to assist walking and cycling (Panter *et al.*, 2008) are all factors that help to promote active travel in children, by creating environments that support safe local walking and cycling, more children may opt to use active travel as an alternative (Hardman *et al.*, 2009). Distance, however, continues to be the main reported difficulty when trying to promote active travel to school (Wong *et al.*, 2011). Consequently, bicycling and walking may not always be an option for young people. Public transport may be a viable option to consider, as according to Voss *et al.* (2015), when incorporated appropriately, it can contribute meaningfully toward daily PA.

Government

In order to effectively promote PA, the involvement and cooperation of all levels of government (national, regional and local) is required (WHO, 2011; Kohl *et al.*, 2012). To enable success, within these divisions, clear roles and responsibilities of different departments are also needed, as existing national sports strategies from across the European Union often tend to refer to sport and PA interchangeably, which can lead to a lack of clarity (WHO 2011).

Local government plays a specific role, as they can not only create environments that are conducive to PA (Edwards and Tsouros, 2006), they can also implement highly targeted, child-focused interventions (Hills *et al.*, 2007). Yet, in order for these to be successful, effective partnerships are vital. Cooperation between urban planners, transport, housing, social services, education, health, sports and the support of both private and voluntary sectors is needed (WHO, 2011). People have been found to be more active when amenities such as shops and schools, for example, are all situated close to an individual's home. Local policy changes, such as reducing speed limits and providing safer routes for walking and cycling in local areas may also have substantial effects on PA levels over the long term (WHO, 2005).

When focusing on bicycle safety alone, educating children and their parents can be beneficial (Carlin *et al.*, 1998); particularly in relation to striking a balance in safety culture (Hills *et al.*, 2007). Yet, until more evidence is available that addresses effective preventive measures of sport and recreational injuries among children in general (MacKay *et al.*, 2004), government initiatives that aim to promote more PA among children and youth may lack effectiveness.

Micro factors

The role of schools

The school environment has the potential to impact siginificantly on child health and presents a number of opportunities for intervention (Lavelle *et al.*, 2012; Kriemler *et al.*, 2011; Vasques *et al.*, 2014; Ward *et al.*, 2007). It is one of the only settings where the full spectrum of socioeconomic positions are represented; children spend a considerable amount of time at school (Garrow, 1991) and the school also provides a context for learning at a time of development that is characterised by high receptiveness (Fox and Harris, 2003). Primary schools are particularly favourable, as children of primary school age can be highly influenced by health promotion initiatives (Fox and Harris, 2003), which can then promote positive behavioural changes that can continue on into adulthood (Bjorntorp *et al.*, 1992). One example of an RCT that assessed the effectiveness of a school playground intervention on the PA levels of primary/elementary school children found making small environmental and policy changes to a school had a promising, significant impact on break-time PA levels of participating children (Parrish *et al.*, 2015). Project Energize (Rush *et al.*, 2014), is another example, which originally began in 2004 as a RCT and has now been expanded across all Waikato region primary schools of New Zealand. Indices of obesity and physical fitness of 2,474 younger (7-year olds) and 2,330 older (10-year olds) children attending 193 of the 235 primary schools were compared with historical measurements and physical fitness was found to be significantly higher and BMI significantly lower among intervention participants children compared to a group of similarly aged children from another region and/or the RCT 'control' participants. As a result, the project was launched overseas in Ireland (Coppinger *et al.*, in 2016) in 2013, with hopes of further expansion.

Although increasing school PE does not increase activity levels enough to meet recommended thresholds (Hardman *et al.*, 2009), Cale and Harris (2005) believe that PE still has an important role to play; particularly as the link between health and education has increasingly been recognised as important by government. In fact, encouraging participation in sport and PA has been a long-standing theme of government policy in recent decades, in relation to how effective PE can be at promoting lifelong participation in sport and PA (Green, 2002). Yet, the ways in which governments support this process varies across countries and few governments dedicate enough compulsory PE time in schools. Findings from a Eurydice report which mapped the state of play of PE and sport activities at schools in 30 European countries found PE to only receive approximately half of the dedicated curricular time compared to that of mathematics, across European countries (Kerpanova and Borodankova, 2013). This is despite increasing evidence that confirms the effectiveness of PA at improving academic performance both in the immediate and long term (Active Living Research, 2015).

School sport; particularly team games, continues to be one of the main foci of PE classes (Kerpanova and Borodankova, 2013; Cale and Harris, 2005), which will have a differing relevance and appeal to youngsters (Green 2002; Fox and Harris, 2003). Green (2002) feels that this strong sporting approach fails to acknowledge participatory trends in young people towards non-competitive, more recreational forms of activity, which could in turn lead to lower participation rates in overall PA. Schools also do not contain homogenous – one size fits all – groups and if they are to continue to be used as a setting for the promotion of PA, it needs to be ensured that any interventions are tailored and targeted to those of particular need.

Neighbourhoods/communities

Increasing children's exposure to the outdoors could be an effective strategy for limiting sedentary behaviour and increasing PA and fitness in children (Ngo et al., 2014; Barber et al., 2013; Gray et al., 2015). One recent nationally representative longitudinal study of 4423 Australian children even found a beneficial effect of green space on children's BMI scores as they aged (Sanders et al., 2015). So much so, a recent Position Statement was commissioned on Active Outdoor Play for children aged 3–12 years (Tremblay et al., 2015), which stated that access to active play in nature and outdoors, with its risks, was essential for healthy child development. The authors recommend, 'increasing children's opportunities for self-directed play outdoors in all settings-at home, at school, in child care, the community and nature' (Tremblay et al., 2015). Despite this, more evidence is amounting to suggest that children are spending less and less time outdoors, and for shorter periods, than previous generations (Bassett et al., 2014; Veitch et al., 2007).

Parent's perceptions of the outdoor environment (Timperio et al., 2004) and heightened safety concerns (Veitch et al., 2006; Valentine et al., 1997; Carver et al., 2008; Clements, 2004; Holt et al., 2015) have an influence over children's opportunities to be physically active in their neighbourhood but evidence also suggests that young people are themselves opting to partake in activities that predominate indoors (Glenn et al., 2013; Miller and Kuhaneck, 2008; Veitch et al., 2007) and, which are more supervised and structured than previous generations (Valentine et al., 1997; Active Health Kids Canada, 2012). Sedentary activities, such as watching television, playing video games, using the Internet, listening to music, art, and reading, are all factors that cause more and more children to be drawn indoors (Larson et al., 2011), which could also be linked to the changing social environments of children that increasingly take place on screens (Skår and Krogh, 2009).

Home

Children's health behaviours develop within an ecological niche (Davison and Birch, 2001), with the family environment playing a key role. Influences on children's PA behaviours within the home environment include access to media, parenting practices, sibling influences and family habits (Jago *et al.*, 2011). Parents alone can also have a strong impact in determining a child's PA (Sallis *et al.*, 2000, Mattocks *et al.*, 2008; Hendrie *et al.*, 2011, Fuemmeler *et al.*, 2011; Yao and Rhodes, 2015), with previous research reporting children who have parents that are regularly active to be six times more likely than their counterparts to take part in PA (Moore *et al.*, 1991). A bi-directional relationship has even been found between parents and children; with both mutually influencing each other's behaviour (Sleddens *et al.*, 2017). Mothers and fathers can provide resources to take part in PA, act as role models (Sallis *et al.*, 1999) and give encouragement and social support to youngsters (O'Loughlin *et al.*, 1999). The level of education or income of parents also plays a role (Tandon *et al.*, 2012); with the more education and higher income a parent has, the greater their awareness of the importance of PA (Borodulin *et al.*, 2008; Mäkinen *et al.*, 2010; Tammelin *et al.*, 2003) and at providing the opportunity for children to be active (Tandon *et al.*, 2012).

Systematic reviews have shown that a child's PA is positively associated with that of their friends (Sawka *et al.*, 2013, Gesell *et al.*, 2012) but the impact of siblings on such behaviour remains limited (Edwards *et al.*, 2015; Liu *et al.*, 2014). One qualitative study of 56 parents in the United Kingdom reported siblings to have an influence over PA behaviour, particularly in relation to informal and spontaneous activities (Edwards *et al.*, 2015). An American study found similar findings, in that a younger sibling's level of PA was positively associated with an older sibling's (Liu *et al.*, 2014) among low income minority youth. Family-based interventions that promote PA in children by establishing positive modeling or by increasing social support from both parents and siblings may therefore be more effective than just focusing on parents alone, but more research is required in the field before any specific recommendations can be made.

Individual factors

A review on the correlates of children's (age range 4–12) PA (Van Der Host *et al.*, 2007) found gender (male), self-efficacy, parental PA (for boys), and parent support to all be positively associated with PA. For adolescents (age range 13–18), gender (male), parental education, attitude, self-efficacy, goal orientation/motivation, physical education/school sports, family influences, and friend support were all found to be factors that supported PA. A more recent umbrella systematic literature review on the behavioural determinants of PA across the lifecourse (Condello *et al.*, 2017) found positive evidence for 'previous PA', 'independent mobility' and 'active transport' as factors determining PA amongst youth. A further umbrella systematic literature review from the same team of researchers that looked at the psychological determinants of PA (Cortis *et al.* (in press) found convincing evidence only for 'self-efficacy' as a determining factor for PA amongst children and adolescents. 'Stress', on the other hand, represented a negative association with PA. An earlier systematic review that looked at both qualitative and quantitative barriers to, and facilitators of, PA among children aged four to 10 years (Brunton et al., 2003) found cost, burden of organising safe transport to facilities, traffic, threat of crime and intimidation by older children to all be barriers to children's PA. Facilitating factors, however, included families with more money and spare time to participate and transport children to activities. This review also went on to suggest that new approaches and interventions that are designed, need to take into account the views of children. Specific recommendations suggest: (i) children should be provided with a wide range of physical activities to choose from, (ii) physical activities that children value should be emphasised (e.g. the chance to spend time with peers), (iii) free or cheap transport and lower costs to activities should be provided and (iv) safer local places where children can play and travel actively should be made available (Brunton et al., 2003). There are few studies, however, that have examined these factors prospectively (Van Der Host et al., 2007), so caution needs to be taken before conclusive statements are made.

What can be done to increase participation in sport and PA?

There are numerous approaches that have been shown to be effective at increasing PA among different age groups from a variety of social groups, communities and countries (Heath et al., 2012). Many initiatives designed to increase PA use community-based informational, environmental, behavioural and social policy approaches (Powell and Paffenbarger, 1985; Pate et al., 1995). Yet, the WHO (2011) believe that there is more scope for organisations to work together to promote health-enhancing PA and sport for all across the globe. For a number of years now, numerous non-governmental organisations have been involved in sport promotion but it has only been in recent years that attention has been made to health as a core objective of these working groups (Kohl et al., 2012). Through utilising skillful practitioners, some promising progress is being made. Examples include trying to combat sporting and PA inequalities, activating disadvantaged groups, those in old age and people with low levels of PA levels, and more attention is being paid to urban planning and how to make the transportation infrastructure more conducive to active transportation. More intersectoral work still needs to be done as the sports sector, in particular, continue to be underutilised with regards their ability to promote PA levels. More support must be given to local authorities and community organisations in order to create safe, accessible local environments that encourage sport and PA and to develop a broader set of activities to reach children and other population groups (WHO, 2007). As it is the intersectoral work at various levels that is seen as the most successful approach to increasing PA in populations (Bauman *et al.*, 2012; Roussos and Fausett, 2000).

In 2011, the International Olympic Committee (IOC) assembled an expert group to discuss the role of PA and sport on the health and fitness of young people and concluded that in order for effective changes to take place, a more coordinated, collaborative, global effort between many stakeholders is required (IOC, 2011). They made specific recommendations for a variety of stakeholders including governments, sporting organisations and healthcare systems.

Recommendations for governments

- Policies need to be developed and implemented that encourage sport and PA participation among youth.
- Political agendas need to put PA and health higher up on the scale.
- Across sectors, more funding needs to be provided to youth sport and PA initiatives.
- To improve PA and sporting opportunities for young people, provision and support needs to be provided for multisectoral partnerships (sport, recreation, health agencies) to be created.
- All providers of government funded recreational programmes need to be educated on the importance of limiting sedentary time in youth.
- PA should be present on any campaign addressing global health.
- Governments should work more closely with international, regional and national PA promotion networks.
- In order to better understand the relationship between PA and health in young people, governments should provide more support of research.

Recommendations for sport organisations

- Youth-oriented activities need to be at the heart of all sport programmes so that young athletes are both engaged and retained.
- Sport organisations should provide more training for sports coaches on how to include suitable growth and maturation health-related fitness training in to sessions.
- They should provide more training for coaches to improve the quality and delivery of sport programmes for young sports participants.
- Continue to both identify and reduce the barriers to sports participation in youth.
- Work closer with young people, parents, school staff and community initiatives to produce better sports programmes that attract and retain young people.
- Create effective, collaborative relationships with international, regional and national PA promotion networks.

- In order to better understand the efficacy and effectiveness of delivery of sport and PA for young people, sport organisations should provide more support of research.

Recommendations healthcare systems

- Ensure that all healthcare professionals receive training and education on the importance of PA during childhood.
- Support closer collaborative networks between healthcare professionals and other providers of PA and sport in the community.
- Change the existing healthcare financing system to allow individuals to be reimbursed for individualised lifestyle counseling and follow-up.

Conclusion

Although the benefits of a physically active lifestyle are numerous, children globally continue to fall below daily PA guidelines recommended for health. Sport, in the context of PA, has the potential to help address this decline, while also providing an effective platform to prevent the global rise in chronic disease. Governments, sporting organisations and health agencies need to recognise this potential through partnerships and collaboration, which can then empower individuals and communities to take action to promote their health.

References

Active Healthy Kids Canada (2012). The Active Healthy Kids Canada 2012 report card on physical activity for children and youth. Toronto, Canada, from https://participaction.com/sites/default/files/downloads/Participaction-2014FullReport Card-CanadaInTheRunning-0.pdf

Active Living Research (2015). Active education: growing evidence on physical activity and academic performance. San Diego, CA. Available at: http://activeliving research.org/sites/default/files/ALR_Brief_ActiveEducation_Jan2015.pdf

Andersen, L. B., Harro, M., Sardinha, L. B., Froberg, K., Ekelund, U., Brage, S., and Anderssen, S. A. (2006). Physical activity and clustered cardiovascular risk in children: a cross-sectional study (The European Youth Heart Study). *The Lancet*, 368(9532), 299–304.

Artero, E. G., Ruiz, J. R., Ortega, F. B., España-Romero, V., Vicente-Rodríguez, G., Molnar, D., and Moreno, L. A. (2011). Muscular and cardiorespiratory fitness are independently associated with metabolic risk in adolescents: the HELENA study. *Pediatric Diabetes*, 12(8), 704–712.

Bailey, R., Hillman, C., Arent, S., and Petitpas, A. (2013). Physical activity: an underestimated investment in human capital? *Journal of Physical Activity and Health*, 10, 289–308.

Balyi, I. (1998). Long-term planning of athlete development: the training to train phase. *The UK's Quarterly Coaching Magazine*, 1, 8–11.

Barber, S. E., Jackson, C., Akhtar, S., Bingham, D. D., Ainsworth, H., Hewitt, C., and Moore, H. J. (2013). 'Pre-schoolers in the playground' an outdoor physical activity intervention for children aged 18 months to 4 years old: study protocol for a pilot cluster randomised controlled trial. *Trials*, *14*(1), 326.

Bar-Or, O. and Baranowski, T. (1994). Physical activity, adiposity, and obesity among adolescents. *Pediatric Exercise Science*, *6*, 348–348.

Bassett, D. R., John, D., Conger, S. A., Fitzhugh, E. C., and Coe, D. P. (2015). Trends in physical activity and sedentary behaviors of US Youth. *Journal of Physical Activity & Health*, *12*(8), 1102–11.

Bauman, A. E., Reis, R. S., Sallis, J. F., Wells, J. C., Loos, R. J. F., and Martin, B. W. (2012). Correlates of physical activity: why are some people physically active and others not? *The Lancet*, *380*(9838), 258–271. doi:10.1016/s0140-6736(12)60735-1

Bergeron, M. (2007). Improving health through youth sports: is participation enough? *New Directions for Youth Development*, *115*, 27–41.

Biddle, S., Gorely, T., Marshall, S., Murdey, I., and Cameron, N. (2004). Physical activity and sedentary behaviours in youth: issues and controversies. *Journal of the Royal Society for the Promotion of Health*, *124*(1), 29–33.

Biddle, S. J. and Asare, M. (2011). Physical activity and mental health in children and adolescents: a review of reviews. *British Journal of Sports Medicine*, *45*, 886–895. doi:10.1136/bjsports-2011-090185

Bjorntorp, P. and Brodoff, B. (1992). *Obesity*. Philadelphia, PA: Lipincott.

Blimkie, C. and Bar-Or, O. (1996). Trainability of muscle strength, power and endurance during childhood. In O. Bar-Or (ed.), *The Child and Adolescent Athlete* (pp. 113–129). Oxford: Blackwell Science.

Bonow, R., Smaha, L., Smith, S., Mensah, G., and Lenfant, C. (2002). World Heart Day 2002: the international burden of cardiovascular disease: responding to the emerging global epidemic. *Circulation*, *106*, 1602–1605.

Boreham, C. and Riddoch, C. (2001). The physical activity, fitness and health of children. *Journal of Sports Sciences*, *19*(12), 915–929.

Borodulin, K., Laatikainen, T., Lahti-Koski, M., Jousilahti, P., and Lakka, T. A. (2008). Association of age and education with different types of leisure-time physical activity among 4437 Finnish adults. *Journal of Physical Activity & Health*, *5*(2), 242.

Bourke, L., Homer, K. E., Thaha, M. A., Steed, L., Rosario, D. J., Robb, K. A., and Taylor, S. J. (2014). Interventions to improve exercise behaviour in sedentary people living with and beyond cancer: a systematic review. *British Journal of Cancer*, *110*(4), 831–841. doi:10.1038/bjc.2013.750

Bourke, L., Rosario, D. J., Steed, L., and Taylor, S. J. (2014). Response to comment on 'Interventions to improve exercise behaviour in sedentary people living with and beyond cancer: a systematic review'. *British Journal of Cancer*, *111*(12), 2378–2379. doi:10.1038/bjc.2014.249

Broderick, J., Hussey, J., and O'Donnell, D. (2014). Comment on 'Interventions to improve exercise behaviour in sedentary people living with and beyond cancer: a systematic review'. *British Journal of Cancer*, *111*(12), 2377–2378. doi:10.1038/bjc.2014.248

Brunton, G., Harden, A., Rees, R., Kavanagh, J., Oliver, S., and Oakley, A. (2003). *Children and Physical Activity: A Systematic Review of Barriers and Facilitators*. London: EPPI-Centre, Social Science Research Unit, Institute of Education, University of London.

Cale, L. and Harris, J. (2005). *Exercise and Young People: Issues, Implications and Initiatives*: Palgrave Macmillan.

Carlin, J. B., Taylor, P., and Nolan, T. (1998). School based bicycle safety education and bicycle injuries in children: a case-control study. *Injury Prevention, 4*(1), 22–27.

Carver, A., Timperio, A., and Crawford, D. (2008). Playing it safe: the influence of neighbourhood safety on children's physical activity—a review. *Health & Place, 14*(2), 217–227.

Caspersen C. J., Powell, K. E., and Christensen G. M. (1985). Physical activity, exercise, and physical fitness: definitions and distinctions for health-related research. *Public Health Reports, 100*, 126–131.

Cavill, N., Biddle, S., and Sallis, J. (2001). Health enhancing physical activity for young people: statement of the United Kingdom Expert Consensus Conference. *Pediatric Exercise Science, 13*, 12–25.

Cavill, N., Kahlmeier, S., and Racioppi, F. (2006). Physical activity and health in Europe: evidence for action. World Health Organization, from http://euro.who.int/__data/assets/pdf_file/0011/87545/E89490.pdf

Center for Disease Control (2015). How much physical activity do children need? From https://cdc.gov/physicalactivity/basics/children/

Cesa, C. C., Sbruzzi, G., Ribeiro, R. A., Barbiero, S. M., de Oliveira Petkowicz, R., Eibel, B., and Pellanda, L. C. (2014). Physical activity and cardiovascular risk factors in children: meta-analysis of randomized clinical trials. *Preventive Medicine, 69*, 54–62. doi:10.1016/j.ypmed.2014.08.014

Chalkley, A., Milton, K., and Foster, C. (2015). Change4Life evidence review: rapid evidence review on the effect of physical activity participation among children aged 5–11 years. London, from https://gov.uk/government/uploads/system/uploads/attachment_data/file/440747/Change4Life_Evidence_review_26062015.pdf

Chinapaw, M. J., Proper, K. I., Brug, J., van Mechelen, W., and Singh, A. S. (2011). Relationship between young peoples' sedentary behaviour and biomedical health indicators: a systematic review of prospective studies. *Obesity Reviews, 12*(7), e621–632. doi:10.1111/j.1467-789X.2011.00865

Clark, J. (2005). From the beginning: a developmental perspective on movement and mobility. *Quest, 57*, 37–45.

Clark, J. and Metcalfe, J. (2002). The mountain of motor development: a metaphor. In J. Clark and J. Humphrey (eds), *Motor Development: Research and Review*, Vol. 2 (pp. 163–190). Reston, VA: National Association for Sport and Physical Education.

Clements, R. (2004). An investigation of the status of outdoor play. *Contemporary Issues in Early Childhood, 5*(1), 68–80.

Cohen, D., Voss, C., and Sandercock, G. (2014). Fitness testing for children: let's mount the zebra! *Journal of Physical Activity and Health, 12*(5), 597–603. doi: 10.1123/jpah.2013-0345

Colley, R. C., Brownrigg, M., and Tremblay, M. S. (2012). A model of knowledge translation in health: the active healthy kids Canada report card on physical activity for children and youth. *Health Promotion Practice, 13*(3), 320–330. doi:10.1177/1524839911432929

Condello, G., Puggina, A., Aleksovska, K., Buck, C., Burns, C., Cardon, G, Carlin, A., Simon C., Ciarapica, D., Coppinger, T., Cortis, C., D'Haese, S., De Craemer, M., Di Blasio, A., Hansen, S., Iacoviello, L., Issartel, J., Izzicupo, P., Jaeschke, L., Kanning, M., Kennedy, A., Chun Man Ling, F., Luzak, A., Napolitano, G., Nazare,

J. A., Perchoux, C., Pesce, C., Pischon, T., Polito, A., Sannella, A., Schulz, H., Sohun, R, Steinbrecher A., Schlicht W., Ricciardi W., MacDonncha C., Capranica L., Boccia, S., and on behalf of the DEDIPAC consortium (2017). Behavioral determinants of physical activity across the life course: a determinants of diet and physical activity (DEDIPAC) umbrella systematic literature review. *International Journal of Behavioral Nutrition and Physical Activity*, 14(58).

Cooper, A. R., Page, A. S., Foster, L. J., and Qahwaji, D. (2003). Commuting to school: are children who walk more physically active? *American Journal Of Preventive Medicine*, 25(4), 273–276.

Coppinger, T., Lacey, S., O'Neill, C., and Burns, C. (2016). Project Spraoi: a randomized control trial to improve nutrition and physical activity in school children. *Contemporary Clinical Trials Communications*, 3, 94–101.

Cortis, C., Puggina, A., Pesce, C., Aleksovska, K., Buck, C., Burns, C., Cardon, G., Carlin, A., Simon, C., Ciarapica, D., Condello, G., Coppinger, T., D'Haese, S., De Craemer, M., *et al.* (2017). Psychological determinants of physical activity across the life course: a 'DEterminants of DIet and Physical ACtivity' (DEDIPAC) umbrella systematic literature review. In Press, PLOS ONE.

Council of Europe (2001). *European Sports Charter* (revised). Brussels. From https://coe.int/t/dg4/epas/resources/texts/Rec(92)13rev_en.pdf

D'Haese, S., Van Dyck, D., De Bourdeaudhuij, I., Deforche, B., and Cardon, G. (2015). The association between the parental perception of the physical neighborhood environment and children's location-specific physical activity. *BMC Public Health*, 15(1), 565.

Davison, K. K. and Birch, L. L. (2001). Childhood overweight: a contextual model and recommendations for future research. *Obesity Reviews*, 2(3), 159–171.

Davison, K. K. and Lawson, C. T. (2006). Do attributes in the physical environment influence children's physical activity? A review of the literature. *International Journal of Behavioral Nutrition and Physical Activity*, 3(1), 19.

De Meester, A., Aelterman, N., Cardon, G., De Bourdeaudhuij, I., and Haerens, L. (2014). Extracurricular school-based sports as a motivating vehicle for sports participation in youth: a cross-sectional study. *International Journal of Behavioral Nutrition and Physical Activity*, 11(48), 11–48.

de Moraes, A. C., Carvalho, H. B., Siani, A., Barba, G., Veidebaum, T., Tornaritis, M., and Moreno, L. A. (2015). Incidence of high blood pressure in children – effects of physical activity and sedentary behaviors: the IDEFICS study: high blood pressure, lifestyle and children. *International Journal of Cardiology*, 180, 165–170. doi:10.1016/j.ijcard.2014.11.175

Department of Health Start Active, Stay Active [SM1](2011). A report on physical activity for health from the four home countries' Chief Medical Officers. *The Department of Health*, from https://gov.uk/government/uploads/system/uploads/attachment-data/file/216370/dh-128210.pdf

de Rezende, L. F., Lopes, M. R., Rey-López, J. P., Matsudo, V. K., and Luiz, O. C. (2014). Sedentary behavior and health outcomes: an overview of systematic reviews. *PloS One*, 9(8), e105620.

Downing, K. L., Hinkley, T., and Hesketh, K. D. (2015). Associations of parental rules and socioeconomic position with preschool children's sedentary behaviour and screen Time. *Journal of Physical Activity & Health*, 12(4), 515–521.

Dwyer, T., Magnussen, C. G., Schmidt, M. D., Ukoumunne, O. C., Ponsonby, A.-L., Raitakari, O. T., and Venn, A. (2009). Decline in physical fitness from childhood to adulthood associated with increased obesity and insulin resistance in adults. *Diabetes Care*, *32*(4), 683–687. doi:10.2337/dc08-1638

Edwards, M., Jago, R., Sebire, S., Kesten, J., Pool, L., and Thompson, J. (2015). The influence of friends and siblings on the physical activity and screen viewing behaviours of children aged 5–6 years: a qualitative analysis of parent interviews. *BMJ Open*, *5*(5), e006593.

Edwards, P. and Tsouros, A. D. (2006). *Promoting physical activity and active living in urban environments: the role of local governments*: WHO Regional Office Europe. From http://euro.who.int/__data/assets/pdf_file/0009/98424/E89498.pdf

Ekelund, U., Brage, S., Froberg, K., Harro, M., Anderssen, S., and Sardinha, L. (2006). TV viewing and physical activity are independently associated with metabolic risk in children: the European Youth Heart Study. *PLoS Medicine*, *3*(12), e488.

Elhakeem, A., Cooper, R., Bann, D., and Hardy, R. (2015). Childhood socioeconomic position and adult leisure-time physical activity: a systematic review. *International Journal of Behavioral Nutrition and Physical Activity*, *12*(1), 92.

Ewing, M., Gano-Overway, L., Branta, C., and Seefeldt, V. (2002). The role of sports in youth development. In M. Gatz, M. Messner and S. Ball-Rokeach (eds), *Paradoxes of Youth and Sport* (pp. 31–47). Albany, NY: State University of New York Press.

Fernandes, R. A. and Zanesco, A. (2010). Early physical activity promotes lower prevalence of chronic diseases in adulthood. *Hypertension Research*, *33*(9), 926–931. doi:10.1038/hr.2010.106

Ferreira, I., van der Horst, K., Wendel-Vos, W., Kremers, S., van Lenthe, F. J., and Brug, J. (2007). Environmental correlates of physical activity in youth – a review and update. *Obesity Reviews*, *8*(2), 129–154. doi:10.1111/j.1467–789X.2006.00264

Fletcher, E., Leech, R., McNaughton, S. A., Dunstan, D. W., Lacy, K. E., and Salmon, J. (2015). Is the relationship between sedentary behaviour and cardiometabolic health in adolescents independent of dietary intake? A systematic review. *Obesity Reviews*. doi:10.1111/obr.12302

Foley, L., Maddison, R., Olds, T., and Ridley, K. (2012). Self-report use-of-time tools for the assessment of physical activity and sedentary behaviour in young people: systematic review. *Obesity Reviews*, *13*(8), 711–722. doi:10.1111/j.1467–789X.2012.00993

Fox, K. and Harris, J. (2003). Promoting physical activity through schools. *Perspectives on Health and Exercise*, 181–202.

Fox, K. and Riddoch, C. (2000). Charting the physical activity patterns of contemporary children and adolescents. *Procedings of the Nutrition Society*, *59*, 497–504.

Fuemmeler, B. F., Anderson, C. B., and Masse, L. C. (2011). Parent-child relationship of directly measured physical activity. *International Journal of Behavioral Nutrition & Physical Activity*, *8*, 17. doi:10.1186/1479–5868-8-17

Gabel, L., Ridgers, N. D., Della Gatta, P. A., Arundell, L., Cerin, E., Robinson, S., and Salmon, J. (2015). Associations of sedentary time patterns and TV viewing time with inflammatory and endothelial function biomarkers in children. *Pediatric Obesity*, *11*(3), 194–201. doi:10.1111/ijpo.12045

Garrow, J. (1991). Importance of obesity. *BMJ, 303*(6804), 704–706.

Gesell, S. B., Tesdahl, E., and Ruchman, E. (2012). The distribution of physical activity in an after-school friendship network. *Pediatrics, 129*(6), 1064–1071.

Glenn, N. M., Knight, C. J., Holt, N. L., and Spence, J. C. (2013). Meanings of play among children. *Childhood, 20*(2), 185–199.

Gordon-Larsen, P., Nelson, M. C., Page, P., and Popkin, B. M. (2006). Inequality in the built environment underlies key health disparities in physical activity and obesity. *Pediatrics, 117*(2), 417–424.

Gray, C., Gibbons, R., Larouche, R., Sandseter, E. B., Bienenstock, A., Brussoni, M., and Tremblay, M. S. (2015). What is the relationship between outdoor time and physical activity, sedentary behaviour, and physical fitness in children? A systematic review. *International Journal of Environmental Research & Public Health, 12*(6), 6455–6474. doi:10.3390/ijerph120606455

Green, K. (2002). Physical education and the 'Couch Potato Society' Part one. *European Journal of Physical Education, 7*(2), 95–107.

Grundy, S. M., Blackburn, G., Higgins, M., Lauer, R., Perri, M. G., and Ryan, D. (1999). Physical activity in the prevention and treatment of obesity and its comorbidities. *Medicine and Science in Sports and Exercise, 31*(11 Suppl), S502–508.

Hallal, P. C., Andersen, L. B., Bull, F. C., Guthold, R., Haskell, W., and Ekelund, U. (2012). Global physical activity levels: surveillance progress, pitfalls, and prospects. The *Lancet, 380*(9838), 247–257. doi:10.1016/s0140-6736(12)60646-1

Hardman, A. E., Stensel, D., and Morris, J. (2009). *Physical Activity and Health: The Evidence Explained*, 2nd edn. Abingdon, UK: Routledge.

Haug, E., Torsheim, T., Sallis, J. F., and Samdal, O. (2010). The characteristics of the outdoor school environment associated with physical activity. *Health Education Research, 25*(2), 248–256.

Healy, G. N., Dunstan, D. W., Salmon, J., Shaw, J. E., Zimmet, P. Z., and Owen, N. (2008). Television time and continuous metabolic risk in physically active adults. *Medicine & Science in Sports & Exercise, 40*(4), 639–645.

Heath, G., Parra, D., Sarmiento, O., Andersen, L., Owen, N., Goenka, S., and Brownson, R. (2012). Evidence-based intervention in physical activity: lessons from around the world. *The Lancet, 380*(9838), 272–281. doi:10.1016/s0140-6736(12)60816-2

Hendrie, G. A., Coveney, J., and Cox, D. N. (2011). Factor analysis shows association between family activity environment and children's health behaviour. *Australian & New Zealand Journal of Public Health, 35*(6), 524–529. doi:10.1111/j.1753-6405.2011.00775

Hills, A. P., Andersen, L. B., and Byrne, N. M. (2011). Physical activity and obesity in children. *British Journal of Sports Medicine, 45*(11), 866–870.

Hills, A. P., King, N. A., and Byrne, N. M. (2007). *Children, Obesity and Exercise: Prevention, Treatment and Management of Childhood and Adolescent Obesity*. Abingdon, UK: Routledge.

Hobbs, M., Pearson, N., Foster, P. J., and Biddle, S. J. (2014). Sedentary behaviour and diet across the lifespan: an updated systematic review. *British Journal of Sports Medicine*. doi:10.1136/bjsports-2014-093754

Holt, N. L., Lee, H., Millar, C. A., and Spence, J. C. (2015). 'Eyes on where children play': a retrospective study of active free play. *Children's Geographies, 13*(1), 73–88.

Hurtig-Wennlof, A., Ruiz, J. R., Harro, M., and Sjostrom, M. (2007). Cardio-respiratory fitness relates more strongly than physical activity to cardiovascular disease risk factors in healthy children and adolescents: the European Youth Heart Study. *European Journal of Cardiovascular Prevention & Rehabilitation*, 14(4), 575–581. doi:10.1097/HJR.0b013e32808c67e3

Imhof, K., Zahner, L., Schmidt-Trucksass, A., Faude, O., and Hanssen, H. (2015). Influence of physical fitness and activity behavior on retinal vessel diameters in primary schoolchildren. *Scandinavian Journal of Medicine & Science in Sports*, 26(7), 731–8. doi:10.1111/sms.12499

Institute for Public Policy Research (2002). Streets ahead: safe and liveable streets for children. London, UK. From http://ippr.org/files/images/media/files/publication/2011/05/streets_ahead_1266.pdf?noredirect=1

International Olympic Committee (2011). Consensus statement on the health and fitness of young people through sport. *British Journal of Sports Medicine*, 45, 839–848 doi:10.1136/bjsports-2011-090228

Jago, R., Davison, K. K., Thompson, J. L., Page, A. S., Brockman, R., and Fox, K. R. (2011). Parental sedentary restriction, maternal parenting style, and television viewing among 10-to 11-year-olds. *Pediatrics*, 128(3), e572–e578.

Janssen, I. and LeBlanc, A. G. (2010). Review Systematic review of the health benefits of physical activity and fitness in school-aged children and youth. *International Journal of Behavioral Nutrition and Physical Activity*, 7(40), 1–16.

Janz, K., Burns, T., and Levy, S. (2005). Tracking of activity and sedentary behaviors in childhood: The Iowa Bone Development Study. *American Journal of Preventive Medicine*, 29, 171–178.

Katzmarzyk, P. T., Church, T. S., Craig, C. L., and Bouchard, C. (2009). Sitting time and mortality from all causes, cardiovascular disease, and cancer. *Medicine & Science in Sports & Exercise*, 41(5), 998–1005.

Katzmarzyk, P. T., Barreira, T. V., Broyles, S. T., Champagne, C. M., Chaput, J. P., Fogelholm, M., and Church, T. S. (2015). Relationship between lifestyle behaviors and obesity in children ages 9–11: results from a 12-country study. *Obesity (Silver Spring)*, 23(8), 1696–1702. doi:10.1002/oby.21152

Kemper, H., Twisk, J., Van Mechelen, W., Post, G., Roos, J., and Lips, P. (2000). A fifteen-year longitudinal study in young adults on the relation of physical activity and fitness with the development of the bone mass: the Amsterdam growth and health longitudinal study. *Bone*, 27(6), 847–853.

Kerpanova, V. and Borodankova, O. (2013). *Physical Education and Sport at School in Europe*. ERIC. From http://eacea.ec.europa.eu/education/eurydice/documents/thematic_reports/150en.pdf

Kohl, H., Craig, C., Lambert, E., Inoue, S., Alkandari, J., Leetongin, G., and Kahlmeier, S. (2012). The pandemic of physical inactivity: global action for public health. *The Lancet*, 380(9838), 294–305. doi:10.1016/s0140-6736(12)60898-8

Kohl, H. and Hobbs, K. (1998). Development of physical activity behaviours among children and adolescents. *Pediatrics*, 101, 549–554.

Kriemler, S., Meyer, U., Martin, E., Van Sluijs, E., Andersen, L., and Martin, B. (2011). Effect of school-based interventions on physical activity and fitness in children and adolescents: a review of reviews and systematic update. *British Journal of Sports Medicine*, 45(11), 923–930.

L'Allemand-Jander, D. (2010). Clinical diagnosis of metabolic and cardiovascular risks in overweight children: early development of chronic diseases in the obese child. *International Journal of Obesity, 34*, S32-S36.

Larouche, R., Saunders, T. J., Faulkner, G. E. J., Colley, R., and Tremblay, M. (2014). Associations between active school transport and physical activity, body composition and cardiovascular fitness: a systematic review of 68 studies. *Journal of Physical Activity & Health, 11*(1), 206–227.

Larson, L. R., Green, G. T., and Cordell, H. (2011). Children's time outdoors: results and implications of the national kids survey. *Journal of Park and Recreation Administration, 29*(2), 1–20.

Lavelle, H., Mackay, D., and Pell, J. (2012). Systematic review and meta-analysis of school-based interventions to reduce body mass index. *Journal of Public Health, 34*(3), 360–369.

LeBlanc, A. G., Katzmarzyk, P. T., Barreira, T. V., Broyles, S. T., Chaput, J.-P., Church, T. S., and Kuriyan, R. (2015). Correlates of total sedentary time and screen time in 9–11-year-old children around the world: the international study of childhood obesity, lifestyle and the environment. *PloS One, 10*(6), e0129622.

LeBlanc, A. G., Spence, J. C., Carson, V., Connor Gorber, S., Dillman, C., Janssen, I., and Tremblay, M. S. (2012). Systematic review of sedentary behaviour and health indicators in the early years (aged 0–4 years). *Applied Physiology Nutrition & Metabolism, 37*(4), 753–772. doi:10.1139/h2012-063

Lee, M. C., Orenstein, M. R., and Richardson, M. J. (2008). Systematic review of active commuting to school and children's physical activity and weight. *Journal of Physical Activity & Health, 5*(6), 930–949.

Liu, G. C., Wiehe, S. E., and Aalsma, M. C. (2014). Associations between child and sibling levels of vigorous physical activity in low-income minority families. *International Journal of Pediatrics and Adolescent Medicine, 1*(2), 61–68. doi: http://dx.doi.org/10.1016/j.ijpam.2014.12.001

Lloyd, M., Colley, R. C., and Tremblay, M. S. (2010). Advancing the debate on 'fitness testing' for children: perhaps we're riding the wrong animal. *Pediatric Exercise Science, 22*(2), 176–182.

Lubans, D. R., Hesketh, K., Cliff, D. P., Barnett, L. M., Salmon, J., Dollman, J., and Hardy, L. L. (2011). A systematic review of the validity and reliability of sedentary behaviour measures used with children and adolescents. *Obesity Reviews, 12*(10), 781–799. doi:10.1111/j.1467-789X.2011.00896

MacKay, M., Scanlan, A., Olsen, L., Reid, D., Clark, M., McKim, K., and Raina, P. (2004). Looking for the evidence: a systematic review of prevention strategies addressing sport and recreational injury among children and youth. *Journal of Science and Medicine in Sport, 7*(1), 58–73. doi:http://dx.doi.org/10.1016/S1440-2440(04)80045-8

Mäkinen, T., Kestilä, L., Borodulin, K., Martelin, T., Rahkonen, O., and Prättälä, R. (2010). Effects of childhood socio-economic conditions on educational differences in leisure-time physical activity. *The European Journal of Public Health, 20*(3), 346–353.

Malina, R. (2001). Tracking of physical activity across the lifespan: President's Council on Physical Fitness and Sports. *Research Digest, 3*(14).

Malina, R. (2006). Weight training in youth-growth, maturation, and safety: an evidence-based review. *Clinical Journal of Sports Medicine, 16*(6), 478–487.

Malina, R. (2012). Sports and children's health. In I. Stafford (ed.), *Coaching Children in Sport* (pp. 241–255). London: Routledge.

Mansoubi, M., Pearson, N., Biddle, S. J., and Clemes, S. (2014). The relationship between sedentary behaviour and physical activity in adults: a systematic review. *Preventive Medicine, 69*, 28–35. doi:10.1016/j.ypmed.2014.08.028

Matthews, C. E., Chen, K. Y., Freedson, P. S., Buchowski, M. S., Beech, B. M., Pate, R. R., and Troiano, R. (2008). Amount of time spent engaging in sedentary behaviours in the United States 2003–2004. *American Journal of Epidemiology, 167*(7), 875–881.

Mattocks, C., Deere, K., Leary, S., Ness, A., Tilling, K., Blair, S. N., and Riddoch, C. (2008). Early life determinants of physical activity in 11 to 12 year olds: cohort study. *British Journal of Sports Medicine, 42*(9), 721–724.

McGill, H. C., McMahan, C. A., Herderick, E. E., Malcom, G. T., Tracy, R. E., and Strong, J. P. (2000). Origin of atherosclerosis in childhood and adolescence. *The American Journal of Clinical Nutrition, 72*(5), 1307s–1315s.

Metcalf, B. S., Hosking, J., Jeffery, A. N., Henley, W. E., and Wilkin, T. J. (2015). Exploring the adolescent fall in physical activity: a 10-yr cohort study (EarlyBird 41). *Medicine & Science in Sports & Exercise*. doi:10.1249/mss.0000000000000644

Miller, E., and Kuhaneck, H. (2008). Children's perceptions of play experiences and play preferences: a qualitative study. *American Journal of Occupational Therapy, 62*(4), 407–415.

Moore, L. L., Lombardi, D. A., White, M. J., Campbell, J. L., Oliveria, S. A., and Ellison, R. C. (1991). Influence of parents' physical activity levels on activity levels of young children. *The Journal of Pediatrics, 118*(2), 215–219.

Must, A., Jacques, P. F., Dallal, G. E., Bajema, C. J., and Dietz, W. H. (1992). Long-term morbidity and mortality of overweight adolescents. A follow-up of the Harvard Growth Study of 1922 to 1935. *New England Journal of Medicine, 327*(19), 1350–1355. doi:10.1056/nejm199211053271904

Must, A. and Tybor, D. (2005). Physical activity and sedentary behavior: a review of longitudinal studies of weight and adiposity in youth. *International Journal of Obesity, 29*, S84–S96.

Muthuri, S. K., Wachira, L. J., Leblanc, A. G., Francis, C. E., Sampson, M., Onywera, V. O., and Tremblay, M. S. (2014). Temporal trends and correlates of physical activity, sedentary behaviour, and physical fitness among school-aged children in Sub-Saharan Africa: a systematic review. *International Journal of Environmental Research and Public Health, 11*(3), 3327–3359. doi:10.3390/ijerph110303327

Nader, P. R., Bradley, R. H., Houts, R. M., McRitchie, S. L., and O'Brien, M. (2008). Moderate-to-vigorous physical activity from ages 9 to 15 years. *The Journal of the American Medical Association, 300*(3), 295–305.

Nelson, T., Stovitz, S., Thomas, S., Lavoi, N., Bauer, K., and Neumark-Sztainer, D. (2011). Do youth sports prevent pediatric obesity? A systematic review and commentary. *Current Sports Medicine Reports, 1*(6), 360–370.

Network, S. B. R. (2012). Letter to the editor: standardized use of the terms 'sedentary' and 'sedentary behaviours'. *Applied Physiologoy Nutrition & Metabolism, 37*, 540–542.

Ngo, C. S., Pan, C. W., Finkelstein, E. A., Lee, C. F., Wong, I. B., Ong, J., and Saw, S. M. (2014). A cluster randomised controlled trial evaluating an incentive-based outdoor physical activity programme to increase outdoor time and prevent myopia in children. *Ophthalmic and Physiological Optics, 34*(3), 362–368.

Nutbeam, D., Aar, L., and Catford, J. (1989). Understanding childrens' health behaviour: the implications for health promotion for young people. *Social Science & Medicine*, 29(3), 317–325.

O'Loughlin, J., Paradis, G., Kishchuk, N., Barnett, T., and Renaud, L. (1999). Prevalence and correlates of physical activity behaviors among elementary schoolchildren in multi-ethnic, low income, inner-city neighborhoods in Montreal, Canada. *Annals of Epidemiology*, 9(7), 397–407.

Owen, N., Bauman, A., and Brown, W. (2009). Too much sitting: a novel and important predictor of chronic disease risk? *British Journal of Sports Medicine*, 43(2), 81–83.

Panter, J. R., Jones, A. P., and van Sluijs, E. M. (2008). Environmental determinants of active travel in youth: a review and framework for future research. *International Journal of Behavioral Nutrition and Physical Activity*, 5(1), 34.

Parrish, A.-M., Okely, A. D., Batterham, M., Cliff, D., and Magee, C. (2015). PACE: a group randomised controlled trial to increase children's break-time playground physical activity. *Journal of Science and Medicine in Sport*. doi:10.1016/j.jsams. 2015.04.017

Pate, R. R., Pratt, M., Blair, S. N., Haskell, W. L., Macera, C. A., and Bouchard, C. (1995). Physical activity and public health. A recommendation from the Centers for Disease Control and Prevention and the American College of Sports Medicine. *Journal of the American Medical Association*, 273(5), 402–407.

Peck, T., Scharf, R. J., Conaway, M. R., and DeBoer, M. D. (2015). Viewing as little as 1 hour of TV daily is associated with higher change in BMI between kindergarten and first grade. *Obesity (Silver Spring)*, 23(8), 1680–1686. doi:10.1002/oby.21132

Physical Activity Guidelines Committee (2008). Physical activity guidelines for Americans advisory committee report. Washington, DC, from https://health.gov/ paguidelines/pdf/paguide.pdf

Powell, K. E., and Paffenbarger, R. S., Jr. (1985). Workshop on epidemiologic and public health aspects of physical activity and exercise: a summary. *Public Health Reports*, 100(2), 118–126.

Prince, S. A., Saunders, T. J., Gresty, K., and Reid, R. D. (2014). A comparison of the effectiveness of physical activity and sedentary behaviour interventions in reducing sedentary time in adults: a systematic review and meta-analysis of controlled trials. *Obesity Reviews*, 15(11), 905–919. doi:10.1111/obr.12215

Raitakari, O., Porkka, K., and Taimela, S., Telama, R., Räsänen, L., and Vllkari, J. S. (1994). Effects of persistent physical activity and inactivity on coronary risk factors in children and young adults. *American Journal of Epidemiology*, 140(3), 195–205.

Riddoch, C. (1998). Relationships between physical activity and physical health in young people. *Young and Active*, 17–48.

Robert Wood Johnson Foundation (2015). Sports and health in America. Harvard, MA. From http://media.npr.org/documents/2015/june/sportsandhealthpoll.pdf

Roussos, S. T. and Fawcett, S. B. (2000). A review of collaborative partnerships as a strategy for improving community health. *Annual Review of Public Health*, 21, 369–402. doi:10.1146/annurev.publhealth.21.1.369.

Ruiz, J. R., Castro-Piñero, J., Artero, E. G., Ortega, F. B., Sjöström, M., Suni, J., and Castillo, M. J. (2009). Predictive validity of health-related fitness in youth: a systematic review. *British Journal of Sports Medicine*. doi:10.1136/bjsm.2008.056499

Rush, E., McLennan, S., Obolonkin, V., Vandal, A. C., Hamlin, M., Simmons, D., and Graham, D. (2014). Project Energize: whole-region primary school nutrition and physical activity programme; evaluation of body size and fitness 5 years after the randomised controlled trial. *British Journal of Nutrition*, 111(2), 363–371. doi:10.1017/S0007114513002316

Sallis, J., Bauman, A., and Pratt, M. (1998). Environmental and policy interventions to promote physical activity. *American Journal of Preventive Medicine*, 15(4), 379–397.

Sallis, J. F. and Owen, N. (1999). *Physical Activity and Behavioral Medicine.* Thousand Oaks, CA: Sage.

Sallis, J. F. and Owen, N. (2008). Ecological models of health behavior. In K. Glanz, B. K. Rimer, and V. K (eds), *Health Behavior and Health Education*, 4th edn (pp. 465–485). Haboken, NJ: John Wiley and Sons.

Sallis, J. F., Prochaska, J. J., and Taylor, W. C. (2000). A review of correlates of physical activity of children and adolescents. *Medicine and Science in Sports and Exercise*, 32(5), 963–975.

Sallis, J. F., Prochaska, J. J., Taylor, W. C., Hill, J. O., and Geraci, J. C. (1999). Correlates of physical activity in a national sample of girls and boys in grades 4 through 12. *Health Psychology*, 18(4), 410.

Sandercock, G., Ogunleye, A., and Voss, C. (2015). Six-year changes in body mass index and cardiorespiratory fitness of English schoolchildren from an affluent area. *International Journal of Obesity*, 39(10), 1504–7. doi:10.1038/ijo.2015.105

Sanders, T., Feng, X., Fahey, P., Lonsdale, C., and Astell-Burt, T. (2015). Greener neighbourhoods, slimmer children? Evidence from 4423 participants aged 6 to 13 years in the Longitudinal Study of Australian children. *International Journal of Obesity*, 39(8), 1224–9. doi:10.1038/ijo.2015.69

Saunders, T. J., Larouche, R., Colley, R. C., and Tremblay, M. S. (2012). Acute sedentary behaviour and markers of cardiometabolic risk: a systematic review of intervention studies. *Journal of Nutrition and Metabolism Volume 2012*, Article ID 712435, 12 pages. From http://dx.doi.org/10.1155/2012/7124352012, 712435

Sawka, K. J., McCormack, G. R., Nettel-Aguirre, A., Hawe, P., and Doyle-Baker, P. K. (2013). Friendship networks and physical activity and sedentary behavior among youth: a systematized review. *International Journal of Behavioral Nutrition & Physical Activity*, 10, 130. doi:10.1186/1479-5868-10-130

Schoeppe, S., Duncan, M. J., Badland, H., Oliver, M., and Curtis, C. (2013). Associations of children's independent mobility and active travel with physical activity, sedentary behaviour and weight status: a systematic review. *Journal of Science & Medicine in Sport*, 16(4), 312–319. doi:10.1016/j.jsams.2012.11.001

Seefeldt, V. and Haubenstricker, J. (1982). Patterns, phases or stages, an analytical model for the study of developmental movement. In J. Kelso and J. Clark (eds), *The Development of Movement Control and Coordination* (pp. 309–318). New York: Wiley.

Seefeldt, V., Malina, R., and Clark, M. (2002). Factors affecting levels of physical activity in adults. *Sports Medicine*, 32(3), 143–168. doi:10.2165/00007256-200232030-00001

Skår, M., and Krogh, E. (2009). Changes in children's nature-based experiences near home: from spontaneous play to adult-controlled, planned and organised activities. *Children's Geographies*, 7(3), 339–354.

Sleddens E., Gubels J., Kremers S., van der Plas E., and Thijs C. (2017). Bidirectional associations between activity-related parenting practices, and child physical activity, sedentary screen-based behavior and body mass index: a longitudinal analysis. *International Journal of Behavioral Nutrition and Physical Activity*, 14(89).

Smith, L., Gardner, B., Aggio, D., and Hamer, M. (2015). Association between participation in outdoor play and sport at 10 years old with physical activity in adulthood. *Preventive Medicine*, 74, 31–35. doi:10.1016/j.ypmed.2015.02.004

Sobol-Goldberg, S., Rabinowitz, J., and Gross, R. (2013). School-based obesity prevention programs: a meta-analysis of randomized controlled trials. *Obesity (Silver Spring)*, 21(12), 2422–2428. doi:10.1002/oby.20515

Sousa Rocha, E. S., Rose, G. J., and Schivinski, C. I. (2014). Level of physical activity and functional in athletes children. *Revista Brasileira de Crescimento e Desenvolvimento Humano*, 24(2), 1–8. 8.

Stalsberg, R. and Pedersen, A. V. (2010). Effects of socioeconomic status on the physical activity in adolescents: a systematic review of the evidence. *Scandinavian Journal of Medicine & Science in Sport*, 20(3), 368–383.

Stodden, D., Lngendorfer, S., and Roberton, M. (2009). The association between motor skill competence and physical fitness in young adults. *Research Quarterly for Exercise & Sport*, 80(2), 223–229.

Taliaferro, L. A., Rienzo, B. A., and Donovan, K. A. (2010). Relationships between youth sport participation and selected health risk behaviors from 1999 to 2007. *Journal of School Health*, 80(8), 399–410.

Tammelin, T., Näyhä, S., Laitinen, J., Rintamäki, H., and Järvelin, M.-R. (2003). Physical activity and social status in adolescence as predictors of physical inactivity in adulthood. *Preventive Medicine*, 37(4), 375–381.

Tanaka, C., Reilly, J. J., and Huang, W. Y. (2014). Longitudinal changes in objectively measured sedentary behaviour and their relationship with adiposity in children and adolescents: systematic review and evidence appraisal. *Obesity Reviews*, 15(10), 791–803. doi:10.1111/obr.12195

Tandon, P. S., Zhou, C., Sallis, J. F., Cain, K. L., Frank, L. D., and Saelens, B. E. (2012). Home environment relationships with children's physical activity, sedentary time, and screen time by socioeconomic status. *International Journal of Behavioral Nutrition & Physical Activity*, 9(88), 10.1186.

Telford, R. M., Telford, R. D., Cochrane, T., Cunningham, R. B., Olive, L. S., and Davey, R. (2015). The influence of sport club participation on physical activity, fitness and body fat during childhood and adolescence: the LOOK Longitudinal Study. *Journal of Science and Medicine in Sport*, 19(5), 400–6. doi:10.1016/j.jsams.2015.04.008

Tew, G. A., Posso, M. C., Arundel, C. E., and McDaid, C. M. (2015). Systematic review: height-adjustable workstations to reduce sedentary behaviour in office-based workers. *Occupational Medicine (Lond)*. doi:10.1093/occmed/kqv044

Teychenne, M., Costigan, S. A., and Parker, K. (2015). The association between sedentary behaviour and risk of anxiety: a systematic review. *BMC Public Health*, 15, 513. doi:10.1186/s12889-015-1843

Timperio, A., Crawford, D., Telford, A., and Salmon, J. (2004). Perceptions about the local neighborhood and walking and cycling among children. *Preventive Medicine*, 38(1), 39–47.

Tortolero, S. R., Taylor, W. C., and Murray, N. G. (2000). Physical activity, physical fitness and social, psychological and emotional health. In N. Armstrong and W. Van Machelen (eds), *Pediatric Exercise and Medicine*. Oxford: Oxford University Press.

Tremblay, M. (2014). 2014 Global Summit on the Physical Activity of Children. *Journal of Physical Activity and Health*, 11(1), S1–S2.

Tremblay, M., Aubert, S., Barnes, J., Saunders, T., Carson, V., Latimer-Cheung, A., Chastin, S., Altenburg, T., Chinapaw, M. and on behalf of SBRN Terminology Consensus Project Participants. Sedentary Behavior Research Network (SBRN) (2017). Terminology Consensus Project process and outcome. *International Journal of Behavioral Nutrition and Physical Activity*, 14(75).

Tremblay, M., LeBlanc, A., Kho, M., Saunders, T., Larouche, R., Colley, R., and Gorber, S. C. (2011). Systematic review of sedentary behaviour and health indicators in school-aged children and youth. *International Journal of Behavioural Nutrition & Physical Activity*, 8, 98. doi:10.1186/1479-5868-8-98

Tremblay, M. S., Colley, R. C., Saunders, T. J., Healy, G. N., and Owen, N. (2010). Physiological and health implications of a sedentary lifestyle. *Appl. Physiol. Nutr. Metab.* 35(6), 725–740.

Tremblay, M. S., Gray, C. E., Akinroye, K., Harrington, D., Katzmarzyk, P. T., Lambert, E. V., Liukkonen, J., Maddison, R., Ocansey, R.T., Onywera, V.O. and Prista, A. (2014). Physical activity of children: a global matrix of grades comparing 15 countries related to the physical activity of children. *Journal of Physical Activity & Health*, 11(Suppl. 1), S113-S125.

Tremblay, M. S., Gray, C., Babcock, S., Barnes, J., Bradstreet, C. C., Carr, D., and Brussoni, M. (2015). Position statement on active outdoor play. *International Journal of Environmental Research and Public Health*, 12(6), 6475–6505. doi:10.3390/ijerph120606475

Treuth, M., Hou, N., Young, D., and Maynard, L. (2005). Accelerometry measured activity or sedentary time and overweight in rural boys and girls. *Obesity Research*, 13(9), 1606–1614.

Treuth, M. S., Baggett, C. D., Pratt, C. A., Going, S. B., Elder, J. P., Charneco, E. Y., and Webber, L. S. (2009). A longitudinal study of sedentary behavior and overweight in adolescent girls. *Obesity (Silver Spring)*, 17(5), 1003–1008.

Troiano, R., Berrigan, D., and Dodd, K. (2008). Physical activity in the United States measured by accelerometer. *Medicine & Science in Sports & Exercise*, 40(1), 81–88.

Tudor-Locke, C., Ainsworth, B. E., and Popkin, B. M. (2001). Active commuting to school. *Sports Medicine*, 31(5), 309–313.

Twisk, J. W. R., Kemper, H. C., and van Mechelen, W. (2000). Tracking of activity and fitness and the relationship with cardiovascular disease risk factors. *Medicine and Science in Sports and Exercise*, 32(8), 1455–1461.

UK Active (2015). Generation inactive: an analysis of the UK's childhood inactivity epidemic and tangible solutions to get children moving. London, UK. From http://ukactive.com/downloads/managed/ON02629_UK_Active_Kids_report_online_spreads_FP.PDF

Valentine, G. and McKendrck, J. (1997). Children's outdoor play: exploring parental concerns about children's safety and the changing nature of childhood. *Geoforum*, 28(2), 219–235.

Van der Horst, K., Paw, M., Twisk, J. W., and Van Mechelen, W. (2007). A brief review on correlates of physical activity and sedentariness in youth. *Medicine and Science in Sports and Exercise*, 39(8), 1241.

Van Mechelen, W. and Kemper, H. (1995). Habitual Physical Activity in Longitudinal Perspective. In H. Kemper (ed.), *The Amsterdam Growth Study: A Longitudinal Analysis of Health, Fitness and Lifestyle*. Champaign, IL: Human Kinetics.

Vasques, C., Magalhaes, P., Cortinhas, A., Mota, P., Leitao, J., and Lopes, V. P. (2014). Effects of intervention programs on child and adolescent BMI: a meta-analysis study. *Journal of Physical Activity & Health*, 11(2), 426–444. doi:10.1123/jpah. 2012-0035

Veitch, J., Bagley, S., Ball, K., and Salmon, J. (2006). Where do children usually play? A qualitative study of parents' perceptions of influences on children's active free-play. *Health & Place*, 12(4), 383–393.

Veitch, J., Salmon, J., and Ball, K. (2007). Children's perceptions of the use of public open spaces for active free-play. *Children's Geographies*, 5(4), 409–422.

Vella, S. A., Cliff, D. P., Magee, C. A., and Okely, A. D. (2015). Associations between sports participation and psychological difficulties during childhood: a two-year follow up. *Journal of Science and Medicine in Sport*, 18(3), 304–309.

Voss, C., Winters, M., Frazer, A., and McKay, H. (2015). School-travel by public transit: rethinking active transportation. *Preventive Medicine Reports*, 2, 65–70. doi:http://dx.doi.org/10.1016/j.pmedr.2015.01.004

Warburton, D. E., Nicol, C. W., and Bredin, S. S. (2006). Health benefits of physical activity: the evidence. *Canadian Medical Association Journal*, 174(6), 801–809.

Ward, D. S., Saunders, R. P., and Pate, R. (2007). Physical activity interventions in children and adolescents. *Pediatric Exercise Science*, 19, 493–494.

Wickel, E. and Eisenmann, J. (2007). Contribution of youth sport to total daily physical activity among 6- to 12-yr-old boys. *Medicine & Science in Sports & Exercise*, 39(9), 1493–1500.

Wong, B. Y.-M., Faulkner, G., and Buliung, R. (2011). GIS measured environmental correlates of active school transport: a systematic review of 14 studies. *International Journal of Behavioral Nutrition & Physical Activity*, 8(39), 1479–5868.

Wong, S. and Leatherdale, S. (2008). Association between sedentary behavior, physical activity, and obesity: inactivity among active kids. *Preventing Chronic Disease*, 6(1), A26.

World Health Organization (2004). *Global Strategy on Diet, Physical Activity and Health: Obesity and Overweight*. Geneva: WHO.

World Health Organization (2005). Preventing chronic diseases: a vital investment: WHO global report. From http://who.int/chp/chronic_disease_report/en/

World Health Organization (2007). Steps to health: a European framework to promote physical activity for health. From http://euro.who.int/__data/assets/pdf_file/0020/101684/E90191.pdf

World Health Organization (2010). Global recommendations on physical activity for health. From http://who.int/dietphysicalactivity/factsheet_recommendations/en/

World Health Organization (2011). Promoting sport and enhancing health in European Union countries: a policy content analysis to support action. From http://euro.who.int/__data/assets/pdf_file/0006/147237/e95168.pdf

World Health Organization (2016). *Report of the Commission on Ending Childhood Obesity*. Geneva: WHO.

Yang, X., Telama, R., Viikari, J., and Raitakari, O. T. (2006). Risk of obesity in relation to physical activity tracking from youth to adulthood. *Medicine & Science in Sports & Exercise*, 38(5), 919–925. doi:10.1249/01.mss.0000218121.19703.f7

Yao, C. A. and Rhodes, R. E. (2015). Parental correlates in child and adolescent physical activity: a meta-analysis. *International Journal of Behavioral Nutrition & Physical Activity*, 12(10). doi:10.1186/s12966-015-0163-y

Chapter 3

Positioning physical activity and sport in a child-friendly manner

Ed Cope

Introduction

The benefits achieved through regular participation in physical activity and sports have been discussed widely and are now well understood, both in the academic literature, and policy and practice. It seems a regular occurrence that some form of evidence is reported, shared, liked, tweeted and retweeted, and discussed on social-networking sites and groups. Building a comprehensive evidence base to prove or disapprove a theory is the basis of good science, and needs to continue. Indeed, this very topic has been eloquently written about in other chapters of this book, also, which again reveals the weight of evidence to support myths or assumptions held of the positive contribution physical activity and sports are able to make to people's lives. However, the extent to which physical activity and sports are capable of making this positive contribution is conditioned by people's level of participation in these.

People's participation in physical activity and sports are founded on the value, enjoyment and pleasure they gain from their engagement in these, with evidence suggesting habits and perceptions towards physical activity are formed in early childhood (Telema *et al.*, 2005). If children experience physical activity, positively, then the likelihood is that they will continue to participate into their adolescent years and beyond, whereas if these early experiences are negative then the chances are children discontinue their participation, and are unlikely to ever re-engage (Telema *et al.*, 2005). The importance of children having early positive experiences during any form of physical activity, then, cannot be understated, given its suggested association to lifelong participation (e.g. Kirk, 2005, Bailey, 2006; Bailey, Cope and Parnell, 2015). Given that the benefits of participation in physical activity and sports have received widespread attention elsewhere this will not be covered here. Instead, the focus of the discussions will be concerned with the need for people to experience physical activity and sports in a positive manner so that the benefits of such can be realised. Therefore, the first section of this chapter will discuss what constitutes positive experiences, with a specific focus placed on what this looks like for children. Second, the available evidence will be reflected upon and a judgement made about what it is that is actually known about what children consider leads to them experiencing physical activity and sports in a positive manner. The aim here is to offer a more critical take on the research evidence than has previously been afforded.

The principles of positive experiences for children

The principles of effective coaching and teaching in the context of physical activity and sports delivery are context and learner dependent (Côté and Gilbert, 2009a; Jones and Ronglan, 2017). This means that making judgements about effective coaching or teaching is only possible if knowledge of context and learner is provided. Saying this, there has been discussed in the research literature a number of general recommendations coaches and teachers should adhere to when delivering some form of sport or physical activity. The first purpose of this part of the chapter is to concentrate on what these principles are, and why they lead to children experiencing sport and physical activity, positively.

While this may seem a rather obvious statement to make, it is a concept lost in a lot of coaching and sport-related research, which is that regardless of the level at which children perform, they are still children. In other words, a 10-year-old is still a 10-year-old whether they play for a local grassroots club, or if they are part of a developmental or high performance programme. The idea of how coaching in these different contexts should alter has been given much thought and reflection, and after much consideration it is felt that it should not change. There is no research evidence that could be found that has identified children's motivations and reasons for taking part in sport or physical activity to change depending on the level at which they compete. For example, just because a child is recruited into an elite development programme does not automatically mean they have different motivations for playing than a child who plays in a recreational context. There should not be confusion in thinking that children want to be treated differently because of the contexts they participate within, or that developmental or high performance sport for children should be the same as it is for adults. Unfortunately, this concept can get all too easily lost in an age when children get recruited into elite sport programmes at younger and younger ages, and the sporting experience they are afforded closely represents that of adults (i.e. structured practices, high training hours).

This has implications for coaches who work in different contexts and the approaches to coaching and teaching that they should adopt. In sticking with the argument that generally, children in different contexts participate for the same or similar reasons, it would be reasonable to suggest that the coaching approaches across contexts should be similar. This isn't to say coaches should be employing one-size-fits-all approaches and treating learners as if they were all the same. Of course, the nature of the sport or form of physical activity will dictate what is delivered, as will the child's stage of development, but the point being made here is how sport and physical activity is positioned to children based on the physical activity or sports context in which they participate. So, if we take the same sport (i.e. soccer), coaching approaches in developmental contexts (i.e. soccer academies) should not be too dissimilar from the coaching approaches within recreational contexts (i.e. grassroots clubs) in the general sense of how coaches behave or how they structure the learning environment. Again, and to reiterate, what is not being suggested is that coaches or teachers of physical activity or sport can follow a step-by-step guide that is independent of context and learner. Each group of children will be different to the next and will have different learning needs and wants (albeit these may only be slight differences), and it is the skill and expertise of the teacher and coach to be able to recognise and attend to this accordingly. However, what is being said is that differences in children's learning needs and wants should not be as an automatic consequence of the broader performance context.

To help think about how physical activity and sports should be delivered to children, the work of influential Brazilian political activist, Paulo Freire is incredibly useful. In 1970, Freire published arguably his most influence text: *the pedagogy of the oppressed*. In this text, Freire proposed an educational system where children were considered active learners, where learning was a co-constructed process between the deliverer (which in the context of this writing is the coach or teacher) and delivered (i.e. child). Therefore, Freire called for education to be re-conceptualised as a process away from being conducted *on* learners to one conducted *with* learners. This is in opposition to traditional educational theory that has gone before, which places the deliverer as the knowledge bearer, and for this knowledge to be transmitted to the delivered. Vygotsky (1980) terms this mode of delivery as the transmission method, as learners are passive recipients, while Freire (1970) terms this the *banking concept of education*, and term those who are being delivered to as the 'oppressed'. In essence, the 'oppressors', which are those people who have control over the learning of others, determine what is to be learned, when it is to be learned, and how it is to be learned. In this system, Freire considers learning a passive exercise, in which the learner is not involved.

Evidence suggests that the teaching/coaching sport and the closely related field of physical education follow a similar pattern to what Freire described as the *banking concept*, or Vygotsky's notion of the transmission method. For example, in physical education, albeit in a secondary school sense (that is not to say this is not the case in a primary physical education it just has not been discussed within this domain) the teaching of this subject has historically been classified as a technically oriented enterprise (Tinning, 1988; Kirk, 1992; 2009). This is where emphasis is placed on the learning of sport-specific skills in a highly structured, highly rigid and technically focused curriculum. In other sporting settings, such as coaching in club environments, a near identical situation exists, where coaching is based on culturally accepted dispositions that prioritise behaviours associated with *control*, such as instruction, management, demonstration, and feedback at the expense of behaviours that potentially enable learners a more prominent voice in their learning, such as questioning and silence (Cushion and Jones, 2006, 2014, Partington and Cushion, 2013). So, in this way, coaching practices are highly structured and prescriptive, with coaches as the primary (and often only) decision maker, placing children as objects, as information is delivered to them, rather than with them (Cope *et al.*, 2015).

Another central concept of Freire's pedagogical theory is that of dialogue between those who educate (i.e. coach/teacher) and those who are educated (learner/child). A truly dialogic relationship is one that is collaborative, as the presence of power is reduced and a primary role of the teacher/coach is focused on understanding the lives of each individual learner, and in the process, ensuring that educational discourse serves the aspirations of those to which it serves. Essentially, Freire advocates an education system that is not imposed onto people in a manner that fails to recognise individual's motives and beliefs, but rather provides learners a freedom and choice, which are grounded in the realities of learners' lives.

For children participating in physical activity and sports, there is much to be learned from the concepts espoused by Freire. Active learning has been suggested to occur when children are listened, and responded to within the context of the sporting environment (Cope *et al.*, 2015). In other words, when children feel as though they are being provided ownership and autonomy, they feel a valued and central part of the learning process. In physical activity and sports, this can happen at both a macro and micro level. On a macro level, children are given autonomy in terms of the activities and sports they wish to engage in, rather than being forced, or feeling they have to partake in a certain activity to please others (i.e. parents or coaches). On a micro level, children are given autonomy over their decision making within specific sports. This includes working problems out for themselves, instead of being provided with answers, as well as having a say in how the practices are structured. However, and re-emphasising a point made in previous work (Cope *et al.*, 2015), listening and responding to children should not be misinterpreted as 'just letting children do what they want'. The person delivering physical activity and sport has to use their knowledge to decide whether what children want to do is always best for their development. This can be a balancing act, but as long as the dialogue remains between teacher/coach and learner/child, the learner/child will continue to have a say in their own development, and feel as though their voice is valued.

Research ideas focused on identifying how the learning environment should be structured for children have received increased interest. The work of Côté *et al.* (Côté, Lidor and Hackfort, 2009c; Côté, Horton, Macdonald and Wilkes, 2009b) have long proposed for an approach to children's sport that enables them the opportunity to sample a range of sports, before moving on to specialise in one or two sports in adolescent hood, and then invest in one sport in adulthood. This model of participant development is built on the premise that children have the opportunity to develop a broad base of fundamental movement skills, which increases children's opportunities to participate in a potentially greater range of sports later in life. For example, being able to catch, throw, kick, bat and move in different ways means children have the skills to play invasion games, striking and fielding games, net/wall games, etc.

Within the sampling phase, Côté *et al.* call for the delivery of sport to be loosely structured, with a focus on ensuring the playing experience is fun and enjoyable with a minimal focus placed on competition, and limited adult involvement. Côté *et al.* term such a learning environment as 'deliberate play', which would appear to be based on the broader concepts of play discussed in the mainstream educational literature. Providing children the opportunity to engage in this form of activity has received a substantive amount of research support because of its potential benefits to children's development. For example, Brockman, Jago and Fox (2011a) suggested some advantages of a play-based learning within the domains of physical activity and sporting environment to include increased opportunities for children to be creative, engagement in higher level of social interaction than in adult-led activity, and conquering fears and building resilience for future challenges.

As well as these highlighted advantages, research would suggest that children perceive play as more enjoyable than more structured physical and sporting activities. Moreover, when an activity has been presented to children so that it represents the same characteristics associated with play, it is perceived by children as being more enjoyable, prevents boredom, has physical and mental health benefits, and children have been observed engaging with activities on a deeper level (Brockman, Fox and Jago, 2011b; Howard and Mcinnes, 2013; Sanders and Graham, 1995). It was also observed that during 'play-like' activities, children were observed moving more freely, and smiling more in comparison to children placed in a 'not like play' group (Howard and Mcinnes, 2013). What was particularly interesting about this study was that the 'play-like' task children were required to engage in was exactly the same as the 'non-play-like' task, with the difference being how children were being asked to engage. It would appear then that how activities are presented to children is of significance. Finally, because children control the direction of the activity when immersed in play, they have greater levels of freedom and autonomy and independence, which lead to increases in their self-esteem and confidence. However, even in light of this evidence, this is not to say structured or organised sport serve no role in children's physical activity or sport, but rather it needs to be considered how children should receive this form of provision.

Based on research evidence there would appear to be a relationship between children's perceptions of their competence and their enjoyment in physical activity and sport. In the sport psychology literature the concepts of mastery and performance orientated learning environments have been widely discussed in relation to children's enjoyment and percepions of competence when participating in physical activity and sport. Essentially, a mastery-oriented environment is one that focuses on individual improvement, where as a performance oriented environment places emphasis on outcomes measures (i.e. winning, test scores, etc.), and comparing performance to others. Children are implicitly mastery-oriented and derive more enjoyment from the thrill and hedonic pleasure an activity brings (Dismore and Bailey, 2011; Wankel and Kriesel, 1985), rather than being concerned with winning or competing against peers. However, adult involvement in these contexts can determine whether children develop mastery or performance orientations, and subsequently whether they develop and sustain high levels of competence, or develop and suffer declining levels of competence.

It has been found that when children are exposed to a consistently high mastery/low performance-oriented environment they decrease their performance-avoidance goals and maintain high level of mastery for physical education (Carr, 2006). Alternatively, when children are subjected to a high performance/low mastery environment, they increase their performance-avoidance goals and decrease their mastery goals for physical education. It has also been identified that children report greater levels of enjoyment when exposed to mastery, rather than performance oriented environment (Theeboom, De Knop and Weiss, 1995). Furthermore, during post intervention skill tests, children in the mastery group have been reported as having more advanced skills than children who were part of the performance group (Theebom et al., 1995). In this study, the mastery group was engaged in activities such as sparring, where as the performance group were required to perform individual drills. Game-like activities, such as the sparring example provided here, have often been cited as more enjoyable and beneficial for the long-term retention of skills (i.e. Renshaw, Chow, Davids, and Hammond, 2010), as well as having a more favorable impact on developing social (i.e. Light and Fawns, 2003), and cognitive skills (Turner and Martinek, 1999).

In summary, the purpose of this section was to highlight some developmentally appropriate principles when delivering physical activity, sport, and/or physical education when the population group is children. The evidence would suggest that less adult involvement, and more opportunities for children to have control and freedom over what types of activities they participate in, as well as choice and freedom when participating, leads to more enjoyable experiences, which in turn increases the likelihood that children will remain actively participating. However, it is important to raise a note of caution here. While the research drawn upon in this section was collected with children and is therefore relevant to the arguments made, this body of literature is undeveloped. As such, these points are more tentative than they are certain, with the next section of this chapter explaining why.

A critical review of the research literature

On first viewing of the research literature, it would be reasonable to think that the evidence base surrounding children's experiences of physical activity and sport is substantial. My aim here is to critique this body of literature in order to determine what is actually known about how children experience sport, and whether the existing literature is sufficient in explaining this. To achieve this aim, there will be a number of sub-discussions. First, an assessment will be made of the number of studies that have actually focused on understanding the views of children. From reviewing the literature to enable the writing of this chapter, it soon became clear that the terms youth, young people, or adolescents are used interchangeably and mean the same population group, when this is often not the case. As will be discussed, this causes some confusion in what can be said about children's experiences, as these are a different population group to the ones mentioned here. Second, the appropriateness of the methodology employed when children are the participants of the study will be reflected on, and third, a judgement concerning the extent to which research findings are relatable across different countries and contexts will be provided.

Number of studies undertaken with children as the focus

What is immediately clear from conducting the review of literature is the lack of recent, relevant evidence on the factors that impact on children's physical activity and sport experiences. While initial evidence searches seemed to provide a wealth of evidence for this topic, closer inspection of studies' abstracts, and in some cases their methodology descriptions, revealed that most of these potential sources were problematic in some way, such as not including children, or the findings being dated and therefore perhaps not representing children's current experiences of physical activity or sport.

This point is supported by systematic reviews undertaken on related topics to the one here. For example, a recent systematic review of literature focusing on dropout from organised sport by children and youth revealed that only one empirical study was solely focused on children as the participants (Crane and Temple, 2015), as they have been written about in this chapter. In addition, a review of qualitative studies that attempted to understand participation in sport and physical activity among children and adults in the United Kingdom revealed only two papers were related to this topic and focused on children between the ages of 5 and 15 between the period of 1990 and 2004 (Allender, Cowburn and Foster, 2006). This led these authors to suggest that there is a limited understanding of why children participate or do not participate in physical activity and/or sport. Although further studies have been conducted since the publication of this review (i.e. McCarthy and Jones, 2007), there remains a paucity of research with children as the participants, despite there being calls for some time for increased attention to be paid to precisely this issue (Hagger, Cale, Almond, and Krüger, 1997; Mulivill, Rivers, and Aggleton, 2000).

The imprecise language often used by researchers in this area does not help matters. The terms 'children', 'adolescents', 'young people' and 'youth' are too-often used interchangeably, with little recognition that these are sometimes different groups of people. In many cases 'children' is the term used in study abstracts as a generic descriptor of a young sample population, even when multiple terms were used when referring to the *same* sample. Why there exists such linguistic ambiguity is not clear, but cultural factors are a plausible reason. Studies conducted in North America, for example, often use the terms 'youth' or 'children' when describing an 'adolescent' population, or when describing anyone within the 5–18-year age range, and therefore not an adult. In the United Kingdom, Australia and most of Europe, however, 'children' are typically of either Primary School age or pre-adolescent. Perhaps, too, a degree of 'laziness' has crept into work in this area. On reflection, what might appear a trivial matter is actually an important one. When researchers use the same term (e.g., youth) to describe anyone from infants to late adolescents, it makes it very difficult to know exactly to whom the implications of the research refer. Clearly, 6-year olds are likely to have different motivations, attitudes and behaviours towards sport and physical activity than 16-year olds, but these differences will become masked by imprecise talk of both groups as 'children'.

This issue also appears in the way in which children are sampled for studies, and there is often little consistency in the age bands used in projects. For example, in some studies the age range is 7–18 years, while in others it is 9–15 years. Quantitative studies, in particular, often seem to rely on a convenience sampling approach in order to get as large a sample size as possible, which invariably means widening the inclusion criteria. In other studies, however, children within a single school year group have been surveyed. The outcome of this is that it is difficult to compare findings from one study with another or to integrate findings from multiple sources.

Appropriateness of the methods employed to generate data

When children are the focus of the research, the use of some methods can be considered more appropriate than others in relation to the research topic posed. In instances where children are required to respond to complex or multifaceted questions with some form of questionnaire or survey, question marks over the reliability and validity of such methods have been raised. When children are the participants of the study, the use of questionnaires as the primary data collection method has received sustained criticism (Christensen and James, 2008; Clark, 2010; Coad and Lewis, 2004; Spyrou, 2011). In particular, the validity of data generated through questionnaires has been questioned when attempting to uncover children's perspectives and experiences (Cope *et al.*, 2015). In some cases, quantitative methods are entirely reasonable, such as when factual information needs to be gathered. However, questions about emotional experiences to specific situations, or personal beliefs about some phenomena are much less easy to reduce to numerical or graded responses, and in these cases, perhaps qualitative methods are better suited. The relevance of research methods is always determined by the question the researchers wish to ask. For example, some studies that have used a questionnaire method have identified issues pertaining to its reliability when completed by children (Sallis *et al.*, 1993; Weiss, Kimmel and Smith, 2001). An associated issue with such methods is that they are concerned with collecting data *on* children, instead of *with* children, which devalues children as active participants in the research process, and as has been discussed in a previous section of this chapter.

Conclusion

The way children experience physical activity early in their lives has a profound impact on their continued participation and enjoyment in these forms of activity. Significant others (primarily coaches and teachers) have a pivotal role to play in ensuring physical activity environments are suitably positioned to children, and thus experienced positively. This chapter has drawn on evidence-based research that specifically relates to children's (those aged 5–11 years of age) experiences and relationship with physical activity and sport. Key messages from this research centre on stimulating children's intrinsic motivations for taking part in activities, which include playing because activities are pleasurable and provide a sense of thrill, wanting to play with friends, and learning and wanting to get better at skills. Generally, what does not interest most children when engaging in sport and physical activity is competing against others and the prioritisation of winning.

Away from adult-led physical activity and sport, child-led play has received support as appropriate for children's development. Suggested advantages are that play provides children with a choice and freedom not afforded to them through adult-led activities, and that children engage in activities that are most meaningful and relevant to their lives given that they have created them. It has been proposed that this leads to increased levels of creativity, autonomy, resilience and the development of social skills. In light of this, it is especially important for parents to consider the extent to which their children are engaged in play-like activities, and for coaches and teachers to consider the extent to which they are allowing children to have some say and choice within their sessions.

Unfortunately, the evidence base drawn upon to form the basis of this chapter is limited and undeveloped. The main reason for this, as has been argued, is that most research in this area has in fact not been conducted with children, but rather adolescents. What has led to much confusion is that the terms children, young people, youth and adolescents are all used interchangeably, yet clearly these are not the same groups of people. Therefore, it is unhelpful to discuss them as though they are. Moving forwards, researchers need to better consider how they are using these terms and ensure they are representative of the groups they are discussing.

Finally, when children are the participants of research studies, there cannot be the assumption that methods used with adults or even adolescents are going to be appropriate when used with children. As has been argued, questionnaire-based approaches are arguably not the most appropriate method to use with children. Just like physical activity and sport needs positioning to children in different ways to adults and adolescents so does the research methods employed with them. Methods are required that break down the power in balance between child and researcher and allow children to more authentically express their perspectives and experiences are what researchers should be striving to achieve.

References

Allender, S., Cowburn, G., and Foster, C. (2006). Understanding participation in sport and physical activity among children and adults: a review of qualitative studies. *Health Education Research*, 21(6), 826–835.

Bailey, R. (2006). Physical education and sport in schools: a review of benefits and outcomes. *Journal of School Health*, 76(8), 397–401.

Bailey, R., Cope, E., and Parnell, D. (2015). Realising the benefits of sports and physical activity: the human capital model. *Retos: Nuevas Tendencias En Educación Física, Deporte Y Recreación*, (28), 147–154.

Brockman, R., Jago, R., and Fox, K. R. (2011a). Children's active play: self-reported motivators, barriers and facilitators. *BMC Public Health*, 11(1), 461.

Brockman, R., Fox, K. R., and Jago, R. (2011b). What is the meaning and nature of active play for today's children in the UK? *International Journal of Behavioral Nutrition and Physical Activity*, 8(1), 15.

Carr, S. (2006). An examination of multiple goals in children's physical education: motivational effects of goal profiles and the role of perceived climate in multiple goal development. *Journal of Sports Sciences*, 24(3), 281–297.

Christensen, P. and James, A. (eds). (2008). *Research with Children: Perspectives and Practices*. London: Routledge.

Clark, A. (2010). Young children as protagonists and the role of participatory, visual methods in engaging multiple perspectives. *American Journal of Community Psychology*, 46(1–2), 115–123.

Coad, J. and Lewis, A. (2004). *Engaging Children and Young People in Research: Literature Review for the National Evaluation of the Children's Fund (NECF)*. London: NECF.

Cope, E., Harvey, S., and Kirk, D. (2015). Reflections on using visual research methods in sports coaching. *Qualitative Research in Sport, Exercise and Health*, 7(1), 88–108.

Côté, J. and Gilbert, W. (2009a). An integrative definition of coaching effectiveness and expertise. *International Journal of Sports Science & Coaching*, 4(3), 307–323.

Coté, J., Horton, S., MacDonald, D., and Wilkes, S. (2009b). The benefits of sampling sports during childhood. *Physical & Health Education Journal*, 74(4), 6.

Côté, J., Lidor, R., and Hackfort, D. (2009c). ISSP position stand: to sample or to specialize? Seven postulates about youth sport activities that lead to continued participation and elite performance. *International Journal of Sport and Exercise Psychology*, 7(1), 7–17.

Crane, J. and Temple, V. (2015). A systematic review of dropout from organized sport among children and youth. *European Physical Education Review*, 21(1), 114–131.

Cushion, C. J. and Jones, R. L. (2014). A Bourdieusian analysis of cultural reproduction: Socialisation and the 'hidden curriculum' in professional football. *Sport, Education and Society*, 19(3), 276–298.

Cushion, C. and Jones, R. L. (2006). Power, discourse, and symbolic violence in professional youth soccer: the case of Albion Football Club. *Sociology of Sport Journal*, 23(2), 142–161.

Dismore, H. and Bailey, R. (2011). Fun and enjoyment in physical education: Young people's attitudes. *Research Papers in Education*, 26(4), 499–516.

Freire, P. (1970). *Pedagogy of the Oppressed*, trans. *Myra Bergman Ramos*. New York: Continuum.

Hagger, M., Cale, L., Almond, L., and Krüger, A. (1997). Children's physical activity levels and attitudes towards physical activity. *European Physical Education Review*, 3(2), 144–164.

Howard, J. and McInnes, K. (2013). The impact of children's perception of an activity as play rather than not play on emotional well-being. *Child: Care, Health and Development*, 39(5), 737–742.

Jones, R. and Ronglan, L. T. (2017) What do coaches orchestrate? Unravelling the 'quiddity' of practice. *Sport, Education and Society*, 1–11.

Kirk, D. (1992). Physical education, discourse, and ideology: bringing the hidden curriculum into view. *Quest*, 44(1), 35–56.

Kirk, D. (2005). Physical education, youth sport and lifelong participation: the importance of early learning experiences. *European Physical Education Review*, 11(3), 239–255.

Kirk, D. (2009). *Physical Education Futures*. London: Routledge.

Light, R. and Fawns, R. (2003). Knowing the game: integrating speech and action in games teaching through TGfU. *Quest*, *55*(2), 161–176.

McCarthy, P. J. and Jones, M. V. (2007). A qualitative study of sport enjoyment in the sampling years. *The Sport Psychologist*, *21*(4), 400–416.

Mulvihill, C., Rivers, K., and Aggleton, P. (2000). Views of young people towards physical activity: determinants and barriers to involvement. *Health Education*, *100*(5), 190–199.

Partington, M. and Cushion, C. (2013). An investigation of the practice activities and coaching behaviors of professional top-level youth soccer coaches. *Scandinavian Journal of Medicine & Science in Sports*, *23*(3), 374–382.

Renshaw, I., Chow, J. Y., Davids, K., and Hammond, J. (2010). A constraints-led perspective to understanding skill acquisition and game play: a basis for integration of motor learning theory and physical education praxis? *Physical Education and Sport Pedagogy*, *15*(2), 117–137.

Sallis, J. F., Buono, M. J., Roby, J. J., Micale, F. G., and Nelson, J. A. (1993). Seven-day recall and other physical activity self-reports in children and adolescents. *Medicine and Science in Sports and Exercise*, *25*(1), 99–108.

Sanders, S. and Graham, G. (1995). Kindergarten children's initial experiences in physical education: the relentless persistence for play clashes with the zone of acceptable responses. *Journal of Teaching in Physical Education*, *14*(4), 372–383.

Spyrou, S. (2011). The limits of children's voices: from authenticity to critical, reflexive representation. *Childhood*, *18*(2), 151–165.

Telama, R., Yang, X., Viikari, J., Välimäki, I., Wanne, O., and Raitakari, O. (2005). Physical activity from childhood to adulthood: a 21-year tracking study. *American Journal of Preventive Medicine*, *28*(3), 267–273.

Theeboom, M., De Knop, P., and Weiss, M. R. (1995). Motivational climate, psychological responses, and motor skill development in children's sport: a field-based intervention study. *Journal of Sport and Exercise Psychology*, *17*(3), 294–311.

Tinning, R. I. (1988). Student teaching and the pedagogy of necessity. *Journal of Teaching in Physical Education*, *7*(2), 82–89.

Turner, A. P. and Martinek, T. J. (1999). An investigation into teaching games for understanding: effects on skill, knowledge, and game play. *Research Quarterly for Exercise and Sport*, *70*(3), 286–296.

Vygotsky, L. S. (1980). *Mind in Society: The Development of Higher Psychological Processes*. Cambridge, MA: Harvard University Press.

Wankel, L. M. and Kreisel, P. S. (1985). Factors underlying enjoyment of youth sports: sport and age group comparisons. *Journal of Sport Psychology*, *7*(1), 51–64.

Weiss, M. R., Kimmel, L. A., and Smith, A. L. (2001). Determinants of sport commitment among junior tennis players: enjoyment as a mediating variable. *Pediatric Exercise Science*, *13*(2), 131–144.

Chapter 4

Older adults, physical activity and public health

Andy Pringle and Stephen Zwolinsky

Introduction

Older Adults (OA) are a key Physical Activity (PA) and Public Health (PH) priority. Linking theoretical principles to practical recommendations using case examples, this chapter covers some of the key considerations when promoting PA with OA. We explore the definitions of OA, the PA recommendations, and levels of PA participation. We make the case for promoting PA with OA including, the health consequences of physical inactivity, alongside the holistic health benefits of becoming and maintaining PA participation. For OA, the adoption of PA is predicated by significant and wide-ranging determinants (*barriers and facilitators*). In this respect, recognising the complex and specific needs that OA have when adopting and maintaining PA, we share the key considerations for implementing PA interventions using case studies that are also framed by key theoretical frameworks and PH guidance referred to in this chapter.

An ageing population

The global population of OA is expected to double from 506 million in 2008 to 1.3 billion in the next 30 years (Hartley and Yeowell, 2015) as increases in life-expectancy result in people living for longer. Recently, we met with one of the UK's leading experts on PA and OA for the last 25 years. He said to me, '*it is no use preparing for the ageing time-bomb now, it is here already!*' People born during the Second World War are already in their 70s and living longer than many in their parent's generation. Hard on their heels are the '*Baby Boomers I and II' (born between 1946–1965)* (Schroer, 2016), many already in retirement age. Baby Boomers represent a group of individuals with multiple chronic conditions and requiring the intervention of health services (Boult and Wolff, 2015). In turn, these groups will be followed by Generation X (1966–1976), then Generation Y (1977–1994) (Schroer, 2016) and then others thereafter. Indeed, thinking about the modern day, it has been reported that two thirds of babies born in 2013 could expect to live to 100 years of age (Bingham, 2013). In short, the nature of ageing has changed.

Changes in the nature of ageing

The nature of ageing and becoming 'old' has changed from that experienced by the parents of today's OA (Laventure, 2016). We illustrate this point using three selected examples. First, retirement has previously been considered a key landmark of the ageing process (Laventure, 2016). Yet in 2016, OA are working beyond the time frames previously considered as 'retirement age'. OA are regularly engaged in paid and voluntary work well beyond 60 and 65 years and in some cases into their, 70s, 80s and even their 90s (Gillan, 2015). This is not only due to personal preferences, but also, changes in personal circumstance and financial necessity – where individuals need to work longer in order that they secure sufficient income to cover the 'costs of their daily living needs' (Gillan, 2015).

Second, the nature of relationships, family and living arrangements has also changed (Laventure, 2016). For example, there has been a rise in the number of OA divorcing and electing to live alone (McVeigh, 2013) and/ or starting new relationships (Alexander, 2015). Third, OA leisure and recreation expectations have also changed, where we see individuals aspiring to pursue existing leisure activities more deeply and for longer, as well as learning new recreational activities and skills (Laventure, 2016). Changes in life expectancy have resulted in a population of OA who aspire to enjoy and wish to participate in activities for longer than their parents did before them. Our selected examples also raise the notion of equity, that some individuals will be 'richer' than others, not only in financial terms (Gillan, 2015), but also from a social (Alexander, 2016), emotional and health perspective (Galenkamp and Deeg, 2016). The challenge for PH is to promote healthy and active ageing. PA comprised incidental human movement, exercise and sport can play an important role in contributing to this aspiration (Department of Health (DH), 2011).

Who are older adults?

One of the points that we impress in this chapter, is that OA are not a single homogenous group (British Heart Foundation (BHF), 2012; Pulkki and Tynkkynen, 2016). Indeed, with OA ranging over 40 years+, it is not appropriate to consider OA as a single group (BHF, 2012). Rather, they represent a diverse group of individuals with varied and often complex PA and/or health needs, diverse PA experiences (Lozano-Sufrategui, Pringle, Carless et al., 2016) and wide ranging skills and abilities to perform and support PA (BHF, 2009; Parnell, Pringle, Zwolinsky et al., 2015).

Chronological definitions of OA and ageing have held sway in both the PH (McCabe, Ling, Wilson *et al.*, 2016) and PA literature and have also guided the foci of PA interventions (Pringle, Marsh, Gilson *et al.*, 2010). It has not been uncommon for interventions to refer to OA as '50 years and over' (Nottingham City Primary Care Trust (PCT, n.d.), the 'over 55s' (Parnell, Pringle, Zwolinsky *et al.*, 2015), '65 plus' (DH, 2011) and so on and so forth. The BHF (2012) define OA as those people who are 65 years and over. Chronological definitions have been supplemented by qualitative or relative definitions of the ageing process which adopt a 'person centred' approach (Pringle, Parnell, Zwolinsky *et al.*, 2014) and which are linked to PA status, needs and health profiles (BHF, 2012) and because of this and in our view, these are more helpful definitions to consider.

This is because these definitions more accurately represent both the felt and expressed accounts of OA called for in PH literature (Bartholomew-Eldredge, Markham, Ruiter *et al.*, 2016). In adopting such an approach, the ageing process is described in a way that is centred on how OA feel. Given that OA are not a homogeneous group, this can vary considerably (BHF, 2012). Moreover, definitions focus on the notions of PA and the needs of OA in performing PA. With those thoughts in mind, the BHF National Centre (2012) provides the readership with a valuable framework for appreciating the relative differences of ageing and how this applies to PA. The BHF use three categories and we summarise these below.

- The Actives – 'those OA already active through leisure-time or occupational PA. This group of OA may benefit from increasing their general PA or introducing PA or an extra activity to improve specific aspects of fitness or function, such as balance.'
- OA in Transition – 'those OA whose physical function is in decline due to a combination of low PA levels and excess sedentary time. They may have lost muscle strength or balance.' In turn, this loss of functional capacity may impact on the ability of the OA to be active.
- Frailer OA – 'those OA who are frail or have very low physical or cognitive function that may have arisen as a result of a chronic disease, such as dementia or arthritis.' This group of OA may require a therapeutic approach when promoting PA 'i.e. interventions that addresses the needs of OA, and their medical condition.'

Membership of each category varies, as constituency is dependent on how OA 'self-rate' their health, wellbeing and PA rather than solely chronological parameters of ageing that has been the focus of interventions in the past (Pringle, Marsh, Gilson *et al.*, 2010). Indeed, reflecting the variation in PA and fitness levels, it is not uncommon for very active and independently dwelling 80- or even 90-year-olds to view themselves 'as actives' and *vice versa* (BHF, 2012). This reinforces the point made at the start of this section, that OA are not a single homogeneous group.

Physical activity recommendations and older adults

The Chief Medical Officer's (CMO) guidelines recommend that OA (classed as adults 65 years and over) accumulate at least 150 minutes of moderate intensity activity per week or around 30 minutes of PA on most days of the week. This can be performed in sessions of 10 minutes or more. For OA who are habitually physically active, similar benefits can be achieved through 75 minutes of vigorous intensity PA, or a combination of moderate and vigorous PA over the course of a week. A key consideration is that OA should also perform activities that help to improve muscle strength on at least 2 days a week. Moreover, OA should reduce the amount of time they spend engaging in sedentary activities, such as prolonged sitting and reclining. Given the potential health risks associated with a sedentary lifestyle (DiPietro, 2015), OA should break-up prolonged sitting or reclining, with light PA. Further, OA who are at risk of falls should incorporate PA that improves balance and coordination on at least 2 days a week (BHF, 2016, DH, 2011).

Physical activity, health benefits and older adults

Increased age is associated with physiological changes that can elicit reductions in functional capacity and negatively influence body composition (Chodzko-Zajko, Proctor, Fiatarone Singh *et al.*, 2009). Furthermore, OAs are considered to be at an increased risk of developing cardiovascular diseases, Type 2 diabetes, cancer and obesity. Simultaneously, the maintenance of physical and cognitive function pose a major challenge with ageing, placing OA at a significantly amplified risk of falling (DH, 2011), while addressing the risk of dementia is a priority for Public Health England (Mitchell, Lucas, Norton and Phillips, 2016). Be that as it may, the health benefits of performing regular PA are well documented and evidence has long supported the beneficial role that PA can have on the management and prevention of more than 20 different conditions (DH, 2004, DH, 2011). Moreover, the health gains of PA are both multi-dimensional and inextricably linked. The following section attempts to outline some examples of the known health benefits of PA for OAs using some selected examples.

Take the illustration of an OA engaging an aerobic exercise programme for >16 weeks, >3 day per week at >60 per cent VO_{2max}, what health benefits might result? Data suggests that this protocol can produce significant increases in aerobic capacity and changes in cardiovascular functioning that are evident at rest and in response to acute exercise. In addition, this type of programme can also induce a variety of favourable metabolic adaptations, including enhanced glycaemic control, increased clearance of postprandial lipids, and reduced total body fat. It can also counteract age-related declines in bone mineral density among postmenopausal women (Chodzko-Zajko *et al.*, 2009).

Next, what if we were to look at PA in relation to a chronic disease? Well, we know that the prevalence of osteoarthritis increases with age (Lawrence *et al.*, 2008) and is a leading cause of functional impairment (Conaghan, Porcheret, Kingsbury *et al.*, 2014; Ettinger *et al.*, 1994; Herbolsheimer, Schaap, Edwards *et al.*, 2016). Further, Hurley and Carter (2016) argue that few people are referred to programmed exercise as structured treatment. Sufferers also consider PA to be harmful and a number will see the onset of pain as 'harming their joints'. Hurley and Carter remind us, that joints enable human movement and a lack of PA results in muscles that atrophise and become weaker, stiffer, exacerbating pain and disability. Yet, programmed PA can help improve muscle function and pain (Uthman, van der Windt, Jordan *et al.*, 2013). As such, Hurley and Carter (2016 p. 67) argue 'muscle function is a modifiable risk factor for osteoarthritis and maintaining well-conditioned muscles might help prevent primary of secondary joint damage'.

Further for OA, high-intensity resistance exercise has also been shown to preserve or improve bone mineral density relative to sedentary participants (Vincent and Braith, 2002). In old age, the risk of impairment and disability occurs partly due to complex changes in the joints, cartilage, bone and tissues (Tanamas *et al.*, 2013) which can lead to reduced mobility. However, by engaging in resistance exercise including isometric, isokinetic, one-repetition maximum, and multiple repetition maximum-effort protocols, OA can expect substantial increases in strength, muscle power, muscle quality and muscle endurance (Chodzko-Zajko *et al.*, 2009). That said, research into the effects of PA needs to be translated into a format which is accessible, achievable and affordable to OA (Lozano-Sufrategui, Pringle, Carless *et al.*, 2016). Gill *et al.* (2016) have proposed that fall prevention programmes incorporating aerobic PA, balance and strength training were more effective when compared with a health education programme in reducing the rate of all serious fall injuries including, fall related fractures and hospital admission in male participants. Moreover, administering strength and balance exercises – such as tai chi – have been shown to be effective in reducing the risk of falls (Li, Harmer, Fisher *et al.*, 2005; Wolf, Sattin, Kutner *et al.*, 2003).

Aside from the well-established physical health benefits, there is now strong evidence that PA can have a beneficial effect on psychological health and wellbeing. For example, habitual PA is associated with significant changes in overall psychological wellbeing (McAuley and Katula 1998, Spirduso, Francis and MacRae, 2005), and physical fitness and aerobic exercise are associated with lower risk for clinical depression and anxiety (Mather, Rodriguez, Guthrie *et al.*, 2002). Joshi *et al.* (2016) studied close to 3,500 adults aged 65–75 for 3 years. Total PA was measured using the Physical Activity Scale for the Elderly (PASE) scale. The mode of PA was assessed using 'a latent class analysis of PASE item responses' (Joshi *et al.*, 2016). The researchers concluded OA who undertook the highest levels of PA and who performed athletic PA had a lower risk for depression.

Herring, Johnson and Connor (2016) investigated the effect of '6 weeks of resistance and aerobic exercise training (AET) on quality of life (QoL) among sedentary adult women with Generalized Anxiety Disorder (GAD)'. In this study, 30 adult women with GAD 'were randomised to either 6 weeks of twice-weekly lower-body weight-lifting or cycling, or waiting list control group. The SF-36 subscales were deployed to assess dimensions of QoL'. Herring *et al.* concluded that the exercise improved QoL dimensions and GAD in adult women.

Dementia is now recognised as a key PH challenge, as well as a leading cause of disability and dependency in OA (Prince, Wimo, Guerchet, *et al.*, 2015). Earlier research concluded there was insufficient evidence to be able to say whether or not PA programmes were beneficial for people with dementia (Forbes *et al.*, 2008). More recently, research has found 'low PA levels to be associated with a higher risk for dementia in OA, thus suggesting that a reduced risk of dementia may be achieved by maintaining PA into old age' (Tan *et al.*, 2016). Indeed, it has been reported that PA has 'the potential to slow the progression of dementia, patient's cognitive and physical decline' (van Alphen, Hortobágyi and van Heuvelen, 2016). Further, Kishimoto *et al.* in a Japanese study, investigated the long-term influence of PA on the risk of dementia in 803 OA without dementia and who were followed prospectively for 17 years. PA was defined as engaging in exercise once weekly. Participants were allocated to an active and inactive group depending on their PA levels. Kishimoto *et al.* concluded that 'PA reduces the long-term risk of dementia, especially Alzheimer's disease, in the general Japanese population' (Kishimoto *et al.*, 2016).

With that in mind, it has been further reported that the pursuit of leisure activities is associated with a reduced risk of developing dementia (Nyman and Szmczynska, 2016) including, the adoption of PA – a key recommendation in PH Guidance (National Institute for Health and Clinical Excellence/National Institute for Health and Care Excellence (NICE), 2015). Johnson *et al.* (2016) found that light PA was associated with higher levels of cognitive functioning in a sample of OA. While higher levels of PA can reduce the risk of cognitive decline and dementia (Ferrucci, Bandinelli, Cavazzini, *et al.*, 2004; Marquis, Moore, Howieson *et al.*, 2002). Research also shows stroke, mid-life hypertension and diabetes increase the likelihood of developing dementia in later life (Alzheimer Disease International, 2014). Mitchell *et al.* (2016) argue that the risk posed by such conditions can be reduced through the adoption of healthy lifestyles, including, PA participation (NICE, 2015).

In spite of all these holistic health benefits, it is important to remember that although health gains accumulate from PA participation, so can the accompanying risks (Zwolinsky, McKenna and Pringle, 2016). While the risks are comparatively small (Department of Health, 2004), they are often related to an OA typical PA levels and any subsequent increase in volume or intensity. Therefore, OAs should take care to gradually introduce small increases in the volume and/or intensity of PA to allow for adaptation and minimise the potential risks (DH, 2011). Moreover, PA participation should be centred on an assessment of the needs of individuals. Helpful guidance is provided in a number of sources including BHF (2009) and a number of health advice websites/GP surgeries.

Physical in/activity levels and older adults

Despite the well-documented health benefits, research indicates that PA participation levels decline with age (DH, 2011) and OA are identified as a PH priority (PHE, 2016, DH, 2011). We have already referred to variations in the PA characteristics of OA and participation levels are just another example where we see huge individual differences. For example, moderate-vigorous PA has been shown to decline by 1 minute per day on average between the ages of 65 and 85 (Hansen, Kolle, Dyrstad et al., 2012). Although age alone is not a sole marker for physical function or exercise capacity, data from the Health Survey for England in 2012 showed that the proportion of OA meeting the PA guidelines was 57 per cent of men and 52 per cent of women (aged 65–74 years), 43 per cent of men and 21 per cent of women (aged 75–84 years), 11 per cent of men and 7 per cent of women (aged 85+ years) (BHF, 2014). When accelerometery reports (Information Centre for Health and Social Care, 2009) are considered, data show that women aged above 75 achieved 2 minutes of moderate-vigorous PA per day. While for men aged above 75, this was as little as 5 minutes. If we further consider the PA levels of Black and Minority Ethnic (BME) populations, participation levels are even lower. Fewer than 11 per cent of South Asian men and 8 per cent of women aged 55 years and over are achieving the recommended PA levels (Sproston and Mindell, 2006). It is then unsurprising that, Horne (2013) reports that South Asian populations were 60 per cent less likely than the White population to meet the PA recommendations.

Physical activity, determinants and older adults

Inactivity is not a prerequisite of getting older. Nevertheless, there is no escaping the fact that a low proportion of OA meet the CMO recommendations (DH, 2011). Given the gaps in the number of OA meeting the PA recommendations, it is no coincidence that OA encounter difficulties which determine if they are able to adopt and sustain PA. Determinants are those influential enablers and inhibitors that prevent and facilitate PA participation. The factors determining PA participation are best understood using a multi-disciplinary framework (Bartholomew-Eldredge et al., 2016). Determinants are discussed here in isolation for means of convenience, but in reality; these can be both complex and interrelated. A useful framework for understanding the multi-level and multi-faceted determinants is Social Ecological Theory (Locher, Bales, Ellis *et al.*, 2011, McLeroy, Bibeau, Steckler *et al.*, 1988. Social Ecological Perspectives have been applied to studies involving OA and PA and (Chaudhury, Campo, Michael *et al.*, 2016) we adapt this framework using three levels (I) *intrapersonal*, (II) *social* and (III) *physical environment*. We use this framework to discuss OA determinants to PA participation which can act in isolation or combine to inhibit PA participation. It is important to understand these factors when planning to intervene on OA PA levels.

- Intrapersonal or individual factors related to PA include demographics and the health profiles of OA. Chaudhury *et al.* (2016) suggest this includes age, gender, educational attainment, physical functioning marital status, self-efficacy and socioeconomic status (SES). We have already discussed age and gender earlier in this chapter. For many OA, ageing coincides with retirement. Research shows that a lack of structure in retirement can act as a barrier to daily PA routines, yet when planned effectively it can contribute to a 'sense of purpose' in the lives of retirees (Kosteli, Williams and Cummings, 2016). Regarding SES, Luten, Reijneveld, Dijkstra *et al.* (2016) identify that OA and people with low SES have unhealthier lifestyle profiles than others. However, OA who were PA and of lower SES had a better chance of 'good health' when compared with OA with higher SES not performing PA (Trachte, Geyer and Sperlich, 2016).
- Linked to low PA are reductions in health status and physical functioning (DH, 2004). It has been suggested that deteriorations in OA level of health condition can act as a risk factor for PA participation. For example, OA with knee osteoarthritis were less likely to follow the PA guidelines and had poorer overall PA profiles than those without (Herbolsheimer *et al.*, 2016). Shankar *et al.* (2017) found that loneliness was associated with an increase in difficulties in performing daily living activities, while Almeida *et al.* (2017) found that non-frail OA men with current or past history of depression, 'demonstrated a greater impairment of physical and functional capacity 9 years later'. Further, deteriorations in cardiovascular health (Kahn, Robertson, Smith *et al.*, 2008), low functional capacity (Hinrichs, Bücker, Wilm *et al.*, 2015), fall-related injuries (Gill *et al.*, 2016), poor mental wellbeing (Becofsky, Baruth, and Wilcox, 2016; Cornwell and Waite, 2009) and cognitive decline (Groot, Hooghiemstra, Raijmakers *et al.*, 2016) represent potentially injurious health consequences of unhealthy ageing which can restrict PA participation (Pringle, Parnell, Zwolinsky *et al.*, 2014).
- Social factors present themselves at a number of different levels, e.g. interpersonal *(friends, family and peers)*, organisational *(workplaces,*

religious settings, clubs) and community (*local community norms and regulations*). These refer to OA social environment that can act to both facilitate and inhibit participation in PA (Chaudhury *et al.*, 2016). At a very simple, but meaningful level, '*not knowing anyone I can go with*' can be a sufficiently influential reason to deter OA from engaging in PA.

Research involving a series of focus groups with OA and conducted by Cohen-Mansfield *et al.* (2016) identified the relationship between loneliness and boredom and inactivity. It is then no surprise that social connectedness and social support are powerful mediators for PA participation (Marcus and Forsyth, 2009, including those with OA (Lozano-Sufrategui, Pringle, Carless *et al.*, 2016).

Support presents itself both in the regularity of social contacts and the quality of help from others (Chaudhury *et al.*, 2016). For instance, support comprises both advice and instruction (*e.g. how, where and when to be PA*), modelling of positive health-enhancing behaviours (*e.g. being PA, what to do, when and how*) (Devereux-Fitzgerald, *et al.*, 2016) and the sharing of important resources (e.g. *knowledge, transport, skills*) which facilitate the adoption of PA (Pringle *et al.*, 2013). Moreover, a group (*e.g. two or more people who meet to go swimming*) creates both momentum and a forum in which other constituents might join, become and stay active (Pringle, Zwolinsky, McKenna *et al.*, 2013). A group also provides the possibility that OA might rehearse behaviours and celebrate their achievements when being active. Such habit formation is part of delivering sustainable behaviour change (Fleig, McCallister, Chen *et al.*, 2016).

- Physical environmental factors not only refer to home environs, but also the local neighbourhood where OA live and work. Central to the interplay between person, place and PA, is OA interaction with their local environment (Laventure, 2016). This includes access to safe facilities for active commuting (e.g. *safe walking routes, street lighting*) and the availability of amenities (e.g. *shops, services and leisure, sporting and community facilities*) which can underpin many daily routines. Research supports that OA typically leave their homes to travel to specific destinations. It has then been argued that local environments that offer a high prevalence of 'destinations' (*e.g. services, amenities and social connections*) may provide OA with an attractive opportunity to actively commute, thus increasing their daily PA levels (Chudyk, Winters, Moniruzzaman *et al.*, 2015).
  Local neighbourhoods exist within climatic conditions and the nature of neighbourhood can change for OA due to seasonal influences (Milton, Pliakas, Hawkesworth, *et al.*, 2015). Severe weather can impact on both health (Hajat, Chalabi, Wilkinson *et al.*, 2016) and PA participation (Kimura, Kobayashi, Nakayama *et al.*, 2015). For example,

ice and snow can result in slippy surfaces resulting in falls and fractures (Hajat *et al.*, 2016). The perceived risk may deter OA from undertaking PA during these conditions. While the UK 'Storms of Christmas 2015' led to persistent rain and severe flooding that restricted access and availability of PA amenities and services (BBC News, 2015 a,b). Autumn and winter months can coincide with shorter daylight hours which in turn, can impact on PA participation. Conversely, some OA might argue these influences provide the 'raison d'être' to keep active. Further, perceptions surrounding threat, personal safety and unsafe neighbourhoods can also serve to impact both PA and health (Cohen-Mansfield *et al.*, 2016). It has been suggested that the perceived barriers for outdoor PA participation precede a decline in the mobility levels in OA within the community (Pringle *et al.*, 2014). As such, addressing concerns of OA regarding safety, distance and access to PA facilities and general amenities is an important PH priority (Rantakokko, Iwarsson, Mänty *et al.*, 2012).

Physical activity interventions for older adults

Milner and Milner (2016 P 1) suggest that

> *Physical inactivity among adults 60 and older is a global health challenge with a significant economic and human cost. Nearly 50 per cent of OA are physically inactive worldwide. To address this challenge, governmental and organizational policy makers have drafted, adopted, and implemented policies to increase physical activity levels, some targeted specifically at the older adult.*

When intervening on PA, the US Centre of Disease Control (CDC), Ransdell *et al.*, 2009) suggests there are five classifications of PA interventions. We discuss these in isolation for means of convenience, but these should be seen as a suite of intervention options.

Policy interventions include those plans, rules or norms that facilitate PA (Ransdell, Dinger, Huberty *et al.*, 2009). For example, a Town or a City may have a policy for PA promotion or rules and laws which make locations more accessible or more amenable for PA. This includes traffic restrictions in city centres or speed limits in neighbourhoods or salt spreading on footpaths during winter months, all interventions which may make the environment more conducive for PA. It may also include a local strategy for PA promotion in a defined area, such as a town or a city or an organisational setting, such as a workplace, club or a church.

- Environmental interventions facilitate changes to the physical infrastructure. This includes traffic-free walking and cycling routes that connect 'destinations' services, leisure facilities. It includes green spaces, such as public gardens and 'Greens' (Kings Fund, 2016) effective street lighting, CCT and provision of PA facilities. We can expect OA in their 70s (Milton *et al.*, 2015) and 80s to be 'out and about' in their local community (Laventure, 2016), so environmental approaches for PA are important for OA and their PA.

- Social change interventions aim to impact on the social environment by targeting the interpersonal (friends, families, peers), organisational (workplaces, churches, clubs) and community level determinants to PA (McLeroy, *et al.*, 1988, Bartholomew-Eldredge *et al.*, 2016) or a combination of the above. Interventions might include those that build social capacity and social connectedness and support such as group-based PA sessions, peer-mentoring, advocacy or a PA buddying system that helps OA learn, start and stick with PA (Pringle *et al.*, 2013).

- Behavioural change interventions target the individual level and/or inter-personal level determinants to PA participation and are central to the design and delivery of interventions to change PA. Behaviour change interventions also aspire to teach behavioural skills to help participants incorporate PA into their daily routines. Interventions can be tailored to participant's specific interests, preferences and readiness for change. Behavioural change techniques can include goal setting, time management, scheduling, counter conditioning and contingency planning and all might be used in programmes, such as motivational interviewing and peer mentoring interventions. Kok *et al.* (2016) provide guidance on behavioural change methods and applications.

- Information interventions typically aim to impact on attitudes, knowledge, awareness and norms about PA (Ransdell *et al.*, 2009). Using a range of media, interventions include mobile apps (Pringle and Pickering, 2015), websites (Marshall, Owen and Bauman, 2004), social media (Thomas, Little and Briggs *et al.*, 2013), brief verbal advice (NICE, 2013) directories and leaflets (Pringle, Marsh, Gilson, *et al.*, 2010) and signage and directions. With OA, the message used, the images included, the theme adopted, the wording, choice of language, the simplicity/complexity and time to process information that is shared through information approaches are important considerations.

- Many interventions will be used as part of an overall strategy or suite of activities to increase awareness, attitudes, knowledge, change behaviours and social and environmental conditions to make PA more conducive. In many cases, interventions will be multi-component (Bartholomew-Eldredge *et al.*, 2016) and have their affiliation in more than one classification. Kok *et al.* (2016) provide useful guidance on change methods and their applications and the reader is directed to their Taxonomy for further guidance.

Tones and Tilford (2001) also provide a hierarchy of interventions and in our example we adapt and apply these descriptions to a geographical context. Three levels of intervention are proposed.

- Micro level: Individual or group interventions delivered at the intra-personal, interpersonal and organisation level.
- Meso level: It is increasingly apparent that strategies to promote PA must be integrated into effective public policy (Chodzko-Zajko, 2014). As such, interventions aimed at increasing PA participation should not exist in isolation, but feed into a more comprehensive strategy for PA and PH, often in place across a city or a county.
- Macro level: Efforts at micro and meso level should contribute towards a strategic context for PA and health such as a national strategy for PA promotion.

We develop this thinking further through the following case study illustrating the relationship between the classifications (Ransdell *et al.*, 2009) and level of interventions (Tones and Tilford, 2001).

Case study: Introduction

The Local Exercise Actions Pilots (LEAP) was a £2.6 million government-funded multi-site evaluation of community PA interventions (Department of Health, 2007). LEAP was based on the 'five a day pilots' which were established for promoting healthy eating recommendations. Centred in local communities, LEAP interventions were delivered in 10 primary-care trusts (PCTs), with at least one pilot site in each of nine NHS regions of England. Pilots aimed to develop and assess the effectiveness of primary-care-led approaches for PA promotion linked to outcomes in key health policy (DH, 2007). It acts as a case example which can inform the implementation of contemporary PA interventions and their evaluations and so has modernity in current efforts to promote PA with OA.

In our case study, a number of LEAP sites focussed solely on OA, identified locally as a PH priority (DH, 2007). For instance, in the East Midlands, the Nottingham LEAP pilot (referred to here as *Get Moving Nottingham* (GMN) was a suite of six interrelated and sequential interventions aimed at increasing the PA levels of OA across the City. Figure 4.1: Intervention 1. An audit, mapping of PA opportunities and consultation with OA, 2. Advertising and promotional campaign for PA and OA, 3. Involving OA in PA (classes and groups), 4. Senior peer mentoring, 5. PA associate advisor and 6. Specialist PA advisors.

Further detailed information about each of these interventions can be found in the published programme evaluation (Nottingham City PCT, n.d., p. 7). This suite of these six interventions (Micro-level) collectively formed

GMN, a city-wide intervention (Meso-level), with the key outcome of increasing the PA levels of OA, including individuals from the most deprived areas in the City (Nottingham City PCT, n.d.). Following the hierarchical model introduced above (Tones and Tilford, 2001), GMN arguably contributed towards a national strategy for PA, *Choosing Activity* (DH, 2005), (Macro-level), a subsidiary of the [then] Choosing Health White Paper (DH, 2004)[1]. It is important to appreciate that the fidelity between the levels and intervention classifications shown here does not always occur in the neat sequential order presented. We will return to this case study later on in this chapter, when we consider how to implement PA interventions with and for OA in line with the key guiding principles and frameworks for promoting PA with OA.

Guiding principles of physical activity promotion with older adults

How an intervention is implemented is an important consideration (Bartholomew-Eldredge *et al.*, 2016, Breitenstein, Gross, Garvey *et al.*, 2010), as it impacts on effectiveness (Pringle, Zwolinsky, McKenna *et al.*, 2014, Zwolinsky, McKenna and Pringle, 2016). In this respect, guidance is available from a number of sources. It is not within the scope of this chapter to comprehensively cover all of these and the reader is referred to these sources for further information. The BHF (2009) *Active for Later Life resource* provides 'a set of guiding principles representing the values, beliefs and philosophical underpinning of OA's beliefs for an active lifestyle and which permeate efforts to increase PA'. Supplementing this is the NICE (2008) Guidance on mental wellbeing in over 65s: occupational therapy and PA interventions. Importantly, guidance subscribes to arguably one of the most important principles, 'placing OA at the centre' of efforts to promote PA. We refer to this guidance in the following sections using the case study we first introduced earlier in this chapter, to illustrate these principles further Table 4.1 summarises the BHF (2009) guiding principles (Adapted from BHF, 2009).

To help the reader understand 'implementation', we provide an organising framework. We frame the key design considerations and guiding principles introduced above using 'Intervention Mapping' (IM). IM is a framework providing a sequential four-stage model (*programme needs, planning, implementation and evaluation*) for putting PA programmes into practice. IM is widely used when planning interventions and further reading can be sourced from Ransdell, Miller, Huberty *et al.* (2009). In the following sections, we show selected examples of the relationship between interventions in our selected case study (GMN) and aspects of the four phases of IM (Figure 4.1) and how these activities meet these guiding principles and other key considerations.

Table 4.1 Summary of the guiding principles for promoting PA with OA

Guiding principle	Check
'PA is essential for daily living and a cornerstone of health and quality of life.'	✓
'Positive attitudes towards ageing, with realistic images that show OA as respected, valued and physically active members of society.'	✓
'OA should be encouraged to participate in decision making and take leadership positions, in all phases of programme development and delivery.'	✓
'Through coordination, collaboration, consistent messages and appropriate programme planning, PA may have positive impacts on individuals and society.'	✓
'Issues, interests and needs of OA in their community must be identified, and accessible, affordable activities must be designed to meet needs.'	✓
'It is recognised that ageing and learning are both lifelong processes, for some, pre-retirement may be a key time to focus on PA and wellbeing.'	✓
'Society should be a society for all ages. It is necessary to develop programmes and services which accommodate OA's choices to be with others.'	✓
'There is a need to identify priorities for research on PA and ageing, and to share research findings.'	✓
'There is a need for education on and promotion of the health benefits of PA as a way of life for both older people and those who work with them.'	✓

Adapted and summarised from British Heart Foundation National Centre (2009) Active for Later Life.

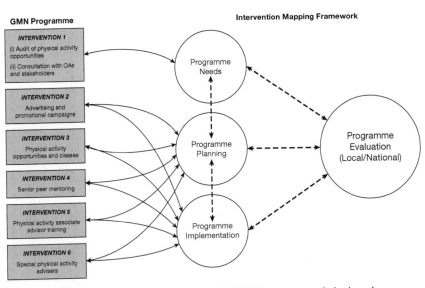

Figure 4.1 Case Study 'Get Moving Nottingham' (GMN) programme linked to the Intervention Mapping Framework

Figure 4.1 shows the relationships between the four phases of intervention mapping and the suite of six interventions that comprise GMN (Nottingham City PCT, n.d.).

Programme needs

Defining health needs is challenging owing to the complexity of the concept, and the diverse determinants which impact on health and behaviour (Asadi-Lari, Packham and Gray, 2003, Bartholomew-Eldredge et al., 2016). In the case of this chapter, 'needs' include, an OA in/activity levels, the barriers and facilitators for PA, sources of PA information, level and PA provision. At the outset, we have impressed upon the reader that OA are not a single, homogeneous group, but a diverse group of individuals (Joseph Rowntree Foundation (JRF), 2014) often with complex needs and varied expertise and experiences. We have also reiterated the importance placing OA at the centre of efforts to help them become and stay active. Indeed, it has been suggested that primary-care services for community dwelling OA need to move from a disease-based and orientated care approach to a person centric, problem focussed and goal-orientated model of integrated health-care (Iliffe, 2016) which embraces innovative approaches (JRF, 2014). PH guidance calls for PA and PH interventions that meet the needs of participants (NICE, 2008).

Central to this aspiration is ensuring OA and their careers are part of this dialogue around PA promotion (BHF, 2009; NICE, 2008). This approach helps secure important information on the activities OA might like to receive, and how these can be best put into practice in a way that meets the needs of OA (Bartholomew-Eldredge et al., 2016). NICE defines health needs assessment as a 'systematic method for reviewing the health issues facing a population, leading to agreed priorities and resource allocation that will improve health and reduce inequalities' (NICE, 2005). Sources of information for needs assessment fall into two categories, (I) primary (II) secondary.

Primary sources of needs assessment are activities performed with stakeholders, in this case, OA their supporters and care givers. Sources of information on health needs include focus groups, community forums, observations, surveys (Ransdell et al., 2009) prototyping and testing. Ransdell, et al. (2009) recommend that the primary sources should be supplemented with secondary sources of needs assessment including, national reports on PA and health profiles e.g. Health Survey for England, Active People Survey, as well as the peer review literature. Further, local resources are also available and these can supplement information secured from primary needs assessment methods and how to subsequently develop action on promoting PA.

Earlier, we referred to the GMN case study (Nottingham City PCT, n.d.), where Intervention 1 an audit and consultation with OA was specifically a needs assessment exercise (Figure 4.1) recommended in guidance and in the literature (Bartholomew-Eldredge *et al.*, 2016). In doing this, aspiring to the principle that OA should be seen as respected, valued and physically active members of society (BHF, 2009). In GMN, local teams set out to audit the existing local PA provision and identify the gaps in PA provision including, those in the most deprived areas of the city. Importantly, over 150 OA were consulted on their PA needs using captive audiences, of OA including, OA who were insufficiently physically active.

In GMN, needs assessments examined OA awareness of the PA recommendations, sources of information, and the opportunities for PA alongside the determinants impacting on PA participation (Nottingham PCT, n.d.). As recommended in guidance, these consultations extended to practitioners who promoted PA with OA (BHF, 2009). Research identifies that healthcare providers play a key role in counselling and encouraging OA to adopt PA (Lobelo and de Quevedo, 2016). Many of these constituents have experiences of working with OA and an understanding why OA may be deterred from taking up existing PA opportunities. Moreover, such individuals can be seen by OA as playing an important 'expert' role in promoting PA (Devereux-Fitzgerald *et al.*, 2016) and the inclusion of these constituents is in line with guidance in the literature (Bartholomew-Eldredge *et al.*, 2016).

In GMN, (Nottingham City PCT, n.d.), outcomes from Intervention 1, the Audit and the Consultation with OA, were framed against information collected from secondary sources including, national data on PA levels and local health and demographic profiles. Franco, Tong, Howard *et al.* (2015) recommends that in order to increase PA in OA, efforts should aim to increase awareness of the benefits and minimise the perceived risks and improve access to PA opportunities. Moreover interventions should address OA concerns surrounding both capability to engage and the necessity of PA participation (Devereux-Fitzgerald *et al.*, 2016), it is then pertinent that outcomes identified from the GMN consultation included the following outcomes:

- OA didn't know what the current PA recommendations were (60 per cent of respondents, 80 per cent in Asian/Asian British groups).
- OA required better information on PA to include, resources that helped OA who were thinking about becoming more active to change their perceptions of PA.
- OA required age-appropriate PA sessions which promote engagement and inclusion.
- OA were more likely to take up opportunities when they were provided within close proximity to their home and local environs and where limited travel was required to participate in PA options (Nottingham City PCT, n.d.).

In our selected case study, the intervention reflects the key guiding principles, that is, OA and their supporters be encouraged to participate in decision-making for service planning for and the design of PA provision (BHF, 2009, NICE, 2008). Moreover, the needs assessment activities deployed here, understood that OA bring important skills and expertise to help facilitate solutions to the health issues they face (JRF, 2014). The insights from OA helped to establish an appreciation by key agencies of the determinants to PA participation. Information was then used to develop multi-level solutions for PA promotion (Mama, McCurdy, Evans et al., 2015). In the following sections, we learn how findings from this intervention, the consultation and audit, were used to shape accessible, acceptable and affordable programmes designed to meet the expressed PA needs of OA.

Programme planning

Programme planning are the preparations that are required to put interventions into practice. It includes, but is not solely limited to reviewing evidence on the effectiveness and implementation of interventions and participant health needs, the setting of aims and objectives in response to identified needs, planning intervention scope, sequence, themes change methods and applications (Bartholomew-Eldredge et al., 2016), securing resources to support these interventions and obtaining the support of various stakeholders, including OA (Ransdell, Dinger, Huberty et al., 2009). In this section, we illustrate 'just one' aspect of how OA were involved in planning the delivery of PA opportunities offered in GMN case study.

Intervention 1 (the audit and consultation of PA opportunities and needs) not only identified gaps in provision, but also OA determinants to participation in PA. Following the completion of needs assessment, a suite of related activities (Interventions 2–6) were designed to address and meet the expressed needs of OA and fill gaps in PA provision (Figure 4.1). One of these interventions, Intervention 3, Getting OA involved in new PA was comprised of two components: (i) Provision of a directory of 160 PA opportunities available to OA. (ii) An opportunity for local groups from areas of deprivation to bid for up to £500 to run PA classes/groups (Nottingham City PCT, n.d.).

These two interventions aimed to increase OA awareness of the health benefits of PA, as well as the number of PA opportunities that were available in the local community. Within Intervention 3, OA were central to the planning of activities (Alsaeed, Davies, Gilmartin et al., 2016) aimed at meeting their PA needs (Franco et al., 2015). OA groups could bid for resources to run their own PA sessions within their communities. Bidding took place through a three-phase process resulting in over 30 applications for funding (Nottingham City PCT, n.d.). Research has identified that individuals residing in the least promising circumstances are often most poorly provided for in terms of access to PA services (Oliver, Hanson, Lyndsey *et al.*, 2016). It is then encouraging to learn that, applications were received from groups located in the 'most deprived wards' in Nottingham. In total, 13 applications were successful in securing 'pump-prime' funding. These included, *'gentle exercises at a local YMCA* and a *walking group at the Muslim Women's Community Centre* (Nottingham City PCT, n.d.). Further information on all the interventions is reported fully elsewhere (Nottingham City PCT, n.d.), but interventions met recommendations to increase engagement in PA, by making PA a fun, sociable, achievable pastime for older adults with an emphasis on the short-term benefits (Devereux-Fitzgerald *et al.*, 2016).

That said and reflecting the importance of performing the evaluation of interventions (Bartholomew-Eldredge *et al.*, 2016), local teams identified a number of challenges with this approach. First, local groups needed intensive support to set up their projects and better pre-planning to achieve sustainability. Second, groups also required help when recruiting 'age-appropriate' instructors. Third, LEAP teams administered advice on operational issues such as, setting an admission fee. Fourth, while Intervention 3 was viewed as less effective at reaching men (Nottingham City PCT, n.d.), often viewed as a hard-to-engage group (Lozano-Sufrategui *et al.*, 2016, Robertson *et al.*, 2016), it was nonetheless successful at engaging women and BME participants. Local evaluations report that over 90 per cent of attendees were women and participants from BME groups (*15 per cent African Caribbean, 12 per cent Pakistani and 12 per cent Indian OA*). Finally, only a handful of the 13 interventions became sustainable. (Nottingham City PCT, n.d.). Limitations were balanced by strengths and these included an increase in PA adoption rates, developing new networks and learning what works, with who and why? Outcomes provide insights and learning for shaping future PA provision (BHF, 2009) and that could inform local policy for PA (Pringle, McKenna, and Zwolinsky, in press).

Despite the relative effectiveness of Intervention 3, process outcomes reflect the importance of adopting 'a person-centred' approach (Alsaeed *et al.*, 2016) that placed 'OA at the heart' of solutions to meet their PA needs (Illfee, 2016). Interventions were located in community facing agencies and groups which many OA were already connected to and familiar with. Given that adopting PA is likely to be challenging in its own right, learning a further set of new protocols for getting to and attending an unfamiliar venue, engaging new behavioural processes, as well as connecting with new people poses further challenges when initiating PA (Pringle, Zwolinsky, McKenna *et al.*, 2014, Pringle, McKenna, and Zwolinsky, in press). Moreover, the involvement of voluntary groups in the delivery of PA opportunities shown here has a new modernity, given the diminishing responsibilities and resources of statutory services, such as local authorities.

Programme implementation

Programme implementation refers to those activities undertaken when putting interventions into practice (Ransdell, Dinger Huberty *et al.*, 2009). This includes implementing the programme theme, scope, sequence, change methods and their applications (Bartholomew-Eldredge *et al.*, 2016). Translating these applications into practice includes a number of considerations including the selection of promotional strategies, intervention venues, instructors, timing, participant group, safety of participants, the Frequency, Intensity, Time and Type (FITT) of the PA sessions among other factors the discussion of which is beyond the scope of this chapter.

Using our case study, we illustrate aspects of how another intervention from GMN (Figure 4.1) was implemented (Nottingham City PCT, n.d.). In doing so, we refer to the guiding principles for promoting PA with OA (BHF, 2009). We have already referred to the outcomes from Intervention 1 which were used to plan and implement PA opportunities for OA. In GMN, OA also identified the need to provide supportive social environments for PA as well as professional education for practitioners. We discuss Intervention 4, Senior Peer Mentoring (SPM) as an example and show selected aspects of 'implementation' further (Nottingham City PCT, n.d.).

We learn from the programme evaluation (Nottingham City PCT, n.d.), that this intervention was based on 'Someone Like Me' a national package of SPM training. This was originally developed in partnership with Later Life Training, the BHF National Centre, Age Concern and Age UK (Later Life Training, 2016). The intervention was not only based on the needs of OA, but also on the principle of effective practice (Ransdell *et al.*, 2011). As such, staff aspired to the notion of 'translation', that is, the model could be adopted, adapted and applied in similar local contexts where it had been used previously.

Importantly, the SPM model was adapted to suit local needs and circumstance – a key implementation issue (DH, 2007). For example, OA from the local area were involved in the development and tailoring of the training which was viewed as providing added value in 'localising' the intervention (Nottingham PCT, n.d.), this can include using knowledge of local issues, use of local venues, promotional images messages/benefits and colloquialisms. Moreover, considering word of mouth is a powerful promotional strategy in PA interventions (Pringle, Zwolinsky, McKenna *et al.*, 2014), many OA had their own person-to-person networks and knowledge of how these worked best for promoting GMN. This approach recognises that OA contribute both important skills and expertise in providing client centred and solution focussed PH interventions.

The SPM provided training to volunteers on the key elements they would need, in order to be a successful mentor. The training also included the CMO guidelines, and the benefits and barriers of PA to OA. Someone Like Me also covered the mechanics of SPM, including, mentoring, communication and deploying motivational skills with mentees. In the understanding that volunteers would need to know about the mentoring opportunities that existed locally, the intervention also outlined mentoring roles that were available and what was required from volunteers who elected to participate, their choices and responsibilities (Nottingham City PCT, n.d.). Given that OA have different learning styles and may require more time and need help with building up confidence to learn new activities and skills (Dunlosky and Hertzog, 1998), involving OA in the 'delivery' process was also important. They understood issues from both the perspective of the mentor and mentee! Engaging key stakeholders is an important ingredient in effective PH practice.

In the spirit of effective practice, the SPM programme included programme content on 'the volunteer policy', a code of 'good practice' that volunteers would aspire to adhere to during their mentoring (Nottingham City PCT, n.d.). Regarding the 'key guiding principles' we introduced earlier in this chapter, the SPM intervention aspired to accommodate OA choices to be with other people, as well as educating OA and their key workers on the benefits and other PA opportunities that existed locally and how these could be accessed (BHF, 2009). In doing so, reflecting the synergies between the different interventions that formed GMN and shown in Figure 4.1. Above all, SPM resulted from an aspiration to assess and meet the PA interests and needs of OA in the City of Nottingham (Nottingham City PCT, n.d.).

Given the restrictions of space, it has not been possible to cover all aspects of SPM and indeed features and issues of the other five interventions from GMN. With this in mind, the reader is directed to the comprehensive programme evaluation where further information, local insights and evaluation outcomes can be found in greater detail from the local LEAP evaluation report (Nottingham City PCT, n.d.). Rather, we have aspired to link key intervention frameworks and essential considerations for promoting PA with OA through a real-life case study.

Programme evaluation

The fourth stage of IM is programme evaluation and describes all those activities designed to assess the impact of interventions and the process by which they were implemented. Evaluation is frequently discussed at the end of interventions when it is too late, and it is important to underscore its importance as a 'front-end' activity which permeates the needs assessment, planning and implementation process (Pringle, McKenna and Zwolinsky, in press) (Figure 4.1).

In Stage 2 of IM, we discussed the importance of setting clear aims and objectives for the intervention. Evaluation is the means of gauging the extent to which programme aims and objectives have been achieved, as well as the means to remodel and refine programme provision (Bartholomew-Eldredge *et al.*, 2016). As such, extensive guidance on monitoring and evaluation is available from a number of sources and we refer the reader to these for more in-depth information. Sources of this information include the Standard Evaluation Framework for PA (National Obesity Observatory (NOO), 2012), the Framework for Programme Evaluation (CDC, 1999), the Learning from LEAP (Sport England, 2006), MRC (Craig, Dieppe, Macintyre *et al.*, 2011) Guidance on Evaluating Complex PH Interventions. A useful checklist is also provided in Pringle *et al.* (2014). Further, specific guidance on evaluating interventions for OA is available at BHF (2009) and (Bartholomew-Eldredge *et al.*, 2016, Pringle, McKenna, and Zwolinsky, in press).

Our experience has led us to conclude that there is variable practice when it comes to evaluating interventions (Pringle, McKenna, Zwolinsky, in press). As we have reported, GMN was part of a multi-level programme evaluation of PA (National Evaluation of LEAP, DH 2007, Pringle *et al.*, 2010). First at a micro/meso level, a local evaluation assessed the impact of interventions against local priorities (*including the profiles of OA recruited, PA levels, health outcomes and experiences and perspectives*) (Nottingham City PCT, n.d.). Impact outcomes from GMN were also included within a national programme evaluation along with those outcomes emerging from the nine other LEAP sites (Pringle *et al.*, 2010). These outcomes included demographic profiles, and pre-/post-intervention PA levels, a cost-effectiveness analysis and a process evaluation which assessed the key design and implementation characteristics of interventions. This included aspects within the four phases of IM, i.e. *programme needs, planning implementation* and *evaluation* discussed earlier (Figure 4.1).

Importantly the national programme evaluation of LEAP provided an opportunity for key stakeholders (participants and deliverers) to provide feedback on the interventions reported elsewhere (DH, 2007). One of the learning points emerging from the National Evaluation of LEAP was that evaluation strategies, including instrumentation (e.g. questionnaires, interviews, applications) and evaluation processes (e.g. consent and participant pre-information), should be accessible to individuals, including OA (Pringle, McKenna, and Zwolinsky, in press). Moreover, evaluation activities should not deter individuals from taking part in interventions, either as a participant or as a volunteer (DH, 2007). During the implementation of LEAP, we learnt that that some volunteers who elected to support PA interventions, through mentoring and advisor roles were also tasked with collecting evaluation data (DH, 2007). Securing participant consent and capturing evaluation information was at times challenging for volunteers and this was off putting to many constituents (DH, 2007). A number of helpers had not volunteered for this specific purpose and threatened to withdraw their services (DH, 2007). Evaluations then need effective planning and need to consider the local context and resources (DH, 2007) in advance of implementation (Pringle, McKenna, Zwolinsky, in press).

It is examples like these that provide helpful learning and outcomes emerging from the LEAP and GMN pilot(s) have been reported elsewhere (Pringle, McKenna, and Zwolinsky, in press; Sport England, 2006; DH, 2007). The local evaluation of GMN specifically reported both the impact and process (Nottingham City PCT, n.d.) and informed future actions for PA promotion locally. The reader is directed to the Programme Evaluation of GMN (Nottingham City PCT, n.d.) for further information on impact and process outcomes, as well as the National Evaluation of LEAP (DH, 2007). Both the local and the national evaluation described in this chapter aspired to meet the BHF (2009) guiding principle that 'identifies priorities for research on PA and ageing, and to share research findings' with a disseminated of stakeholders in order that translational lessons can be shared (Mansfield and Piggin, 2016).

Conclusion

The benefits of PA for OA are well documented (BHF, 2016). Yet, the number of OAs failing to meet PA guidelines is a cause for concern, as such, OA are a PH priority (DH, 2011). We have tried to underscore that OA are not a single homogeneous group, but a diverse group of individuals who present with varied and sometimes complex health and PA needs. A diverse range of interrelated determinants impact on PA participation. In response to this challenge, there is a need for a sophisticated suite of PA interventions which reflect needs, differentiation, choice and access (Laventure, 2016). When developing and implementing interventions designed to meet the PA needs of OA, a number of guiding principles and helpful frameworks and useful guidance is available in this respect. We have tried to show how these frameworks and guiding principles can be put into practice using an applied case study from the PH literature.

Declarations of interest

Co-Author A. Pringle led the National Evaluation of the Local Exercise Action Pilots across 10 English PCTs and featured as a Case Study in this chapter. Leeds Beckett University received funding to undertake the National Evaluation of the Local Exercise Action Pilots. We gratefully acknowledge the contribution of all individuals and organisations involved in this research.

Note

1   Choosing Health has subsequently been replaced by Healthy Lives Healthy People.

References

Alexander, R. (2015) Getting divorced after 60. *BBC Magazine*. Available at http://bbc.co.uk/news/magazine-34767821 (accessed 20 June 2016).

Almeida, O. P., Hankey, G. J., Yeap, B. B., Golledge, J., Hill, K. D., and Flicker, L. (2017). Depression among non-frail old men is associated with reduced physical function and functional capacity after 9 years follow-up: the health in men cohort study. *Journal of the American Medical Directors Association*, 18(1), 65–69.

Alsaeed, D., Davies, N., Gilmartin, J. F. M., Jamieson, E., Kharicha, K., Liljas, A. E., Raimi-Abraham, B. T., Aldridge, J., Smith, F. J., Walters, K., and Gul, M. O. (2016). Older people's priorities in health and social care research and practice: a public engagement workshop. *Research Involvement and Engagement*, 2(1), 1.

Alzheimer's Disease International (2014). *World Alzheimer Report 2014: Dementia and Risk Reduction*. Alzheimer's Disease International. Available at www.alz.co.uk/research/WorldAlzheimerReport2014.pdf

Asadi-Lari, M., Packham, C., and Gray, D. (2003) Unmet health needs in patients with coronary heart disease: implications and potential for improvement in caring services. *Health and Quality of Life Outcomes*, 1(1), 1.

Bartholomew-Eldredge, L. K, Markham, C. M., Ruiter, R. A, Fernandez, M. E., Kok, G., and Parcel, G. (2016). *Planning Health Promotion Programmes: An Intervention Mapping Approach*. London, Wiley.

BBC News (2015a). UK floods: homes evacuated amid heavy rain. Available at http://bbc.co.uk/news/uk-35181139 (accessed 13 January 2016).

BBC News (2015b). UK floods: water levels continue to rise in York. Available at http://bbc.co.uk/news/uk-35185228 (accessed 13 January 2016).

Becofsky, K., Baruth, M., and Wilcox, S. (2016) Physical activity mediates the relationship between program participation and improved mental health in older adults. *Public Health*. http://dx.doi.org/10.1016/j.puhe.2015.07.040

Bingham, J. (2013) Two thirds of babies could live to 100. *The Telegraph*, December 12. Available at http://telegraph.co.uk/news/health/news/10511865/Two-thirds-of-todays-babies-could-live-to-100.html (accessed 23 June 2016).

Boult, C. and Wolff, J. L. (2015). 'Guided Care' for People with Complex Health Care Needs. In *Geriatrics Models of Care* (pp. 139–145). Springer International Publishing.

Breitenstein, S. M., Gross, D., Garvey, C. A., Hill, C., Fogg, L., and Resnick, B. (2010) Implementation fidelity in community-based interventions. *Research in Nursing & Health*, 33(2), 164–173.

British Heart Foundation, National Centre (2009). Active for later life resource. Available at http://bhfactive.org.uk/older-adults-resources-and-publications-item/78/index.html (accessed 1 April 2016).

British Heart Foundation, National Centre (2012). Interpreting the UK physical activity guidelines for older adults (65+). Guidance for those working with older adults described as in transition. Available at www.ssehsactive.org.uk/files/4170/transitionolderadults.pdf

British Heart Foundation, National Centre (2014). Current levels of physical activity in older adults. Available at www.bhfactive.org.uk/files/1171/Physical%20Activity%20Older%20Adults%20AW.pdf

British Heart Foundation, National Centre (2016). Physical activity guidelines for older adults. Available at http://bhfactive.org.uk/olderadultsguidelines/index.html (accessed 30 March 2017).

Centers for Disease Control and Prevention (1999). Framework for program evaluation in public health. *Morbidity Mortality Weekly Reports*, 48(RR-11). A811.pdf.

Chaudhury, H., Campo, M., Michael, Y., and Mahmood, A. (2016) Neighbourhood environment and physical activity in older adults. *Social Science & Medicine*, 149, 104–113.

Chodzko-Zajko, W. J. (2014). Exercise and physical activity for older adults. *Kinesiology Reports*, 3(1), 101–106.

Chodzko-Zajko, W., Proctor, D., Fiatarone Singh, M., Minson, C., Nigg, C., Salem, G., and Skinner, J. (2009) Exercise and Physical Activity for Older Adults. *Medicine and Science in Sports Exercise*, 41(7), 1510–1530.

Chudyk, A. M., Winters, M., Moniruzzaman, M., Ashe, M. C., Gould, J. S., and McKay, H. (2015). Destinations matter: the association between where older adults live and their travel behaviour. *Journal of Transport & Health*, 2(1), 50–57.

Cohen-Mansfield, J., Hazan, H., Lerman, Y., and Shalom, V. (2016). Correlates and predictors of loneliness in older-adults: a review of quantitative results informed by qualitative insights. *International Psychogeriatrics*, 28(4), 557–576.

Conaghan, P. G., Porcheret, M., Kingsbury, S. R., Gammon, A., Soni, A., Hurley, M., Rayman, M. P., Barlow, J., Hull, R.G., Cumming, J. and Llewelyn, K. (2015). Impact and therapy of osteoarthritis: the Arthritis Care OA Nation 2012 survey. *Clinical Rheumatology*, 34(9), 1581–1588.

Cornwell, E. and Waite, L. (2009). Social disconnectedness, perceived isolation and health among older adults. *Journal of Health and Social Behaviour*, 50, 31–48.

Craig, P., Dieppe, P., Macintyre, S., Michie, S., Nazareth, I., and Petticrew, M. (2011). *Developing and Evaluating Complex Interventions*. London: Medical Research Council, available at www.mrc.ac.uk/documents/pdf/complex-interventions-guidance

Department of Health (2004). *At Least Five a Week: Evidence on the Impact of Physical Activity and its Relationship to Health*. London: Department of Health.

Department of Health (2004). *Choosing Health: Making Healthy Choices Easier*. London: Department of Health.

Department of Health (2005). *Choosing Activity: A Physical Activity Action Plan*. London: Department of Health.

Department of Health (2007). *National Evaluation of the Local Exercise Action Pilots*. London: Department of Health. Available at http://dh.gov.uk/en/Publications andstatistics/Publications/PublicationsPolicyAndGuidance/DH_073600 (accessed 4 April 2016).

Department of Health (2011). *Start Active Stay Active: A Report for the Four Home Countries Medical Officers*. London: Department of Health.

Devereux-Fitzgerald, A., Powell, R., Dewhurst, A., and French, D. P. (2016). The acceptability of physical activity interventions to older adults: a systematic review and meta-synthesis. *Social Science & Medicine*, 158, 14–23.

DiPietro, L. (2015). Physical activity in older people. Commentary. Washington, DC: Institute of Medicine, available at http://nam.edu/wp-content/uploads/2015/06/PAandolderpeople (accessed 31 October 2016).

Dunlosky, J. and Hertzog, C. (1998). Training programs to improve learning in later adulthood: helping older adults educate themselves. *Metacognition in Educational Theory and Practice*, 249, 276.

Ettinger, W. H., Davis, M. A., Neuhaus, J. M., and Mallon, K. P. (1994). Long-term physical functioning in persons with knee osteoarthritis from NHANES I: effects of comorbid medical conditions. *Journal of Clinical Epidemiology*, 47(7), 809–815.

Ferrucci, L., Bandinelli, S., Cavazzini, C., Lauretani, F., Corsi, A., Bartali, B., Cherubini, A., Launer, L., and Guralnik, J. M. (2004). Neurological examination findings to predict limitations in mobility and falls in older persons without a history of neurological disease. *The American Journal of Medicine*, 116(12), 807–815.

Fleig, L., McAllister, M. M., Chen, P., Iverson, J., Milne, K., McKay, H. A., Clemson, L., and Ashe, M. C. (2016). Health behaviour change theory meets falls prevention: feasibility of a habit-based balance and strength exercise intervention for older adults. *Psychology of Sport and Exercise*, 22, 114–122.

Forbes, D., Forbes, S., Morgan, D.G., Markle-Reid, M., Wood, J., and Culum, I. (2008). *Physical Activity Programs for Persons with Dementia*. The Cochrane Library.

Franco, M. R., Tong, A., Howard, K., Sherrington, C., Ferreira, P. H., Pinto, R. Z., and Ferreira, M. L. (2015). Older people's perspectives on participation in physical activity: a systematic review and thematic synthesis of qualitative literature. *British Journal of Sports Medicine*, pp.bjsports-2014.

Galenkamp, H. and Deeg, D. J. (2016). Increasing social participation of older people: are there different barriers for those in poor health? Introduction to the special section. *European Journal of Ageing*, 13(2), 87–90.

Gill, T. M., Pahor, M., Guralnik, J. M., McDermott, M. M., King, A. C., Buford, T. W., Strotmeyer, E. S., Nelson, M. E., Sink, K. M., Demons, J. L., and Kashaf, S. S. (2016). Effect of structured physical activity on prevention of serious fall injuries in adults aged 70–89: randomized clinical trial (LIFE Study). *British Medical Journal*, 352, i245.

Gillan, A. (2015). Not the retiring type: meet the people still working in their 70s, 80s and 90s. *The Guardian*, 1 August. Available at http://theguardian.com/lifeandstyle/2015/aug/01/still-working-aged-in-70s-80s-90s (accessed 20 June 2016).

Groot, C., Hooghiemstra, A. M., Raijmakers, P. G. H. M., van Berckel, B. N. M., Scheltens, P., Scherder, E. J. A., van der Flier, W. M., and Ossenkoppele, R. (2016). The effect of physical activity on cognitive function in patients with dementia: a meta-analysis of randomized control trials. *Ageing Research Reviews*, 25, 13–23.

Hajat, S., Chalabi, Z., Wilkinson, P., Erens, B., Jones, L., and Mays, N. (2016). Public health vulnerability to wintertime weather: time-series regression and episode analyses of national mortality and morbidity databases to inform the Cold Weather Plan for England. *Public Health*, doi:10.1016/j.puhe.2015.12.015

Hansen, B. H., Kolle, E., Dyrstad, S. M., Holme, I., and Anderssen, S. A. (2012). Accelerometer-determined physical activity in adults and older people. *Medicine and Science in Sports and Exercise*, 44(2), 266–272.

Hartley, S. E. and Yeowell, G. (2015). Older adults' perceptions of adherence to community physical activity groups. *Ageing and Society*, 35(8), 1635–1656.

Herbolsheimer, F., Schaap, L. A., Edwards, M. H., Maggi, S., Otero, Á., Timmermans, E. J., Denkinger, M. D., van der Pas, S., Dekker, J., Cooper, C.,

Dennison, E. M., van Schoor, N. M., Peter, R., and the Eposa Study Group. (2016). Physical activity patterns among older adults with and without knee osteoarthritis in six European countries. *Arthritis Care Research*, 68, 228–236.

Herring, M. P., Johnson, K. E., and O'Connor, P. J. (2016). Exercise training and health-related quality of life in generalized anxiety disorder. *Psychology of Sport and Exercise*, 27, 138–141.

Hinrichs, T., Bücker, B., Wilm, S., Klaaßen-Mielke, R., Brach, M., Platen, P., and Moschny, A. (2015). Adverse events in mobility-limited and chronically ill elderly adults participating in an exercise intervention study supported by general practitioner practices. *Journal of the American Geriatrics Society*, 63(2), 258–269.

Horne, M. (2013). Promoting active ageing in older people from black and minority ethnic groups. *Journal of Health Visiting*, 1(3), 148–155.

Hurley, M. and Carter, A. (2016). ESCAPE-into the community: a community-based rehabilitation programme for elderly people with chronic joint pain. *Perspectives in Public Health*, 136(2), 67–69.

Iliffe, S. (2016) Community-based interventions for older people with complex needs: time to think again? *Age Ageing*, 45(1), 2–3. doi:10.1093/ageing/afv185

Information Centre for Health and Social Care (2009). *Health Survey for England. Physical Activity and Fitness: Summary of Key Findings, 2008*. London: The Information Centre for Health and Social Care. Available at https://catalogue.ic. nhs.uk/publications/public-health/surveys/heal-surv-phys-acti-fitn-eng-2008/heal-surv-phys-acti-fitn-eng-2008-rep-v1.pdf (accessed 14 March 2016).

Johnson, L. G., Butson, M. L., Polman, R. C., Raj, I. S., Borkoles, E., Scott, D., Aitken, D., and Jones, G. (2016). Light physical activity is positively associated with cognitive performance in older community dwelling adults. *Journal of Science and Medicine in Sport*. doi:10.1016/j.jsams.2016.02.002

Joseph Rowntree Foundation (2014). At a glance 65: a better life for older people with high support needs: the role of social care. Available at http://scie.org.uk/publications/ataglance/ataglance65.asp (accessed 14 March 2016).

Joshi, S., Mooney, S. J., Kennedy, G. J., Benjamin, E. O., Ompad, D., Rundle, A. G., Beard, J. R., and Cerdá, M. (2016). Beyond METs: types of physical activity and depression among older adults. *Age and Ageing*, 45(1), 103–109.

Kahn, R., Robertson, R. M., Smith, R., and Eddy, D. (2008). The impact of prevention on reducing the burden of cardiovascular disease. *Diabetes Care*, 31(8), 1686–1696.

Kimura, T., Kobayashi, H., Nakayama, E., and Kakihana, W. (2015). Seasonality in physical activity and walking of healthy older adults. *Journal of Physiological Anthropology*, 34(1), 1.

Kings Fund (2016). *Gardens and Health: Implications for Policy and Practice*. London: Kings Fund.

Kishimoto, H., Ohara, T., Hata, J., Ninomiya, T., Yoshida, D., Mukai, N., Nagata, M., Ikeda, F., Fukuhara, M., Kumagai, S., and Kanba, S. (2016). The long-term association between physical activity and risk of dementia in the community: the Hisayama Study. *European Journal of Epidemiology*, 31(3), 267–274.

Kok, G., Gottlieb, N. H., Peters, G. J. Y., Mullen, P. D., Parcel, G. S., Ruiter, R. A., Fernández, M. E., Markham, C. and Bartholomew, L. K. (2016). A taxonomy of behaviour change methods: an Intervention Mapping approach. *Health Psychology Review*, 10(3), 297–312.

Kosteli, M. C., Williams, S. E., and Cumming, J. (2016). Investigating the psycho-social determinants of physical activity in older adults: a qualitative approach. *Psychology & Health*, 1–20.

Later Life Training (2016). *Someone Like Me*. Available at http://laterlifetraining. co.uk/courses/someone-like-me/ (accessed 29 April 2016).

Laventure, R. (2016). Active ageing: the best is yet to come. The Centre for Trans-lational Research in Public Health, Newcastle University, 17 May. Available at http://fuse.ac.uk/events/fusephysicalactivityworkshops/presentations/sixthfusepa workshop/Bob%20Laventure%20-%20presentation.pdf (accessed 20 June 2016).

Lawrence, R. C., Felson, D. T., Helmick, C. G., Arnold, L. M., Choi, H., Deyo, R. A., Gabriel, S., Hirsch, R., Hochberg, M. C., Hunder, G. G., and Jordan, J. M. (2008). Estimates of the prevalence of arthritis and other rheumatic conditions in the United States: Part II. *Arthritis & Rheumatism*, 58(1), 26–35.

Li, F., Harmer, P., Fisher, K. J., McAuley, E., Chaumeton, N., Eckstrom, E., and Wilson, N. L. (2005). Tai Chi and fall reductions in older adults: a randomized controlled trial. *The Journals of Gerontology Series A: Biological Sciences and Medical Sciences*, 60(2), 187–194.

Lobelo, F. and de Quevedo, I. G. (2016). The evidence in support of physicians and health care providers as physical activity role models. *American Journal of Lifestyle Medicine*, 10(1), 36–52.

Locher, J. L., Bales, C. W., Ellis, A. C., Lawrence, J. C., Newton, L., Ritchie, C. S., Roth, D. L., Buys, D. L., and Vickers, K. S. (2011). A theoretically based behavi-oural nutrition intervention for community elders at high risk: the B-NICE randomized controlled clinical trial. *Journal of Nutrition in Gerontology and Geriatrics*, 30(4), 384–402.

Lozano-Sufrategui, L., Pringle, A., Carless, D., and McKenna, J. (2016). 'It brings the lads together': a critical exploration of older men's experiences of a weight management programme delivered through a Healthy Stadia project. *Sport in Society*, 1–13.

Luten, K. A., Reijneveld, S. A., Dijkstra, A., and de Winter, A. F. (2016). Reach and effectiveness of an integrated community-based intervention on physical activity and healthy eating of older adults in a socioeconomically disadvantaged community. *Health Education Research*, 31(1), 98–106.

Mama, S. K., McCurdy, S. A., Evans, A. E., Thompson, D. I., Diamond, P. M., and Lee, R. E. (2015). Using community insight to understand physical activity adop-tion in overweight and obese african american and hispanic women a qualitative study. *Health Education and Behavior*, 42(3), 321–328.

Mansfield, L. and Piggin, J. (2016). Sport, physical activity and public health. *International Journal of Sport Policy and Politics*, 8(4), 533–537, doi:10.1080/ 19406940.2016.1254666

Marcus, B. and Forsyth, L. (2009). *Motivating People to be Physically Active*, 2nd edn. Champaign, IL: Human Kinetics.

Marquis, S., Moore, M. M., Howieson, D. B., Sexton, G., Payami, H., Kaye, J. A. and Camicioli, R. (2002). Independent predictors of cognitive decline in healthy elderly persons. *Archives of Neurology*, 59(4), 601–606.

Marshall, A. L., Owen, N., and Bauman, A. E. (2004). Mediated approaches for influencing physical activity: update of the evidence on mass media, print, telephone and website delivery of interventions. *Journal of Science and Medicine in Sport*, 7(1), 74–80.

Mather, A. S., Rodriguez, C., Guthrie, M. F., McHarg, A. M., Reid, I. C., and McMurdo, M. E. (2002). Effects of exercise on depressive symptoms in older adults with poorly responsive depressive disorder: randomised controlled trial. *The British Journal of Psychiatry*, 180(5), 411–415.

McAuley, E. and Katula, J. (1998). Physical activity interventions in the elderly: influence on physical health and psychological function. *Annual Review of Gerontology and Geriatrics*, 18(1), 111–154.

McCabe, K., Ling, J., Wilson, B., Crossland, A., Kaner, E. A. S., and Haighton, C. (2016). Alcohol services provision for older people in an area experiencing high alcohol use and health inequalities. *Perspectives in Public Health*, 136(2), 83–85.

McLeroy, K. R., Bibeau, D., Steckler, A., and Glanz, K. (1988). An ecological perspective on health promotion programs. *Health Education & Behavior*, 15(4), 351–377.

McVeigh, T. (2013). Divorcing baby boomers seize the moment to go it alone. *The Guardian*. Available at http://theguardian.com/lifeandstyle/2013/jun/29/divorcing-baby-boomers-go-it-alone (accessed 20 June 2016).

Milner, C. and Milner, J. (2016). Impact of policy on physical activity participation and where we need to go. *Annual Review of Gerontology and Geriatrics*, 36(1), 1–32.

Milton, S., Pliakas, T., Hawkesworth, S., Nanchahal, K., Grundy, C., Amuzu, A., Casas, J. P., and Lock, K. (2015). A qualitative geographical information systems approach to explore how older people over 70 years interact with and define their neighbourhood environment. *Health & Place*, 36, 127–133.

Mitchell, S., Lucas, C., Norton, M., and Phillips, L. (2016). Dementia risk reduction it's never too early, it's never too late. *Perspectives in Public Health*, 136(2), 79–80.

National Institute for Health and Care Excellence (2013). *Physical Activity: Brief Advice for Adults in Primary Care*. London: National Institute for Health and Care Excellence.

National Institute for Health and Care Excellence (2015). *Dementia, Disability and Frailty in Later Life – Mid-Life Approaches to Delay or Prevent Onset*. London: National Institute for Health and Care Excellence.

National Institute for Health and Clinical Excellence (2005). *Health Needs Assessment: A Practical Guide*. London: National Institute for Health and Clinical Excellence.

National Institute for Health and Clinical Excellence (2008). *Mental Wellbeing in Over 65s: Occupational Therapy and Physical Activity Interventions*. London: National Institute for Health and Clinical Excellence.

National Obesity Observatory (2012). *Standard Evaluation Framework for Physical Activity Interventions*. National Obesity Observatory.

Nottingham City Primary Care Trust (n.d.). Get moving Nottingham: physical activity for the over 50s: final report. Nottingham City PCT.

Nyman, S.R. and Szymczynska, P. (2016). Meaningful activities for improving the wellbeing of people with dementia: beyond mere pleasures to meeting fundamental psychological needs. *Perspectives in Public Health*, 136(2), 99–107.

Oliver, E. J., Hanson, C. L., Lindsey, I. A., and Dodd-Reynolds, C. J. (2016). Exercise on referral: evidence and complexity at the nexus of public health and sport policy. *International Journal of Sport Policy and Politics*, 8(4), 731–736.

Parnell, D., Pringle, A., McKenna, J., Zwolinsky, S., Rutherford, Z., Hargreaves, J., Trotter, L., Rigby, M., and Richardson, D. (2015). Reaching older people with PA delivered in football clubs: the reach, adoption and implementation characteristics of the Extra Time Programme. *BMC Public Health*, 15(1), 1.

Prince, M., Wimo, A., Guerchet, M., Ali, G. C., Wu, Y.T., and Prima, M. (2015). *World Alzheimer Report 2015: The Global Impact of Dementia: An Analysis of Prevalence, Incidence, Costs and Trends*. London: Alzheimer's Disease International.

Pringle, A. R. and Pickering, K. (2015). Smarter running: shaping the behavioural change interventions of the future! *Perspectives in Public Health*, 135(3), 116–116.

Pringle, A., Hargreaves, J., Lozano, L., McKenna, J. and Zwolinsky, S. (2014). Assessing the impact of football-based health improvement programmes: stay onside, avoid own goals and score with the evaluation! *Soccer & Society*, 15(6), 970–987.

Pringle, A., Marsh, K., Gilson, N., McKenna, J., and Cooke, C. (2010). Cost effectiveness of interventions to improve moderate physical-activity: a study in nine UK sites. *Health Education Journal*, 69(2), 211–224.

Pringle, A., McKenna, J., and Zwolinsky, S. (in press). Linking Physical Activity & Health Evaluation to Policy: Lessons from UK Evaluations. In J. Piggin, L. Mansfield, and M. Weed (eds), *Routledge Handbook of Physical Activity Policy and Practice*. London: Routledge.

Pringle, A., Parnell, D., Zwolinsky, S., Hargreaves, J., and McKenna, J. (2014). Effect of a health-improvement pilot programme for older adults delivered by a professional football club: the Burton Albion case study. *Soccer & Society*, 15(6), 902–918.

Pringle, A., Zwolinsky, S., McKenna, J., Robertson, S., Daly-Smith, A., and White, A. (2014). Health improvement for men and hard-to-engage-men delivered in English Premier League football clubs. *Health Education Research*, 29(3), 503–520.

Pringle, A., Zwolinsky, S., McKenna, J., Smith, A., Robertson, S., and White, A. (2013). Delivering men's health interventions in English Premier League football clubs: key design characteristics. *Public Health*, 127(8), 716–726.

Public Health England (2016). Public Health Matters. Available at https://publichealthmatters.blog.gov.uk/author/kevin-fenton/ (accessed 4 April 2016).

Pulkki, J. and Tynkkynen, L. K. (2016). 'All elderly people have important service needs': a study of discourses on older people in parliamentary discussions in Finland. *Ageing and Society*, 36(01), 64–78.

Ransdell, L. B., Dinger, M. K., Huberty, J., and Miller, K. H. (2009). Developing effective physical activity programs. Champaign, IL: Human Kinetics, pp. 11–23.

Rantakokko, M., Iwarsson, S., Mänty, M., Leinonen, R., and Rantanen, T. (2012). Perceived barriers in the outdoor environment and development of walking difficulties in older people. *Age and Ageing*, 41(1), 118–21.

Robertson, S., Woodall, J., Henry, H., Hanna, E., Rowlands, S., Horrocks, J., Livesley, J., and Long, T. (2016). Evaluating a community-led project for improving fathers' and children's wellbeing in England. *Health Promotion International*, p.daw090.

Schroer, W. J. (2016). Generation X, Y, Z and the others. Available at http://socialmarketing.org/archives/generations-xy-z-and-the-others/ (accessed 23 June 2016).

Shankar, A., McMunn, A., Demakakos, P., Hamer, M., and Steptoe, A. (2017). Social isolation and loneliness: prospective associations with functional status in older adults. *Health Psychology*, 36(2), 179.

Spirduso, W. W., Francis, K. L., and MacRae, P. G. (2005). *Physical Dimensions of Aging*. Champaign, IL: Human Kinetics.

Sport England (2006). *Learning from LEAP*. London: Sport England.

Sproston, K. and Mindell, J. E. (2006). Health Survey for England 2004. The Health of Minority Ethnic Groups.

Tan, Z. S., Spartano, N. L., Beiser, A. S., DeCarli, C., Auerbach, S. H., Vasan, R. S., and Seshadri, S. (2016). Physical activity, brain volume, and dementia risk: the Framingham Study. *The Journals of Gerontology Series A: Biological Sciences and Medical Sciences*, p.glw130.

Tanamas, S. K., Wluka, A. E., Davies-Tuck, M., Wang, Y., Strauss, B. J., Proietto, J., Dixon, J. B., Jones, G., Forbes, A., and Cicuttini, F. M. (2013). Association of weight gain with incident knee pain, stiffness, and functional difficulties: a longitudinal study. *Arthritis Care & Research*, 65(1), 34–43.

Thomas, L., Little, L., Briggs, P., McInnes, L., Jones, E., and Nicholson, J. (2013). Location tracking: views from the older adult population. *Age and Ageing*, 42(6), 758–763.

Tones, K. and Tilford, S. (2001). *Health Promotion: Effectiveness, Efficiency and Equity*. Cheltenham, UK: Nelson Thornes.

Trachte, F., Geyer, S., and Sperlich, S. (2016). Impact of physical activity on self-rated health in older people: do the effects vary by socioeconomic status? *Journal of Public Health*, p.fdv198.

Uthman, O. A., van der Windt, D. A., Jordan, J. L., Dziedzic, K. S., Healey, E. L., Peat, G. M., and Foster, N. E. (2013). Exercise for low limb osteoarthritis: systematic review incorporating trial sequential analysis and network meta analysis. *British Medical Journal*, 347, f5555.

van Alphen, H. J., Hortobágyi, T., and van Heuvelen, M. J. (2016). Barriers, motivators, and facilitators of physical activity in dementia patients: a systematic review. *Archives of Gerontology and Geriatrics*, 66, 109–118.

Vincent, K. R. and Braith, R. W. (2002). Resistance exercise and bone turnover in elderly men and women. *Medicine and Science in Sports and Exercise*, 34(1), 17–23.

Wolf, S. L., Sattin, R. W., Kutner, M., O'Grady, M., Greenspan, A. I., and Gregor, R. J. (2003). Intense tai chi exercise training and fall occurrences in older, transitionally frail adults: a randomized, controlled trial. *Journal of the American Geriatrics Society*, 51(12), 1693–1701.

Zwolinsky, S., McKenna, J., and Pringle, A. (2016). How can the health system benefit from increasing participation in sport, exercise and physical activity? In D. Conrad and A. White (eds), *Sports-Based Health Interventions: Case studies from Around the World* (pp. 29–52). London: Springer.

Chapter 5

Health through state supported voluntary sport clubs

Søren Bennike, Lone Friis Thing and Laila Ottesen

Introduction

This chapter will discuss how state-supported sport clubs, including sports participation is linked to health. We will present a case, building on football, highlighting how this link is very present and influential and we will finish with a short closing discussion on future perspectives regarding sport clubs and health.

We will take our point of departure in recreational, voluntary-organised state-supported sport clubs in Denmark, though simultaneously provide comments regarding more global perspectives. Especially in relation to the European countries. Going back more than 150 years, sport (including gymnastics) in Denmark has traditionally been organised by voluntary associations (Kaspersen and Ottesen, 2001), labelled sport clubs in the following. These clubs are an important part of the public sphere, as many people spend numerous hours of their life there (Kaspersen and Ottesen, 2001). They do so as members, athletes, coaches, volunteers, parents and so forth. This is likewise the case in several other European countries. It will unfold in the following, but briefly stated the sport clubs of Denmark are situated in what Pestoff (1992) defines as the *'third sector'*, which plays a unique role in the Scandinavian welfare state model (Klausen and Selle, 1996). See Breuer *et al.* (2015) for a portrait and cross-national comparison of the characteristics of sport clubs and their embedding in society in 20 European countries, among these Norway, The Netherlands, Germany, Italy, France and England. The authors conclude that sport clubs, organised traditionally as non-profit organisations, are to be found all over Europe and takes on an important role as the main provider of sporting activities for the population. One perspective of interest to this chapter is that the connection between the state and sport clubs differs as a result of historical, ideological, political and religious background (Hoekman *et al.*, 2015).

Denmark is among the countries in the European Union with the highest level of sports participation. According to the Eurobarometer (European Commission, 2014) Denmark is the second most 'active' country (European

Commission, 2014) and also the second most 'sport club active' country (European Commission, 2014). According to a national survey 61 per cent of the adult (16+) population is active of which 39 per cent are active in sport clubs (Pilgaard and Rask, 2016). The latter is more than doubled when considering children (age 7–15), as 83 per cent are active, of which between 8 and 9 out of every 10 children will have participated in sports in a sport club setting within the last year (Laub, 2013; Pilgaard and Rask, 2016). The total number of sport clubs in Denmark is estimated to 16,000 corresponding to one pr. 350 inhabitants as the total poulation is approx. 5.6 million (Ibsen *et al.*, 2015) and Denmark is among the countries in the world with the highest number of sports facilities per capita (Rafoss and Troelsen, 2010). These facilities are often used by sport clubs. In 2003 Ibsen and Ottesen highlighted that there is a football pitch for every 1,000 people, a sports hall for every 4,000 and swimming facilities for every 12,000.

Health, the voluntary-organised sport clubs and sports participation

Health and sport clubs – the early days

To fully understand the voluntary state supported sport clubs in Denmark, or any other country, one needs to reflect on history. It becomes important especially as state support is linked to societal development and societal challenges of different kinds – health included. In some eras of time this link is more obvious and explicit than others. In the following we will provide the reader with a few purposefully selected examples.

We will begin at the 'Constitution' of 1849, which is of crucial importance to the development of sport clubs and the recreational sport in Denmark (Kaspersen and Ottesen, 2001). In the constitution 'freedom of association' and 'freedom of assembly' was established and in the time to come many sport clubs were formed. The first sport clubs were established in relation to the Danish-German conflict in the mid-/late-nineteenth century and the activities organised included shooting and gymnastics (Ibsen and Ottesen, 2003). In fact, the sport club history in many other European countries was at first linked to the military (Hoekman *et al.*, 2015). In the following time to come more clubs were formed around English sports such as cricket, football, rowing and tennis (Ibsen and Ottesen, 2003). Clubs conducting shooting and gymnastics activities organised themselves in what later became the Danish Gymnastics and Sports Associations (DGI) and clubs conducting different kind of sports, such as the English, organised themselves in the Sports Confederation of Denmark (DIF), which today holds the National Olympic Committee. This organisational form of building on two strong national sports organisations[1] still persists and is a unique trait of the Danish sports structure (Thing and Ottesen, 2010; Ibsen *et al.*, 2015). Today both DGI and

DIF are organising numerous sports activities, many of them the same, which makes them seem alike. Nevertheless they have different organisational structures and different cultural and political traditions (Ibsen, 1999).

The present structural position for sport clubs in the national sport structure is as follows; with the point of departure in DIF[2], it is not possible for a sport club to be a member of DIF, as was the case in the very early days. The sport clubs are members of a specific sporting organisation (SSO) which look after general interests of the specific sport[3]. This SSO (e.g. the Danish Football Association (DFA)) is then a member of DIF. With the point of departure in DGI, the structure is different. The DGI is divided into regional county units, looking after the interest of all sports activities in that specific region. The sport club is a member of the regional county unit, and the regional county unit is a part of DGI. Many sport clubs are organised both in DGI and DIF. It is not either or. To oversimplify DIF is a strong organisation in competitive sport and DGI is a strong organisation in sport for all.

An important point in the early years of the more formalised organisation of sport is that the shooting and gymnastic activities received state support because a physically strong and 'ready-to-shoot' population (men) would contribute to a stronger defence and simultaneously create a more productive, healthy and efficient work force (Kaspersen and Ottesen, 2001). The organisation of other sports were, in contrast to gymnastics and shooting, not (significantly) financially supported by the state until well into the 1900s (Ibsen and Ottesen, 2003).

In 1930, a law on education (The Act on Adult Education) was passed, where a number of new subjects were approved as education and thereby entitled to state support. This applied, among other things, to cooking, sewing, singing, and not least important in this context, gymnastics. The role of sport (including gymnastics) in the education system became stronger and in 1937, a new school law required the municipalities to provide public schools of a certain size with a ball-playing field and to make these facilities available to the local sport clubs after school hours. With the school law of 1937 the link between state and sport clubs became clearer. At this time sport clubs were seen as institutions that contributed to the formation of democratic structures, practices, and ideals (Gundelach and Torpe, 1999) and at the same time sport, especially gymnastics, were educating the population in health and hygiene.

Building on theories from political science one can argue that the financial support and state recognition of sport clubs creates an 'associative democracy' as a parallel form of government to 'representative democracy' forming a dual strategy, called 'the double democratic principle' (Kaspersen and Ottesen, 2001). The state uses infrastructural power (Mann, 1990) as a strategy in parallel with the representative democracy. Central to infrastructural power is the state's ability and wish to exercise its power in dialogue with society's institutions, such as sports organisations (e.g. DGI,

DIF and DFA). Inversely despotic power (Mann, 1990) is used by the state when it intervenes directly in society without dialogue with the society's agents.

Health and sport clubs – the presence

In 1948 the state support to voluntary sport clubs increased heavily as the Danish parliament passed a State Football Pool (Tipsloven), which among others secured sport organisations (DGI and DIF) a relatively big part of the national monopolistic betting profits (including the national lottery profits in 1989). Today this law is called the 'Act of Allocation' (Udlodningsloven, 2015). This led to a professionalisation of the sports organisations in the years to follow (Ottesen, 2012). They expanded with large administrations and well-educated personnel, both of which made DGI and DIF into somewhat official institutions that could contribute to the construction and reestablishment of the post-war welfare state. In 1968 yet another law was passed (The Leisure Act), which provided favourable conditions for sport clubs. This law made sure that municipal support was given to all leisure-time activities within associations, including sport clubs. Today this law is called the 'Act of Enlightenment' (Folkeoplysningsloven, 2011). The leisure time was considered as a welfare benefit, and the culture and leisure-time policy became significant for building municipal welfare (Ottesen, 2012). By this time exists a subsidise structure, which is present today; the state supports the work of the main sports organisations, the municipalities support citizens' voluntary self-organised sport clubs activities and the citizens pay (affordable) membership fees to the sport clubs (Kaspersen and Ottesen, 2001). In other words, the state uses infrastructural power, as an 'arms-length distance' strategy. It is a model of two (or three) parallel state and municipal (and individual membership) flows of support. See Figure 5.1.

The sport clubs and the sports organisations are deeply dependent of the state and municipals, having favourable but also dependent conditions. Ibsen and Eichberg (2012) argues that the sports organisations of today have become a sector in the state intervention, among others as the state support make up just over 9/10 of the income (Ibsen and Ottesen, 2003). In relation to sport clubs about half the income (facilities included) of the sport clubs are based on municipal support (Ibsen and Ottesen, 2003). In addition to the municipal funding, membership fees do stand as a strong financial income for sport clubs (Ibsen et al., 2015). In a European perspective non-profit sport clubs in most countries do get some support from the state, especially related to facilities (Breuer et al., 2015).

In our present time the welfare state do not have the same amount of financial capacity as earlier, due to numerous factors, related to expenditures and world economy recession. As a result in a time of austerity policy (Blyth,

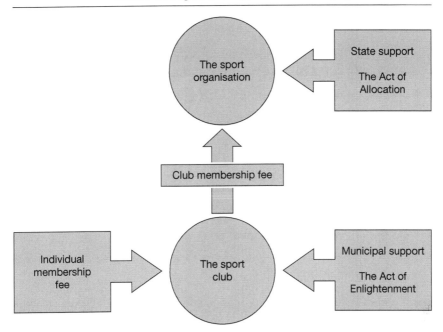

Figure 5.1 The financial support system of voluntary organised sport in Denmark

2013), the support for sport club activities is being questioned and challenged (Parnell *et al.*, 2016) under a lens of greater scrutiny (See KUM, 2014). A clear tendency to evaluate the support for sport clubs according to criteria of cost-utility is present (Ibsen and Ottesen, 2003). The state asks: Are sport clubs value for money? How do they contribute to society? Health is a strong yardstick among others. Policy makers are increasingly recognising the value of advocating sport as a means of enhancing the overall health of the population (Thing and Ottesen, 2010). The increasing interest coming from governmental and municipal departments involved in health is also detected in other European countries (Houlihan, 2005; Bergsgard *et al.*, 2007; Bloyce and Smith, 2010). By all means sport organised by sport clubs seems to be in a position where it has to legitimise state subsidy more than ever due to limited state resources. This goes especially for the sport organisations, such as DGI and DIF but also, for example, the DFA, which serves as a SSO and a member of DIF. While it is not revolutionary for sport clubs and sports organisations to be used to achieve non-sporting objectives, as showed in the previous, the role of sport in for example enhancing public health seems to have progressed from passive and symbolic to more explicit and ambitious. From the state/municipal perspective this is to make the most from the support. From the sport organisation perspective this is to legitimise support.

With the point of departure in recreational football Bennike (2016) shows how health has a very central position in the latest strategy of the DFA (DFA, 2012). The creation and introduction of Football Fitness (FF), which is a new initiative coming from the DFA is an illustrative example, and will be introduced in the following. Another example to underline the present issue of legitimacy is a joint vision from DGI and DIF launched in 2013. They will work together for a common end, and make sure that in the year of 2025, 50 per cent of the Danish population will be active in a sport club and 75 per cent will be active regardless of organisational form (DIF and DGI, 2014). This is ambitious and it is remarkable that it also targets possible participants outside the sport clubs, even though the DGI and DIF are professional bodies of interest to sport clubs. They are sending a clear message to the state, that they will contribute even more strongly to raise the activity level of the nation regardless of organisational form, with the outcomes attached to this (e.g. a healthier population). If the state cut budget for the DGI and DIF, these goals can 'of course not be met'. DGI and DIF are securing funding by 'promising' that they will contribute to a more physically active population. A similar situation is seen in England, where Sport England in a press release (Sport England, 2016a) concerning a new strategy 2016–2021 states that they will spend £250 million to raise the activity level, with health beneficial outcomes. The strategy is called 'Towards an active nation' (Sport England, 2016b). An important note to make is that quite often the creation of new sporting programmes highlighting beneficial outcomes of sport, such as health, presented by policy makers and sports organisations are without reflections towards possible negative sides, such as issues related to the competitive nature of sport, gender, inequality and marginalisation, which actually can work against the high hopes of getting more people active (Sanders, 2016). This discussion, though being rather big, will continue closing this chapter.

Health and the participants in sport

As is the case of the organisation of recreational sport the participants are likewise affected by society. The population is not active in the same form as when the first sport clubs were formed. The activity patterns are influenced by factors, such as demographics, trends and facilities, and it is assumed that the opportunities for participating in sports activities are closely linked to the way sport is organised, which again is closely linked to the state and society as such (Ibsen and Ottesen, 2003). In this section we will not take the reader back to 1849, but begin our analysis from 1964 and pay attention to adult sports participants, as these data are the most extensive and from a 'health and sport clubs – perspective' interesting changes are worth paying attention to.

This short section is based on statistics from the national sports participation survey (Laub, 2013; Pilgaard and Rask, 2016), which shows a steady
increase in the proportion of adult sports active from 15 per cent in 1964
to 61 per cent in 2016. See Figure 5.2. Sport has not only become more
prevalent over time, it has also become more diverse in terms of activity form
and more democratic in terms of gender and age group. Men and women
of all ages are doing numerous kinds of different sports. In 1964, there was
a clear relationship between age and sports participation, as sports activity
level declined with age. This correlation has evened out throughout the
years, and the least active group of today ranging from 16 to 69 years of
age is people from 30 to 39 years of age (57 per cent is active). This means
that an increasing number of elderly people have become active. Of particularly interest to this chapter, the number of people being active in sport clubs
has not met the increasing tendencies of people doing more sports, regardless
of organisational form, lowering the market share of the state supported
sport. See Figure 5.2.

By reference to Figure 5.2 the increase in sports activity outside sport clubs
relative to the sports activity in sport clubs started in 1987. From this time
on the commercial for-profit sports market, for example fitness centres, is
increasingly growing (Steen-Johnsen and Kirkegaard, 2010) providing
new possibilities for people to be active outside sport clubs. Even though
sport clubs are central for many adults' sports participation a still larger
part of the number doing sports can be found outside the sport clubs. See

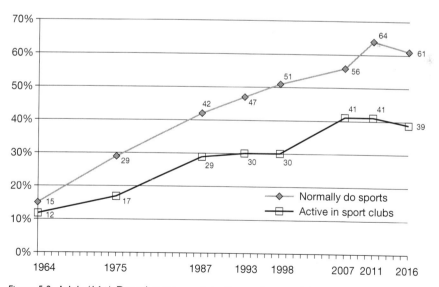

Figure 5.2 Adult (16+) Danes' sports participation and sport club activity

Adapted from Laub, 2013; Pilgaard and Rask, 2016

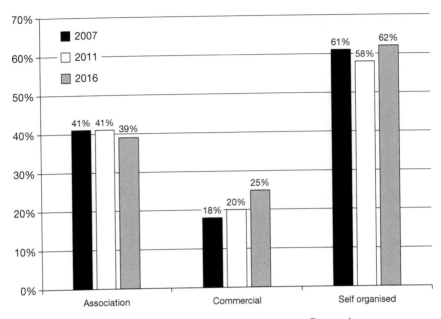

Figure 5.3 The organisational setting of sports participation in Denmark

Adapted from Pilgaard and Rask, 2016

Figure 5.3. This adds fuel to the debate regarding the *'are sport clubs value for money – question'* posed by the state. Moreover the share of people being sport club active is decreasing with age, especially during adolescence, where the number of sport clubs participants drop from 80 per cent among the age group 13–15 to 53 per cent among the age group 16–19 and further to 37 per cent among the age group 20–29 (Pilgaard and Rask, 2016). In the same age spans (13–29) we see an increase in self- and commercially-organised sports activity.

If we look closer to the numbers of specific sports it becomes clear that individual sports often self- or commercially-organised is increasing in popularity. From 1964 to 1993 gymnastics, football and swimming, mainly organised by sport clubs where the most popular activities (Pilgaard, 2009). From 1998 and onward strength training, jogging/running and walking/ hiking have gained increasing popularity and is the most popular sports of today. In recent years yoga has become more popular than football. All of these four sports are mainly organised outside the sport clubs. We will argue that these activities more than, for example, football are focused on health-related outcomes (Thing and Ottesen, 2013). This transformation in sports participation is also taking place elsewhere in Europe (see e.g. Scheerder *et al.*, 2011; European Commision, 2014; Lamprecht *et al.*, 2014; Tiessen-

Raaphorst and van den Dool, 2015). The proportion of European citizens who are not members of any sport club increased from 67 per cent in 2009 to 74 per cent in 2013[4], and the most common reason for engaging in sport or physical activity is to improve health (European Commission, 2014).

If you look to the Danish sports participation patterns (Pilgaard and Rask, 2016), gender differences are present, whereas significantly more women than men take part in walking/hiking, aerobics, yoga, Pilates and gymnastics. Significantly more men than women play football, badminton and do road cycling, of which football has the strongest domination by men. It is moreover the case that more women than men are involved in activities organised in a private centre and the other way around more men than women are involved in activities organised in sport clubs. If our assumptions on which sports have a stronger focus on health-related outcomes are true, women are more attracted by these.

Health through recreational football – the case of Football Fitness

The above sections clearly show a changing landscape of recreational sport in Denmark, which is present in many other European countries. The sporting activity patterns of the citizens are changing (Laub, 2013; Ibsen et al., 2015; Pilgaard and Rask, 2016), the funding of voluntary sport is being questioned (KUM, 2014) and political focus on sport due to the health-related outcomes of participation is rising (Thing and Ottesen, 2010). From the perspective of sport clubs, these changes are becoming difficult to ignore and the heavily state-funded sports organisations are positioning the role of sport clubs in order to legitimise future funding. In connection to the above-mentioned changes, studies published in 2010 highlighting recreational small-sided football as a highly beneficial health-enhancing activity led to the development of Football Fitness (FF), a football-based health-related initiative launched by the DFA in 2011. Krustrup et al. (2010a, 2010b) highlights beneficial physiological health effects from small sided football and Ottesen et al. (2010) highlights football's potential for accumulating social capital (Putnam, 2000). Ottesen et al. (2010) compared to a running group (N:25) and a football group (N:25) engaging in the already mentioned activities training two times a week for 16 weeks. Both groups consisted of inactive women. The study showed that the football group was able to create more internal bonding than the running group. The runners stayed focused on health-related aspects of running, whereas the football players were smitten by the fun and ludic aspects of football. An interesting aspect of the study, was that prior to a lottery, dividing them in two groups, most participants viewed running as the preferred activity over football because it was a flexible activity they could continue after the intervention, whereas playing football was considered inconceivable.

One year after the intervention nine women were playing football together in a sport club and in contrast only very few of the runners have been running together after the intervention period and only one has joined a sport club. Football showed to have an advantage over running as a more broad-spectred beneficial activity for improving cardiovascular and metabolic health (Bangsbo *et al.*, 2010) and as a better sport to create adherence in the physical activity as a group.

In the following we will explore the initiative of FF, which serves as a case to understand how state-funded sports organisations respond to the already-mentioned changes in the landscape of sport clubs. We will analyse the initiative from an organisational perspective (Bennike *et al.*, 2014, Ottesen *et al.*, 2017) and also pay attention to female participants (Thing *et al.*, 2016), which are highest in numbers. We will ask; what defines FF and what is the organisation of FF? And we will explore FF from the female participants' point of view.

What defines Football Fitness?

Shortly FF is a football-based activity with a focus on health and enjoyment rather than skills and tactics. It has no tournament structure, providing some kind of flexibility. As a participant you are not involved in matches in the weekend, and the team is not dependent on you training to improve to do better in the league tables. The target group is adults (25+) of both gender and the clubs can organise FF in a form they feel suitable, providing another kind of flexibility.

Building on the changing landscape of sport, where a growing number of adults are active outside the sport clubs in more flexible and health-orientated activities, FF is trying to meet these changes. Most other initiatives for health in the context of football compromise time limited interventions with a particular focus on the health of men and/or as community activities conducted by professional football clubs, especially in Great Britain (See e.g. Robertson, 2003; Brown *et al.*, 2006; Spandler and McKeown, 2012; Robertson *et al.*, 2013; Hunt *et al.*, 2014; Lansley and Parnell, 2016; Parnell and Pringle, 2016). Some of these interventions are specifically targeting fans of professional football clubs and playing football is not the only or main intervention activity (See e.g. Pringle *et al.*, 2013; Gray *et al.*, 2013). This is not the case with FF, which is an activity aimed at both men and women and conducted by municipally supported football clubs. It is not intended to exist only for a limited timeframe, as the DFA wants it to become a long-standing football activity organised in football clubs, just as they organise 'normal' recreational 11 a-side football. FF is top-down developed by the DFA and the Sports Confederation of Denmark (DIF) and managed voluntarily (non-profit) at a local level by the clubs.

It is created to (DFA, 2010a):

'. . . promote football as a health-beneficial activity', 'to create an interest in football for fitness and exercise', and 'to support football clubs in creating more flexibility in relation to adult players, primarily over the age of 25'.

Key factors are that FF (DFA, 2010b):

'. . . have a focus on health and enjoyment', 'is offered at a reduced membership fee compared to regular club members', 'teams do not engage in a tournament structure' and 'clubs can present the concept in a local way and adapt to the participants'.

FF is hugely inspired by the English form of 5-a-side Football, which in contrast to FF very often is influenced by the market and can be defined as 'pay-per-play concepts' (see e.g. Pitch Invasion, Goals Soccer Centres and Lucozade Powerleague). A representative of the FF steering committee states:

'We went to England to see this five-a-side, a big trend and very commercial, where companies build courts. . . . Where they rent out the courts and run small tournaments. . . . We looked at this and wondered if this could be an alternative way for clubs to arrange the game for busy family dads who don't have time for weekly training sessions and 11-a-side matches at the weekend. They could offer some flexibility, and from that came FF.'

Both FF and commercial 5-a-side Football are more organisationally flexible than the 'regular' form of football, and they both meet new demands for flexibility not present in the 11 versus 11 game. But in contrary to the commercial 5-a-side football in England FF is without a tournament structure. As part of its National Game Strategy 2011–2015, the English Football Association (EFA) states in *'Developing football for everyone'* (EFA, 2011) that a specific challenge is to provide:

'. . . local and flexible formats of football to suit changing consumer lifestyles.'

Similarly to the EFA, the DFA states in the *Strategy for development 2015* (DFA, 2012) that:

'. . . the game of football has to maintain and strengthen its position through continuous development in accessibility and flexibility regardless of the skills and ambitions of the participants'.

To sum up, the definition of FF includes a strong focus on health and flexibility and the target group is adult participants. These are all factors hugely involved in the changing activity pattern of the population and the increasing political health focus on sport clubs.

How is Football Fitness organised?

To fully understand FF and outline how the organisation of football is changing, among others due to a significant focus on the healthy outcomes of football, this section will compare the initiative to the activities normally conducted by the DFA, namely recreational football and professional football. This comparison is summarised in Figure 5.4, also illustrating the distinction, which is unfolded in the following. We aim to show how FF differs in the organisational and sporting form and pin point how health is a decisive factor. But before we can make use of this distinction, it is necessary to define recreational and professional football.

Recreational football, as it is used below can be traced back to the constitution, as recreational football is organised by sport clubs. As an outcome of the strong associative history of sport benefitting from state and municipal support, football as recreation, represented in the middle column of Figure 5.4, is in a strong, tradition-bound position playing a key role in Danish football. To benefit from municipal support (cf. Figure 5.1), clubs must be open to everyone (members pay a membership fee), function as non-profit and have a democratic legal structure (management), including a voluntary member-elected board. The teams, which are playing football as a hobby, fit into a tournament structure following a rulebook, pretty much identical to the international rules. In contrast to other countries, there

Ways in which football is organised by the Danish Football Association	Professional Football	Recreational Football	Football Fitness
Characteristics of the organisation	For-profit organisation Private support Hierarchical management No membership fee	Non-profit organisation Public support Democratic management Membership fee	Non-profit organisation Public support Democratic management Reduced membership fee
Characteristics of the game	Football as a job Improving skills and tactics International rules	Football as a hobby Improving skills and tactics National rules	Football as a means for health Improving fitness Local rules

Figure 5.4 Three types of adult football organised by the Danish Football Association

existed a long-standing ideal to keep the football game free from economic interests. This ideal of amateurism existed until 1978, when the DFA cancelled the amateur code (Grønkjær and Olsen, 2007). This was epoch making and resulted in a radical change in the organisation of Danish football and laid the foundation of professional football, represented in the left column. The clubs competing at the highest level gradually changed their organisational system and today these are profit driven and privatised, with a hierarchical bureaucratic structure. The players are employed on contracts (workers) and have no say in the management of the clubs unlike the players (members) of recreational football. The game is basically like that seen in recreational football, while the organisational structure of the club is strikingly different.

With the introduction of FF, we experience another change in the organisation of football. This change is not strong in the characteristics of the organisation, as was the case with the introduction of professional football. However FF brings a change in the characteristics of the game. It brings an explicit focus on health and improvement of fitness. At the same time it provides a possibility for local clubs to incorporate an increasing variety of organised football. One FDO states:

> 'It (FF) is a concept that fits in with a lot of target groups and can be managed in many different ways. Some teams do ordinary fitness exercises, and some just play football. Others mix and match from activities that they are fond of. It is up to the clubs.'

Allowance for local input, with FF being tailored to the local community and the culture of the organising club, is possible because FF is not part of a season-long tournament structure where the game has to be somehow controlled and the object is to 'do well'. One FF administrator states:

> 'The flexible format is where FF and traditional football differ. FF is played under different conditions. You don't have to train twice a week and play matches at the weekend. It's more that you play whenever you have the opportunity.'

The rules for playing FF are not fixed, which means the teams themselves control the format, providing local rules. There are no restrictions regarding format, gender, age or skills, which allows men and women to play together, just as players of different ages and different skills can play together. This is a new approach to the game, which is highly social and non-competitive, albeit there are most often two teams of players trying to score, playing on a rectangular field with two goals, unable to use their hands, and with free-kicks awarded for overenthusiastic tackles.

Football Fitness from a female participant's point of view

As previously discussed it is highlighted that women are overrepresented in activities carrying a more flexible organisational form and underrepresented in activities organised in sport clubs. Interestingly, and not expected by the DFA, FF is played by more women than men (Bennike *et al.*, 2014). See Figure 5.5.

Especially women in the age groups 25–39 and 40–59 are participating in FF, which is interesting as only few women in these age groups play football as recreation. Several factors are possible explanations, whereas work and family life balance is plausible. Thing *et al.* (2016) interviewed 32 female FF participants (aged 27–56) in six focus groups with the purpose to investigate how women who often have obligations to family and work life manage their time to make room for leisure as sport and how they experienced FF. Twenty-two of them were both working and raising children. In general the women expressed that it is difficult for them to prioritise leisure activities, because work and family are a high priority. On that note it is an important point, that FF has a 'flexible ideology'. You don't have to attend matches in the weekends and if family and/or work life is busy it is ok to come and go as they please. It is a form of un-organising the normally much organised game of recreational football. In the focus group interviews, the football activity

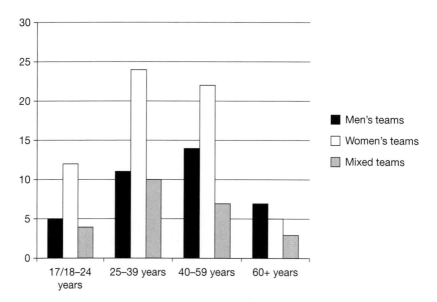

Figure 5.5 Football Fitness teams broken down in numbers by gender and age of participants

Adapted from Bennike *et al.*, 2014

stands out as a 'free space' – here the women can, according to themselves, let loose. FF serves as a space to 'breathe' in their everyday life. When they play they step out of their mom role and they experience recognising themselves from before they were mothers. This is experienced as being pleasurable and adhere their commitment to the game. Three FF participants states:

'*I am a completely different person, when I'm at football practice; I become that person like before I was a mom.*' (Anja, 41 years old)

'*My family they also said to me: "Haven't you started to go out quite a lot after you started with that football?" (laugh). I haven't been out since I became a mom, so now it's my time. Because we have so much fun together, we have a good time, when we are out, so I can't help but say yes, if there is an event.*' (Louise, 49 years old)

'*Well in my case, I have had a very hard time focusing on myself, getting my "alone time", and I have become really good at that these last couple of years. I am really trying to be a mom, I am trying to be a wife, but I also really need to be Tina, I do. Then I can be happy.*' (Tina, 39 years old)

Thing *et al.* (2016) concludes that FF can be described as an enabling opportunity for women, who want to play football, not for the aspect of competition but because it is rewarding for their 'selves' to participate.

Closing discussion

As mentioned, we experience a change in the surrounding landscape of sport clubs towards a focus on health, including flexibility, which seems to be of high priority for sports participants. The case of FF, an initiative launched by the DFA directly generated by these changes and designed to promote health is an illustrating example. One should be careful with predicting the future, but if these trends of health and flexibility will continue, it could prove highly decisive for sport clubs to adapt to the new situation, as is the case with FF. Future will call the success of FF, but at the moment the number of participants are rising indicating that the initiative seems to be long lasting. Yet implementation difficulties are present (Bennike and Ottesen, 2016) as FF is challenging the inertia of recreational football. From a research perspective as well as a policy maker point of view, especially if working in countries in which an associative-based sports system similar to the Danish, it will become interesting to follow the continuous diffusion and influence of the FF concept. At this moment the Handball and Badminton Federations in Denmark are organising respectively Handball Fitness and Badminton Fitness.

Henderson (2009) states that most theory regarding how to get people to participate in healthy behaviour relates to individual behaviour and cognition, concluding that identifying additional ways to more fully connect health and sport is essential. With the example of FF, a top down initiative created by the DFA, we argue that it can be helpful to ground this connection in the sport clubs. FF is one example in a Danish context of how football, one of the biggest sports in the world, given the sociocultural changes and political focus on health, can encourage greater physical activity by changing its form. Sanders (2016) highlights that there appears to be a lack of initiatives that reform the social structures, within sport itself, which have created tendencies such as social inequality, gender stereotypes and rigid masculinities. This goes also for the recent drop in sports participation and club-based sport in particular. An interesting aspect of FF is that it challenges the organisational structure of football and the consumeristic and private market tendencies often being strongly present in activities related to health, as FF is organised in non-profit associations. It is down-toning competition and it is played by more women than men. Vail (2007) demonstrates how top-down initiatives that ignore community needs have failed to succeed in sustaining sports participation. Though FF is a top-down initiative, it makes room for local input and bottom-up activities, as the clubs can organise it in a form which fits the club, team and the community needs which Vail asks for. Given a large number of football clubs throughout Denmark and the fact that they are locally embedded, this concept has the potential to combine a political focus on health with a local focus within the clubs, organising football for health in a sustainable way. If the concept proves long standing, it will become self-governing as an activity for health managed by volunteers in democratic organised non-profit sport clubs with a local focus and with state support pursuant to the legislation benefitting the sport clubs.

In the public health programme 'A healthier life for all' (Danish Government, 2014) the state sets the scene for increasingly involving the civil society, such as the sports organisations and sport clubs. This goes especially when it comes to raising the physical activity level of the population, with a healthy outcome. This goal of interest can be implemented via infrastructural power or via despotic power of earlier explanation. If the state chooses to maintain to work in the infrastructural way (which seems to be the case), it will entail that the sports organisations and sport clubs can and will voluntarily take part in working with health, to a bigger extend than today. In the public health programme the civil society is mentioned several times in relation to 'social inequality', 'mental health', 'obesity', 'population activity level' and 'prevention of sickness' (Danish Government, 2014). FF is an illustrative example, showing that the organisations and the clubs has the will to be innovative and make changes in order to get the inactive part of the population to be active. If the sports organisations and sport clubs do not realise the necessity of contributing to health in a more explicit form than today, the state's possible use of despotic power in the sports area will increase or organised sports will be marginalised and thereby probably lose both funding and political recognition (Ottesen, 2012).

There is no doubt that there exists a pressure, not just in Denmark, on the sports organisations and sport clubs of today to transform themselves so they can contribute to tackle the state's health-related challenges, which makes the link between health and sport clubs even stronger in the future. In this moment the DFA is creating partnerships with municipalities, in which FF is to be organised among others for vulnerable groups in a joint collaboration between municipality, sports organisation and sports club. It is also the case that FF in collaboration with other state-support dependent actors, such as patients associations have led to teams of prostate cancer patients called FC Prostate (Bruun *et al.*, 2014) and a team of former breast cancer patients called Football Fitness ABC, which is short for After Breast Cancer. To include the civil society and its non-profit associations/organisations and incorporate the broader concept of sport as a ludic play element in health promotion, prevention and treatment has great potential, being in Europe, China, South America or United States, though due to different state and sports systems you cannot expect it to adapt the same form.

Notes

1   The Danish Company Sports Association is a third sports organisation which is worth mentioning. DIF organises 9,287 clubs with 1.9 million members, DGI organises 6,331 clubs with 1.5 million members and the Danish Company Sport Association organises 244 clubs, all connected to workplaces, with 350,000 members (Ibsen *et al.* 2015)
2   It is not mandatory for a sport club to be a member of DIF and/or DGI, but it is often the case.
3   If the sport is big in participation numbers the SSO will often be divided into regional county SSOs.
4   Note that the proportion of European citizens that never exercises or plays sport increased from 39 per cent to 42 per cent in the same period.

References

Bangsbo, J., Nielsen, J. J., Mohr, M., Randers, M. B., Krustrup, B. R., Brito, J., Nybo, L., and Krustrup, P. (2010). Performance enhancements and muscular adaptations of a 16-week recreational football intervention for untrained women. *Scandinavian Journal of Medicine & Science in Sports*, 20(suppl. 1), 24–30. doi: 10.1111/j.1600-0838.2009.01050.x

Bennike, S. (2016). Fodbold Fitness – implementeringen af en ny fodboldkultur. PH.D. Afhandling. University of Copenhagen. Faculty of Science. [Football Fitness – the implementation of a new football culture. PH.D thesis]. SL grafik, Frederiksberg C, Denmark.

Bennike, S. and Ottesen, L. (2016b). How does interorganisational implementation behaviour challenge the success of Football Fitness? *European Journal for Sport and Society*, 13(1), 19–37. doi:10.1080/16138171.2016.1153879

Bennike, S., Wikman, J. M., and Ottesen, L. (2014). Football Fitness – a new version of football? A concept for adult players in Danish football clubs. *Scand J Med Sci Sports*, 24(suppl. 1), 138–146. doi:10.1111/sms.12276

Bergsgard, N. A., Houlihan, B., Mangset, P., Nødland, S. V., and Rommetvedt, H. (2007). *Sport Policy – A Comparative Analysis of Stability and Change*. London: Elsevier.

Bloyce, D. and Smith, A. (2010). *Sport Policy and Development – An Introduction*. Abindon, UK: Routledge.

Blyth, M. (2013). *Austerity: The History of a Dangerous Idea*. Oxford: Oxford University Press.

Breuer, C., Hoekman, R., Nagel, S., and van der Werf, H. (2015). *Sport Clubs in Europe: A Cross-National Comparative Perspective*. Neuchâtel, Switzerland: Springer. doi:10.1007/978-3-319-17635-2

Brown, A., Crabbe, T., and Mellor, G. (2006). English professional football and its communities. *International Review of Modern Sociology*, 32(2), Special Issue (Autumn 2006), 159–179.

Bruun, D. M., Bjerre, E., Krustrup, P., Brasso, K., Johansen, C., Rørth, M., and Midtgaard, J. (2014). Community-based recreational football: a novel approach to promote physical activity and quality of life in prostate cancer survivors. *International Journal of Environmental Research and Public Health*, 11, 5567–5585. doi:10.3390/ijerph110605567

Danish Government (2014). Et sundere liv for all – Nationale mål for danskernes sundhed de næste 10 år. [A healthier life for all – national goals for the health of the Danes in the coming 10 years]. Copenhagen, Denmark: Ministeriet for Sundhed og Forebyggelse.

DFA (2010a). Fodbold Fitness (motionsfodbold) [Football Fitness (Exercise football)]. (internal document).

DFA (2010b). Fodbold som fitness [Football as fitness]. DBU press release. (Downloaded 6.11.2013) http://dbu.dk/Nyheder/2010/December/fodbold_som_fitness.aspx

DFA (2012). *Passion Udvikling Fællesskab – Strategi for videreudviklingen af dansk fodbold frem til 2015*. [Passion Development Community – Strategy for further development of Danish football until 2015] Brøndby: DBU. (Downloaded 6.11.2013) http://dbu.dk/~/media/Files/DBU_Broendby/publikationer/PUF_folder.pdf

DIF & DGI (2014). Vision 25, 50, 75 – Visionsgruppens afsluttende rapport. [Vision 25, 50, 75 – The visiongruops final report]. DIF & DGI.

EFA (2011). English Football Association. *'Developing football for everyone' – National game strategy 2011–15*. (Downloaded 30.10.2013). Wembley Stadium. Wembley. Middlesex HA9 OWS. http://thefa.com/~/media/Files/PDF/Get%20into%20Football/1134_FA_NGS_200x260_Booklet_07.ashx

European Commission (2014). *Sport and Physical Activity*. Conducted by TNS Opinion & Social.

Folkeoplysningsloven (2011). Bekendtgørelse af lov om støtte til folkeoplysende voksenundervisning, frivilligt folkeoplysende foreningsarbejde og daghøjskoler samt Folkeuniversitet (folkeoplysningsloven). [Act on support for adult education, Voluntary Association work and day high schools and University Extension (Act of Enlightenment)]. Kulturministeriet. LBK nr. 854 af 11/07/2011.

Goals Soccer Centres (website visited 30.5.2016): https://goalsfootball.co.uk/

Grey, C.M., Hunt, K., Mutrie, N., Anderson, A.S., Leishman, J., Dalgarno, L., and Wyke, S. (2013). Football fans in training: the development and optimization of an intervention delivered through professional sports clubs to help men lose weight, become more active and adopt healthier eating habits, *BMC Public Health*, 13, 232. http://biomedcentral.com/1471-2458/13/232

Grønkjær, A. and Olsen, D.H. (2007). *Fodbold, fairplay og forretning* [Football, fairplay and business]. Århus, Denmark: Turbineforlaget.

Gundelach, P. and Torpe, L. (1999). Befolkningens fornemmelse for demokrati: foreninger, politisk engagement og demokratisk kultur. In T. B. Jørgensen, P. M. Christensen, L. Togeby, J. G. Andersen, and S. Vallgårda (eds), *Den demokratiske udfordring* (pp. 70–91). Copenhagen, Denmark: Hans Reitzels.

Henderson, K.A. (2009). A paradox of sport management and physical activity interventions. *Sport Management Review*, 12 (2009) 57–65. doi:10.1016/j.smr.2008.12.004

Hoekman, R., van der Werff, H., Nagel, S., and Breuer, C. (2015). A Cross-National Comparative Perspective on Sport Clubs in Europe. In C. Breuer, R. Hoekman, S. Nagel, and H. van der Werff (eds), *Sport Clubs in Europe: A Cross-National Comparative Perspective* (pp. 419–435). Neuchâtel, Switzerland: Springer. doi:10.1007/978-3-319-17635-2

Houlihan, B. (2005). Public sector sport policy. *International Review for the Sociology of Sport*, 40, 163–185. doi:10.1177/1012690205057193

Hunt, K., Wyke, S., Gray, C. M., Anderson, A. S, Brady, A., Bunn, C., Donnan, P. T, Fenwick, E., Grieve, E., Leishman, J., Miller, E., Mutire, N., Rauchhaus, P., White, A., and Treweek, S. (2014). A gender-sensitised weight loss and healthy living programme for overweight and obese men delivered by Scottinsh Premier League football clubs (FFIT): a pragmatic randomised controlled trial. *The Lancet*, 282, 1211–21.

Ibsen, B. (1999). Structure and development of sports organisations in Denmark. In K. Heinemann (ed.), *Sport Clubs – in Various European Countries*, Vol. 1 (pp. 241–268). The Club of Cologne: Hofmann Verlag, Schattauer, Schorndorf.

Ibsen, B., and Eichberg, H. (2012). Dansk idrætspolitik – mellem frivillighed og statslig styring. In H. Eichberg, *Idrætspolitik i komparativ belysning – national og international* (s. 147–209). Odense, Denmark: Syddansk Universitetsforlag 2012.

Ibsen, B., and Ottesen, L. (2003). Sport and welfare policy in Denmark: the development of sport between state, market and community. In K. Heinemann (ed.), *Sport and Welfare policies – Six European Case Studies*, Vol. 3 (pp. 31–86). The Club of Cologne: Hofmann, Reinheim.

Ibsen, B., Østerlund, K., and Laub, T. (2015). Sport clubs in Denmark. In C. Breuer, R. Hoekman, S. Nagel, and H. van der Werff (eds), *Sport Clubs in Europe: A Cross-National Comparative Perspective* (pp. 85–109). Neuchâtel, Switzerland: Springer. doi:10.1007/978-3-319-17635-2

Kaspersen, L. B. and Ottesen, L. (2001). Associationalism for 150 years and still alive and kicking: some reflections on Danish civil society. *Critical Review of International Social and Political. Philosophy*, 4, 105–130, doi:10.1080/1369823 0108403340

Klausen, K. K. and Selle, P. (1996). The third sector in Scandinavia. *Voluntas: International Journal of Voluntary and Nonprofit Organizations*, 7(2), 99–122.

Krustrup, P., Aagaard, P., Nybo, L., Petersen, J., Mohr, M., and Bangsbo, J. (2010b). Recreational football as a health promoting acitivity: a topical review. *Scand J Med Sci Sports*, 20, 1–13. doi:10.1111/j.1600-0838.2010.01108.x

Krustrup, P., Dvorak, J., Junge, A., and Bangsbo, J. (2010a). Executive summary: the health and fitness benefits of regular participation in small-sided football games. *Scand J Med Sci Sports*, 20, 132–135. doi:10.1111/j.1600-0838.2010.01106.x

KUM (2014). Udredning af idrættens økonomi og struktur. Analyse. [Clearing sport economy and structure. Analysis]. Af: Kulturministeriet, Idrættens analyseinstitut og KPMG.

Lamprecht, M., Fischer, A., and Stamm, H. (2014). Sport Schweiz 2014: Sportaktivität und Sportinteresse der Schweizer Bevölkerung [Sport Switzerland 2014: sport activity and sport interest of the Swiss population]. Observatorium Sport und Bewegung Schweiz c/o Lamprecht & Stamm Sozialforschung und Beratung AG. Available at www.sportobs.ch/fileadmin/sportobs-dateien/Downloads/Sport_Schweiz_2014_d.pdf

Lansley, S. and Parnell, D. (2016). Football for health: getting strategic. *Soccer & Society*, 17(2), 259–266. doi:10.1080/14660970.2015.1082764

Laub, T. B. (2013). Sports participation in Denmark 2011 – National survey – English version. Copenhagen: Danish Institute for Sports Studies.

Lucozade Powerleague (website visited 30.5.2016): https://powerleague.co.uk/lucozade

Mann, M. (1990). *The Rise and Decline of the Nation-State*. Oxford: Blackwell.

Ottesen, L. (2012). Idrætspolitik i et velfærdsperspektiv. In L. Thing and U. Wagner (eds), *Grundbog i idrætssociologi*. Munksgaard, København.

Ottesen, L., Bennike, S., and Thing, L. F. (2017). The emergence of the Danish Football Fitness concept. *Proceedings of the 8th World Congress on Science and Football*.

Ottesen, L., Jeppesen, R. S., and Krustrup, B. R. (2010). The development of social capital through football and running: studying an intervention program for inactive women. *Scand J Med Sci Sports*, 20, 118–131. doi:10.1111/j.1600-0838.2010.01123.x

Parnell, D. and Pringle, A. (2016). Football and health improvement: an emerging field. *Soccer & Society*, 17(2), 171–174, doi:10.1080/14660970.2015.1082753

Parnell, D., Spracklen, K., and Millward, P. (2016). Introduction: sport management issues in an era of austerity. *European Sport Management Quarterly*, Special Issue. doi:10.1080/16184742.2016.1257772

Pestoff, V. A. (1992). Third sector and co-operative services – an alternative to privatization. *Journal of Consumer Policy*, 15, 21–45.

Pilgaard, M. (2009). *Sport og motion i danskernes hverdag*. [Sport and exercise in the everyday life of the Danes]. Idrættens Analyseinstitut. Buchs.

Pilgaard, M. and Rask, S. (2016). *Danskernes motions- og sportsvaner 2016*. [Sports participation in Denmark 2016]. Idrættens Analyseinstitut.

Pitch invasion (website visited 30.5.2016). http://pitchinvasion.net/

Pringle, A., Zwolinsky, S., McKenna, J., Daly-Smith, A., Robertson, S., and White, A. (2013). Effect of a national programme of men's health delivered in English Premier League football clubs. *Public Health*, 127: 18–26.

Putnam, R. D. (2000). *Bowling Alone – The Collapse and Revival of American Community*. New York: Simon & Schuster.

Rafoss, K. and Troelsen, J. (2010). Sports facilities for all? The financing, distribution and use of sports facilities in Scandinavian countries. *Sport in Society*, 13(4), 643–656, doi:10.1080/17430431003616399

Robertson, S. (2003). 'If I let a goal in, I'll get beat up': contradictions in masculinity, sport and health. *Health Education Research*, 18(6), 706–716, doi:10.1093/her/cyf054

Robertson, S., Zwolinsky, S., Pringle, A., McKenna, J., Daly-Smith, A., and White, A. (2013). 'It is fun, fitness and football really': a process evaluation of a football-based health intervention for men. *Qualitative Research in Sport, Exercise and Health*, 5(3), 419–439.

Sanders, B. (2016). An own goal in sport for development: time to change the playing field. *Journal of Sport for Development*, 4(6), 1–5.

Scheerder, J., Vandermeerschen, H., Van Tuyckom, C., Breedveld, K., and Vos, S. (2011). *Understanding the Game: Sport Participation in Europe. Facts, Reflections and Recommendations (Sport Policy & Management 10)*. Leuven, Belgium: Katho lieke Universiteit Leuven.

Spandler, H., and McKeown, M. (2012). A critical exploration of using football in health and welfare programs: gender, masculinities, and social relations. *Journal of Sport & Social Issues*, 36(4), 387–409. doi:10.1177/0193723512458930

Sport England (2016a). New strategy to tackle inactivity – We'll spend £250 million to combat inactivity as part of five-year strategy. Sport England Press release. (Downloaded 30.5.2016). https://sportengland.org/news-and-features/news/2016/may/19/sport-england-triples-investment-in-tackling-inactivity/

Sport England (2016b). Sport England: towards an active nation – strategy 2016–2021. Available at www.sportengland.org/media/10629/sport-england-towards-an-active-nation.pdf

Steen-Johnsen, K., and Kirkegaard, K. L. (2010). The history and organization of fitness exercise in Norway and Denmark. *Sport in Society*, 13, 609–624.

Thing, L. F. and Ottesen, L. (2010). The autonomy of sports: negotiating boundaries between sports governance and government policy in the Danish welfare state. *International Journal of Sport Policy and Politics*, 2, 223–235, doi:10.1080/19406940.2010.488070

Thing, L. F. and Ottesen, L. (2013). Young people's perspectives on health, risks and physical activity in a Danish secondary school. *Health, Risk & Society*. doi:10.1080/13698575.2013.802294

Thing, L. F., Hybholt, M. G., Jensen, A. L., and Ottesen, L. S. (2016). 'Football Fitness': constraining and enabling possibilities for the management of leisure time for women. *Annals of Leisure Research*, 1–19. doi:10.1080/11745398.2016.1178153

Tiessen-Raaphorst, A. and van den Dool, R. (2015). Sportdeelname [Sport participation]. In A. Tiessen-Raaphorst (ed.), *Rapportage Sport 2014* [Sport Report 2014]. The Hague: The Netherlands Institute for Social Research.

Udlodningsloven (2015). Bekendtgørelse af lov om udlodning af overskud fra lotteri samt heste-og hundevæddemål (udlodningsloven) [Act on distribution of profits from lotteries, horse racing and dog racing (distribution law)]. LBK nr. 115 af 31/01/2015.

Vail, S. E. (2007). Community development and sport participation. *Journal of Sport Management*, 21, 571–596.

Chapter 6

Psychological benefits of team sport

Johan M. Wikman, Peter Elsborg and Knud Ryom

Introduction

It is commonly accepted that participation in physical activity, exercise or sport is followed by a wide array of positive consequences, both physical and psychological in nature (Biddle, Mutrie, and Gorely, 2015). Research in the last decade has suggested that these consequences depend on the nature of the physical activity, exercise or sport. Notably, team sports seem to offer better physical benefits than many individual exercise activities, due to the intermittent nature of team sports (Krustrup *et al.*, 2009, 2010). Naturally, one can wonder: Do team sports offer positive psychological consequences above and beyond those followed by participation in individual exercise?

This chapter will investigate the possible positive psychological consequences of participation in team sports, above and beyond those achieved by participation in physical activity. After a discussion of the team concept, the psychological health outcomes of participation in physical activity as well as team sports will be discussed, followed by a review of the motivational considerations in conjunction with participation in general physical activity and team sports, respectively. Challenges of team sports will also be addressed, and implications for practice, research and governance are discussed.

What is team sports?

In order to explore the positive psychological consequences of team sports, we must first define what exactly this term entails. We will define the words team and sports individually, and consider the word team first.

Wenger (2000) has introduced the term community of practices, which can be seen as a definition of team. Though Wenger (Wenger and Snyder, 2000) works within an organisational perspective and not sport per se, the term also reflects team sport: *'Since the beginning of history, human beings have formed communities to share cultural practices reflecting their collective learning . . . Participating in these "communities of practice" is essential to our learning. It is at the very core of what makes us human beings capable of meaningful knowing'* (Wenger, 2000: 229). For a team to thrive, three elements are of concern; *mutual engagement, a joint enterprise* and *a shared repertoire* (Wenger, 2000). *Mutual engagement* exits due to team members' engaging with each other and negotiate meaning together. The engagement is built upon the participants' ability to supplement each other, while they each have overlapping competencies making them able to take part in the community of practice. Hence, in order for a team to exist, the members of a team must meet and interact. This implies that for a community of pratice to exist, members of it have to interact and learn together, but this doesn't have to be on a daily basis (Wenger, 2011). *A joint enterprise* creates unity and cohesion, which should be founded by a collective negotiation, with all team members involved and committed to deliver his or her opinion. All team members are ultimately responsible for the current situation. Consequently, the team needs a common goal for their activities. *A shared repertoire* involves routines, verbal concepts, tools, strategies, narratives, gestures, symbols, actions, concepts and specific ways to act. Thus, the team has common practice and communication, only fully understood by the members of this team. As Wenger sees participation as fundamental to the success of a community, teams require involvement and participation to thrive (Wenger, 2000). Usually different levels of participation exist within a team, meaning that participants can have different involvement and thus produce different learning outcome (Wenger, 2011).

A similar position is taken by Carron and Hausenblas (1998). Here, team is defined as *'a collection of two or more individuals who possess a common identity, have common goals and objectives, share a common fate, exhibit structured patterns of interaction and modes of communication, hold common perceptions about group structure, are personally and instrumentally interdependent, reciprocate interpersonal attraction, and consider themselves to be a group'* (Carron and Hausenblas, 1998, pp. 13–14). Carron's work incorporates the team definition in defining cohesion as *'a dynamic process that is reflected in the tendency for a group to stick together and remain united in the pursuit of its instrumental objectives and/or for the satisfaction of member affective needs'* (Carron, Brawley, and Widmeyer, 1998, p. 213).

Although originating from different perspectives, the above definitions of team seem similar. In this chapter we take the position that a team is a group of individuals who share practice as well as communication, and who must work together to achieve a common goal.

With a definition of team, we turn to the term sport. In this chapter, we define sport as a sub-component of exercise whereby the activity is rule-governed, structured, competitive, and involves gross motor movement characterised by physical strategy, prowess and chance (Rejeski and Brawley,

1988). The competitive nature of sport has sometimes been difficult to clarify. Indeed the Sports Councils in the United Kingdom (for example, 'Sport England') have jurisdiction over activities that are non-competitive (for example, keep-fit and yoga), and 'Sport for All' campaigns have often included a wider range of activities than 'traditional' competitive sports (Biddle and Mutrie, 2008). Moreover, not all sports will necessarily contribute to the physiological side of health. For example, playing darts or pool may be enjoyable and require great skill, but provide minimal physical activity.

Joining the terms team and sport, a fitting definition for team sport can be: *a physical activity, in which the individuals in at least one group consisting of two or more, work together to achieve a common goal, in spite of resistance embedded in the rules of that activity.* Hence, the most activities normally considered team sport by the layman are included in this definition. How the intricacies of the definition affect the activity, the cooperation, the outcome, or the effects of the activity is beyond the scope of this chapter.

However, some general conclusions about the psychological effects of team sport will be addressed. Here, we loosely define psychological effects as the effects on an individual's mental health, quality of life and motivation, as these are generally agreed upon to be very important, and are affected positively by physical activity and team sports.

With our definition of team sport and psychological effects, we can now review if team sports posit additional positive consequences from participation, over and beyond those achieved from participation in general physical activity.

What positive consequences for mental health and quality of life, above and beyond those offered by physical activity, do team sports offer?

It is a prevalent opinion in the general population as well as in the academic community that regular physical activity is beneficial for mental health. A vast amount of research has supported exercise participation as a valid method for battling psychiatric illnesses. Exercise has been shown to positively affect individuals suffering from diseases such as anxiety and depression (De Moor *et al.*, 2006; Petruzzello *et al.*, 1991; Stephens, 1988; Wipfli *et al.*, 2008; Krogh *et al.*, 2010). While a small number of studies have shown no effect of exercise, the vast majority of the studies provide a strong evidence-based argument for exercise being as effective as other treatment offers for both these illnesses, while it is argued that it may be important to differentiate between the types of exercise activities. Petruzzello *et al.* (1991) concluded in their meta-analysis that aerobic exercise activities had a positive effect on anxiety, whereas for anaerobic forms of exercise there either was a small negative effect or no relation was found. Regular physical activity has also been linked to positive mental health development in the non-ill population. Meta-analyses have provided strong indication that regular physical activity has significant positive effects on body image (Campbell and Hausenblas, 2009; Hausenblas and Fallon, 2006; Reel et al., 2007) and research showing a positive link between cognitive functioning and regular exercise participation is well established (e.g. Brisswalter, Collardeau, and René, 2002; Tomporowski, 2003). Exercise participation has also been linked with improved quality of life in general. A thorough meta-analysis on exercise interventions showed that the exercise interventions had positive effects in the healthy population on both the physical and psychological aspects of quality of life (Gillison et al., 2009). In accordance with these results, sedentary behaviour has been shown to correlate with poor mental health outcomes such as health related quality of life (Heath and Brown, 2009) anxiety and depression (Petruzzello et al., 1991). In sum, massive amounts of research supporting the positive relation between participation in regular physical activity and mental health exists.

What does team sports offer in addition to the positive effects of physical activity on mental health and quality of life? Some studies have found little or no evidence for differences between team sports and individual exercise. For example, McGale, McArdle and Gaffney (2011) compared a team sport intervention, an individual exercise intervention and a control group on depression and perceived social support in a population of young men. While intervention groups developed better scores than the control group, McGale, McArdle and Gaffney found no noteworthy differences between intervention groups, lending support to the notion that no differences can be found between team sports and individual exercise. However, the general body of evidence points to an additional positive effect of team sports. Eime et al. (2013a, 2013b) conducted reviews of the psychological benefits of participation in sport, in both youth and adult populations, and found that club- or team-based participation seems to be associated with improved psychological health outcomes. Similarly, a longitudinal study with 840 Canadian adolescents explored how having participated in individual sports such as track and field, swimming or judo during school affected their depression levels when compared to having participated in team sports such as basketball, football or soccer (Sabiston et al., 2016). Results showed that having participated in team sport during school had a protecting effect on the average number of exhibited depression symptoms with a small but significant effect size, while the effect of individual sport participation was observed as non-significant. In line with this, Edwards, Edwards and Basson (2004) investigated the differences in psychological wellbeing and self-perception between participants in a team sport (hockey), physical activity in a fitness centre, and a control group. They found that both groups of exercisers had higher psychological wellbeing and self-perception than non-exercisers, and above and beyond these differences, hockey players scored higher on the subscales relations with others, sports competence and sports importance than the exercisers in the fitness centres.

All in all, there seems to be support for the notion that team sports offer positive psychological effects above and beyond those offered by individual physical activity, and it seems that one deciding difference between team sports and physical activity is, not surprisingly, that team sports require some sort of social interaction. Many studies in the sport and exercise context have found that social variables have a positive effect on the psychology of the participants. For example, the concept of cohesion seems to be associated with numerous positive effects, such as positive youth development (Bruner, Eys, Wilson, and Côté, 2014), positive affect (Loughead, Patterson, and Carron, 2008) and satisfaction (Evans and Eys, 2015). Similarly, social influences can affect intervention effects of a weight-loss programme (Leahey et al., 2012), sport satisfaction (Hoffmann and Loughead, 2016), self-confidence (Jackson et al., 2014), as well as negatively associated with substance abuse (Terry-McElrath and O'Malley, 2011) and burnout (DeFreese and Smith, 2013; Smith, Gustafsson, and Hassmén, 2010). Looking at the social variable in exercise, Gillison et al. (2009) performed a review on exercise interventions and quality of life and concluded that exercise interventions in a group setting improved quality of life more than interventions in an individual setting, again supporting the social aspect as an important factor for mental health and quality of life in physical activity. There is indeed initial evidence supporting the importance of social aspects for mental health and quality of life in sport and exercise participation. However, more research is needed, both to confirm this, and to uncover the mediating and moderating variables in the causal relationship between social interaction and mental health/quality of life in physical activity (Biddle and Mutrie, 2008).

The social perspective of team sport has attracted some interest. For instance, Ottesen, Jeppesen and Krustrup (2010) investigated a team sport activity (football) compared to an individual physical activity in groups (running) and looked at the social capital gained from these activities. Social capital, roughly understood as trust, norms and networks which promote cooperation between participants and thereby enhance society's efficiency, is deemed very important, because it is related to individual health (Putnam, 2000). Ottesen et al. used a combination of focus group interviews, participant observations and a questionnaire, and found that team sports, such as football, may have an advantage over individual sports in the development of social capital. The runners primarily discussed health-related stories in their group, while the footballers reported an interest in the fun and ludic aspects. This contrast gave football an advantage over running, because the participants were able to develop we-stories, which moved them personally closer together. So even though both groups positively developed social capital, the team sport seemed to hold an immediate advantage. An advantage over time was also noted, as the football group still playing together 1 year after the intervention stopped.

All in all, the presented studies suggest that team sports offer psychological benefits above and beyond those offered by individual sports, although more research is needed in order to fully understand this. They also indicate that the social component is very important for mental health and quality of life.

Do team sports offer more motivation?

Despite the positive health outcomes of physical activity described above, physical inactivity is increasing and is considered a pandemic (Kohl *et al.*, 2012). Therefore, the question of how to facilitate adherence to physical activity has been investigated in a number of research studies. Numerous strategies has been developed and applied in interventions aiming to increase physical activity (Artinian *et al.*, 2010). However, despite the prevalent knowledge, interventions aiming at increasing physical activity have only had a moderate effect size (Conn, Hafdahl, and Mehr, 2011). Therefore, it is of importance to address continuation not only through interventions, but also through the individual motivation of participants. In the following we will address the potential for team sport as a tool in promoting motivation and adherence to exercise.

Many motivational theories suggest that team sports can elicit more motivation than individual physical activity. The Self-Determination Theory (Deci and Ryan, 1985) advances a position on wellbeing and intrinsic as well as extrinsic motivation that suggests a possible advantage for team sports. Intrinsic motivation is motivation to participate in a physical activity for the sake of the activity itself, for the enjoyment of the activity. Extrinsic motivation is the motivation to participate in a physical activity for the positive consequences of that activity, such as losing weight or gaining better health. There is abundant research support for the claim that intrinsic motivation is a better predictor for continuation in physical activity (Moller *et al.*, 2013; Ntoumanis, 2005; Ryan and Deci, 2007). The notion of intrinsic motivation in the Self-Determination Theory rests on the assumption that all normal and healthy individuals have three basic psychological needs that should be satisfied for the individual to be psychologically healthy and motivated. These are the needs for autonomy, for competence, and for relatedness to others. The latter, the need for relatedness to others, is of special interest to our chapter of the psychological benefits of participation in team sports. In short, an individual has a need to engage in positive and authentic relationships with other human beings to be psychologically healthy, and, more importantly, if a physical activity helps to satisfy this need, the individual is more intrinsically motivated for the activity.

Looking at the definition of team sport in the beginning of this chapter, it is clear that team sport involves quite a bit of interaction and cooperation by its very nature. It seems plausible that this necessary interaction and cooperation in team sports can satisfy the need for relatedness to others to a higher degree than individual physical activities, hence giving team sports an advantage over individual physical activities.

The theoretical position that social aspects are important is supported by research. Social aspects seems to be linked to motivation (DeFreese and Smith, 2013; Evans, Eys, and Wolf, 2013), and predict continuation in the activity (Jõesaar and Hein, 2011; Stults-Kolehmainen, Gilson, and Abolt, 2013) as well as intention to return to sport (Spink *et al.*, 2015).

However, if we want to determine if the proposed advantage of team sports compared to individual sports is to be reckoned with, it is needed to compare team and individual sports. A few new studies have done just that. Turning to the experiences of participants in team and individual sports, respectively, Elbe *et al.* (Elbe *et al.*, 2010; Elbe *et al.*, 2016) investigated the flow experiences in team sport (football) participants and individual sport (running and Zumba, respectively) in two studies. Using two intervention groups and distribution of flow questionnaires at the end of selected training sessions, both studies found that flow elicitation in both team and individual sport participants were medium to high (4.99 to 6.01 and 3.50 to 4.25, respectively, on a scale from 1 to 7, with flow values over 5 being characterised as high [Reinhardt *et al.*, 2006; Reinhardt *et al.*, 2008]), and that flow elicitation was similar in individual and team sports. These results do not support the notion that flow can be easier elicited from team sports. Although more research is needed to confirm this, it seems that participation in team sports do not elicit higher levels of flow compared to individual physical activities in groups. Elbe *et al.* (2010; 2016) results suggest that high levels of flow can be elicited from both team sports and individual physical activity, and that flow is connected to continuation (Elbe *et al.*, 2010).

In contrast to this, studies on intrinsic motivation suggest that team sports hold an advantage over individual physical activity. Nielsen *et al.* (2014) investigated motivational differences between team and individual sports in elderly men. Two groups, who had participated in interventions with football or a mix of cross-fit and spinning, respectively, showed remarkable differences in continuation after the intervention had ended, with almost all participants continuing in the football group, and almost none in the cross-fit/spinning group. Nielsen *et al.* conducted focus group interviews to discover the differences between the two forms of activities that could lead to such differences in continuation. While both groups stressed the health benefits and the physical wellbeing that followed the training participation, this was not in itself enough to elicit continuation. However, when turning to the experiences of the activities, the football participants voiced having fun and enjoying the activity. Nielsen *et al.* used the Self-Determination Theory (Deci and Ryan, 1985) as a framework for analysing the interviews. The football participants experienced a very high satisfaction of the needs for relatedness to others, through the interactive nature of the game, and for competence, through the technical and tactical challenge in the game and the successful feelings through accomplishment of these challenges. The overall conclusion was that the satisfaction of the basic psychological needs for relatedness and competence that caused the enjoyment, experienced by the football participants, followed by intrinsic motivation. In line with this, a recent study (Wikman *et al.*, in review) used questionnaires to compare motivation levels between floorball and spinning, and found that intrinsic motivation for the activity was higher in the floorball group. Although more research is needed to confirm this, it seems that team sports elicit higher levels of intrinsic motivation compared to individual physical activity, perhaps due to greater satisfaction of the needs for relatedness and competence (Nielsen *et al.*, 2014).

However, the motivational climate should be considered as a challenge of team sports. Most team sports are automatically placed in a sporting and competitive logic (Nielsen *et al.*, 2014). This creates a performance climate, in which the emphasis is put on performance outcomes (winning or losing in training or match) and between-player rivalries, is common among team sports (Ames, 1992; Ntoumanis and Biddle, 1999; Duda and Balaguer, 2007) and notoriously linked with team sport (Nesti, 2010). The performance climate is detrimental to participant motivation (Ntoumanis and Biddle, 1999), and can negate the motivational advantages of team sports. Therefore, it should be attempted to create a mastery climate instead, in which skill development and effort are important, and mistakes are perceived as part of the learning process (Duda and Balaguer, 2007).

Accordingly, rethinking team sport has been deemed necessary. The new concept of football fitness (Bennike *et al.*, 2014) is a type of football designed with a focus on health and enjoyment (over competition), without a tournament structure, reduced member fee and is adjustable to local context and participants. Football fitness is managed by local football clubs and has attracted new target groups, such as middle-aged women, normally not participating in competitive football. Thus, less competitive team sports seems to be a possible way of increasing motivation and participation in physical activity on a larger scale, and initiatives such as football fitness should serve as an inspiration when offering team sports to the public.

To conclude on this section, social interactions and perhaps feelings of competence during the activity in team sports seem to be central to the participants' motivation, as opposed to extrinsic perspectives of improved health. If enjoyment is the focus of sport participation, individuals or groups are more likely to maintain future interest in physical activity (Biddle *et al.*, 2015). Team sport can in this regard be a positive arena for sport participation and maintenance for many individuals, provided that they are organised in a way that emphasises enjoyment and health. The foresight of Carron, Hausenblas and Estabrook, combined with the knowledge presented in this chapter, makes a strong argument of the positive aspects of developing team sport in regards to health: *'the need for interpersonal attachment is a fundamental human motive – a fact that has important implications for promoting adherence in exercise and physical activity'* (Carron, Hausenblas, and Estabrooks, 1999, p. 4).

Implications for practice and research

Turning to practical implications, the physical inactivity pandemic (Kohl *et al.*, 2012) is a serious threat to health and quality of life. Individual exercise trends have in the past decade flourished with popularity of running/ jogging and strength training (Ibsen and Seippel, 2010). To ensure continued participation in physical activity, however, it seems beneficial to focus on participation in team sport, rather than the individual gym-based exercise activities in exercise on prescription (Willemann, 2004) or offered by municipalities' health centres (Sørensen and Pfister, 2008; Toft, 2013). Team sport seem to offer better psychological effects of participation, and, not least, higher motivation, which leads to continuation. However, as team sport have more logistic challenges (e.g. a minimum number of participants, a space in which the team sport can be played), it should be considered how these logistic challenges can be overcome. Also, many team sports are automatically placed in a sporting and competitive logic, which can deter many participants from partaking (Nielsen *et al.*, 2014), and practitioners should consider how the competitive element of team sport can be removed or de-emphasised, perhaps through an emphasis on mastery climate. As the motivational climate of a team highly relies on the coach efforts, emphasis, skills and orientation in organising and managing the team (Balaguer *et al.*, 2012), the coaches and leaders should be a focus point in creating motivating team sport activities. Evidence-based education of team sport leaders should be an ambition at political and societal level, based on current research such as empowering coaching (Duda, 2013), life skills and positive youth development research (Gould and Carson, 2008).

Throughout this chapter we have presented research that underlines the potential of team sport and how team sport could play a significant role in the important task of increasing mental health as well as heightening motivation for physical activity in the broad population. However, the research on this area is still at a point of departure and most literature has only investigated team sport either implicitly or as a secondary outcome. There is indeed a need for high quality studies with a clearly defined research question investigating the differences in mental health effects of teams sports compared to individual sports and physical activity. There is a need for studies comparing team sports' effect on motivation to individual sports'. There is a need for studies investigating what particular mechanisms in team sport that especially affect mental health and motivation. And finally, there is a need for studies investigating how to efficiently implement team sport as a promotion tool for both mental health and motivation towards physical activity in society. Such knowledge would be of great importance to practitioners on all levels through individuals, sport clubs, corporations, organisations, communities and societies.

Conclusion

Team sport has existed for more than a century in an organised form, and is in modern society mainly a venue for competition and increasing performance, illustrated in its purest form as professional team sport. However, recent research suggests that team sport, when organized correctly, can offer more psychological benefits of participation as well as more motivation and hence participation than individual physical activity. While research needs to confirm and elaborate on this statement, we propose that team sport should be considered and used as a way of increasing physical activity to a larger extent than is the case today. We acknowledge the hard work ahead, but given the many positive benefits working with team sports earlier presented, we firmly believe that team sport is a fertile future path in the area of sport and health.

References

Ames, C. (1992). Achievement goals, motivational climate, and motivational processes. In G. C. Roberts (ed.), *Motivation in Sport and Exercise* (pp. 161–176). Champaign, IL: Human Kinetics.

Artinian, N. T., Fletcher, G. F., Mozaffarian, D., Kris-Etherton, P., Van Horn, L., Lichtenstein, A. H., Kumanyika, S., Kraus, W. E., Fleg, J. L., Redeker, N. S., and Meininger, J.C. (2010). Interventions to promote physical activity and dietary lifestyle changes for cardiovascular risk factor reduction in adults: a scientific statement from the American Heart Association. *Circulation*, *122*(4), 406–441. doi:10.1161/CIR.0b013e3181e8edf1

Balaguer, I., Gonzáles, L., Fabra, P., Castillo, I., Mercé, and Duda, J. L. (2012) Coaches' interpersonal style, basic psychological needs and the well-being of young soccer players: a longitudinal analysis. *Journal of Sports Sciences*, *30*, 1619–1629.

Bennike, S., Wikman, J. M., and Ottesen, L. S. (2014). Football Fitness – a new version of football? A concept for adult players in Danish football clubs. *Scandinavian Journal of Medicine & Science in Sports*, *24*, 138–146. doi:10.1111/sms.12276

Biddle, S. J. H. and Mutrie, N. (2008). *Psychology of Physical Activity: Determinants, Well-Being and Interventions*, 2nd edn. Abingdon, UK: Routledge.

Biddle, S. J. H., Mutrie, N., and Gorely, T. (2015). *Psychology of Physical Activity: Determinants, Well-Being and Interventions*, 3rd edn. New York: Routledge.

Bowling, A. and Stenner, P. (2011). Which measure of quality of life performs best in older age? A comparison of the OPQOL, CASP-19 and WHOQOL-OLD. *Journal of Epidemiology and Community Health*, 65(3), 273–280. doi:10.1136/jech.2009.087668

Brisswalter, J., Collardeau, M., and René, A. (2002). Effects of acute physical exercise characteristics on cognitive performance. *Sports Medicine*, 32(9), 555–566.

Bruner, M. W., Eys, M. A., Wilson, K. S., and Cote, J. (2014). Group cohesion and positive youth development in team sport athletes. *Sport, Exercise, and Performance Psychology*, 3(4), 219–227. doi:10.1037/spy0000017

Campbell, A. and Hausenblas, H. A. (2009). Effects of exercise interventions on body image: a meta-analysis. *Journal of Health Psychology*, 14(6), 780–793. doi:10.1177/1359105309338977

Carron, A. V. and Hausenblas, H. A. (1998). *Group Dynamics in Sport*, 2nd edn. Morgantown, WV: Fitness Information Technology.

Carron, A. V., Hausenblas, H. A., and Estabrooks, P. A. (1999) Social influence and exercise involvement. In S. J. Bull (ed.), *Adherence Issues in Sport and Exercise* (pp. 1–17). Chichester: Wiley.

Carron, A.V., Brawley, L. R., and Widmeyer,W. N. (1998). The measurement of cohesiveness in sport groups. In J. L. Duda (ed.), *Advances in Sport and Exercise Psychology Measurement* (pp. 213–226). Morgantown, WV: Fitness Information Technology.

Conn, V. S., Hafdahl, A. R., and Mehr, D. R. (2011). Interventions to increase physical activity among healthy adults: meta-analysis of outcomes. *American Journal of Public Health*, 101(4), 751–758. doi:10.2105/AJPH.2010.194381

De Moor, M. H. M., Beem, A. L., Stubbe, J. H., Boomsma, D. I., and De Geus, E. J. C. (2006). Regular exercise, anxiety, depression and personality: a population-based study. *Preventive Medicine*, 42(4), 273–279. doi:10.1016/j.ypmed.2005.12.002

Deci, E. L. and Ryan, R. M. (1985). *Intrinsic Motivation and Self-Determination in Human Behavior*. New York: Plenum Publishing.

DeFreese, J. D. and Smith, A. L. (2013). Teammate social support, burnout, and self-determined motivation in collegiate athletes. *Psychology of Sport and Exercise*, 14(2), 258–265. doi:10.1016/j.psychsport.2012.10.009

Duda, J. L. and Balaguer, I. (2007) Coach-created motivational climate. In S. Jowett and D. Lavallee (eds), *Social Psychology in Sport* (pp. 117–130), Champaign, IL: Human Kinetics.

Duda, J. L. (2013) The conceptual and empirical foundations of Empowering Coaching: setting the stage for the PAPA project. *International Journal of Sport and Exercise Psychology*, 11(4), 311–318.

Edwards, D. J., Edwards, S. D., and Basson, C. J. (2004). Psychological well-being and physical self-esteem in sport and exercise. *International Journal of Mental Health Promotion*, 6(1), 25–32. doi:10.1080/14623730.2004.9721921

Eime, R. M., Young, J. A., Harvey, J. T., Charity, M. J., and Payne, W. R. (2013a). A systematic review of the psychological and social benefits of participation in sport for adults: informing development of a conceptual model of health through sport. *International Journal of Behavioral Nutrition and Physical Activity*, 10, 135. doi:10.1186/1479-5868-10-135

Eime, R. M., Young, J. A., Harvey, J. T., Charity, M. J., and Payne, W. R. (2013b). A systematic review of the psychological and social benefits of participation in sport for children and adolescents: informing development of a conceptual model of health through sport. *International Journal of Behavioral Nutrition and Physical Activity*, 10, 98. doi:10.1186/1479-5868-10-98

Elbe, A.-M., Barene, S., Strahler, K., Holtermann, A., and Krustrup, P. (2016). Experiencing flow in a work place physical activity intervention: a longitudinal comparison between a Football and Zumba intervention. *Women in Sport and Physical Activity Journal*, 24, 70–77.

Elbe, A.-M., Strahler, K., Krustrup, P., Wikman, J., and Stelter, R. (2010). Experiencing flow in different types of physical activity intervention programs: three randomized studies. *Scandinavian Journal of Medicine & Science in Sports*, 20, 111–117. doi:10.1111/j.1600-0838.2010.01112.x

Evans, B., Eys, M., and Wolf, S. (2013). Exploring the nature of interpersonal influence in elite individual sport teams. *Journal of Applied Sport Psychology*, 25(4), 448–462. doi:10.1080/10413200.2012.752769

Evans, M. B. and Eys, M. A. (2015). Collective goals and shared tasks: interdependence structure and perceptions of individual sport team environments. *Scandinavian Journal of Medicine & Science in Sports*, 25(1), e139–e148. doi:10.1111/sms.12235

Gillison, F. B., Skevington, S. M., Sato, A., Standage, M., and Evangelidou, S. (2009). The effects of exercise interventions on quality of life in clinical and healthy populations; a meta-analysis. *Social Science & Medicine*, 68(9), 1700–1710. doi:10.1016/j.socscimed.2009.02.028

Gillison, F. B., Skevington, S. M., Sato, A., Standage, M., and Evangelidou, S. (2009). The effects of exercise interventions on quality of life in clinical and healthy populations; a meta-analysis. *Social Science & Medicine*, 68(9), 1700–1710. doi:10.1016/j.socscimed.2009.02.028

Gould, D. and Carson, S. (2008) Life skills development through sport: current status and future directions. *International Review of Sport and Exercise Psychology*, 1(1), 58–78.

Hausenblas, H. A. and Fallon, E. A. (2006). Exercise and body image: a meta-analysis. *Psychology & Health*, 21(1), 33–47. doi:10.1080/14768320500105270

Heath, G. W. and Brown, D. W. (2009). Recommended levels of physical activity and health-related quality of life among overweight and obese adults in the United States, 2005. *Journal of Physical Activity & Health*, 6(4), 403–411.

Hoffmann, M. D. and Loughead, T. M. (2016). A comparison of well-peer mentored and non-peer mentored athletes' perceptions of satisfaction. *Journal of Sports Sciences*, 34(5), 450–458. doi:10.1080/02640414.2015.1057517

Ibsen, B. and Seippel, Ø. (2010). Introduction: sport in Scandinavian societies. *Sport in Society*, 13(4), 563–566.

Jackson, B., Gucciardi, D. F., Lonsdale, C., Whipp, P. R., and Dimmock, J. A. (2014). 'I think they believe in me': the predictive effects of teammate- and classmate-focused relation-inferred self-efficacy in sport and physical activity settings. *Journal of Sport and Exercise Psychology*, 36(5), 486–505. doi:10.1123/jsep.2014-0070

Jõesaar, H. and Hein, V. (2011). Psychosocial determinants of young athletes' continued participation over time. *Perceptual and Motor Skills*, 113(1), 51–66. doi:10.2466/05.06.13.PMS.113.4.51-66

Kohl, H. W., Craig, C. L., Lambert, E. V., Inoue, S., Alkandari, J. R., Leetongin, G., Kahlmeier, S., Lancet Physical Activity Series Working Group. (2012). The pandemic of physical inactivity: global action for public health. *The Lancet, 380*(9838), 294–305. doi:10.1016/S0140-6736(12)60898-8

Krogh, J., Nordentoft, M., Sterne, J. A. C., and Lawlor, D. A. (2010). The effect of exercise in clinically depressed adults: systematic review and meta-analysis of randomized controlled trials. *The Journal of Clinical Psychiatry, 72*(4), 529–538. doi:10.4088/JCP.08r04913blu

Krustrup, P., Hansen, P. R., Randers, M. B., Nybo, L., Martone, D., Andersen, L. J., Bune, L. T., Junge, A., and Bangsbo, J. (2010). Beneficial effects of recreational football on the cardiovascular risk profile in untrained premenopausal women. *Scandinavian Journal of Medicine & Science in Sports, 20*, 40–49. doi:10.1111/j.1600-0838.2010.01110.x

Krustrup, P., Nielsen, J. J., Krustrup, B. R., Christensen, J. F., Pedersen, H., Randers, M. B., Aagaard, P., Petersen, A. M., Nybo, L., and Bangsbo, J. (2009). Recreational soccer is an effective health-promoting activity for untrained men. *British Journal of Sports Medicine, 43*(11), 825–831. doi:10.1136/bjsm.2008.053124

Leahey, T. M., Kumar, R., Weinberg, B. M., and Wing, R. R. (2012). Teammates and social influence affect weight loss outcomes in a team-based weight loss competition. *Obesity, 20*(7), 1413–1418. doi:10.1038/oby.2012.18

Loughead, T. M., Patterson, M. M., and Carron, A. V. (2008). The impact of fitness leader behavior and cohesion on an exerciser's affective state. *International Journal of Sport and Exercise Psychology, 6*(1), 53–68. doi:10.1080/1612197X.2008.9671854

McGale, N., McArdle, S., and Gaffney, P. (2011). Exploring the effectiveness of an integrated exercise/CBT intervention for young men's mental health. *British Journal of Health Psychology, 16*(3), 457–471.

Moller, A. C., Buscemi, J., McFadden, H. G., Hedeker, D., and Spring, B. (2013). Financial motivation undermines potential enjoyment in an intensive diet and activity intervention. *Journal of Behavioral Medicine.* doi:10.1007/s10865-013-9542-5

Nesti, M. (2010). *Psychology in Football: Working with Elite and Professional Players.* London: Routledge.

Nielsen, G., Wikman, J. M., Jensen, C. J., Schmidt, J. F., Gliemann, L., and Andersen, T. R. (2014). Health promotion: the impact of beliefs of health benefits, social relations and enjoyment on exercise continuation. *Scandinavian Journal of Medicine & Science in Sports, 24*, 66–75. doi:10.1111/sms.12275

Ntoumanis, N. (2005). A prospective study of participation in optional school physical education using a self-determination theory framework. *Journal of Educational Psychology, 97*(3), 444–453. doi:10.1037/0022-0663.97.3.444

Ntoumanis, N. and Biddle, S. J. H. (1999) A review of motivational climate in physical activity. *Journal of Sport Sciences, 17*, 643–665.

Ottesen, L., Jeppesen, R. S., and Krustrup, B. R. (2010). The development of social capital through football and running: studying an intervention program for inactive women. *Scandinavian Journal of Medicine & Science in Sports, 20*, 118–131. doi:10.1111/j.1600-0838.2010.01123.x

Petruzzello, S. J., Landers, D. D. M., Hatfield, B. D., Kubitz, K. A., and Salazar, W. (1991). A meta-analysis on the anxiety-reducing effects of acute and chronic exercise. *Sports Medicine, 11*(3), 143–182. doi:10.2165/00007256-199111030-00002

Putnam, R. D. (2000). *Bowling Alone. The Collapse and Revival of American Community*. New York: Simon & Schuster Paperbacks.

Reel, J. J., Greenleaf, C., Baker, W. K., Aragon, S., Bishop, D., Cachaper, C., Handwerk, P., Locicero, J., Rathburn, L., Reid, W. K., and Hattie, J. (2007). Relations of body concerns and exercise behavior: a meta-analysis. *Psychological Reports*, 101(3), 927–942. doi:10.2466/pr0.101.3.927-942

Reinhardt, C., Lau, A., Hottenrott, K., and Stoll, O. (2006). Flow-Erleben unter kontrollierter Beanspruchungssteuerung – Ergebnisse einer Laufbandstudie [Flow experiences under controlled load – results of a treadmill study]. *Zeitschrift für Sportpsychologie*, 4, 140–146.

Reinhardt, C., Wiener, S., Heimbeck, A., Stoll, O., Lau, A., and Schliermann, R. (2008). Flow in der Sporttherapie der Depression – ein beanspruchungsorientierter Ansatz [Flow in the sport therapy of depression – an approach based on load]. *Bewegungstherapie und Gesundheitssport*, 4, 147–151.

Rejeski, W. J. and Brawley, L. R. (1988). Definding the boundaries of sport psychology. *The Sport Psychologist*, 2, 231–242.

Ryan, R. M. and Deci, E. L. (2007). Self-determination theory and the promotion and maintenance of sport, exercise, and health. In M. S. Hagger and N. L. D. Chatzisarantis (eds), *Intrinsic Motivation and Self-Determination in Exercise and Sport* (pp. 1–20). Champaign, IL: Human Kinetics.

Sabiston, C. M., Jewett, R., Ashdown-Franks, G., Belanger, M., Brunet, J., O'Loughlin, E., and O'Loughlin, J. (2016). Number of years of team and individual sport participation during adolescence and depressive symptoms in early adulthood. *Journal of Sport and Exercise Psychology*, 38(1), 105–110. doi:10.1123/jsep.2015-0175

Smith, A. L., Gustafsson, H., and Hassmén, P. (2010). Peer motivational climate and burnout perceptions of adolescent athletes. *Psychology of Sport and Exercise*, 11(6), 453–460. doi:10.1016/j.psychsport.2010.05.007

Sørensen, M. R. and Pfister, G. (2008). *Ældre og fysisk aktivitet – muligheder for idræt og motion i København [Elderly and physical activity – possibilities for sports and exercise in Copenhagen]*. Copenhagen: Department for Sport and Exercise Sciences, Faculty of Science, University of Copenhagen.

Spink, K. S., Ulvick, J. D., McLaren, C. D., Crozier, A. J., and Fesser, K. (2015). Effects of groupness and cohesion on intention to return in sport. *Sport, Exercise, and Performance Psychology*, 4(4), 293–302. doi:10.1037/spy0000043

Stephens, T. (1988). Physical activity and mental health in the United States and Canada: evidence from four population surveys. *Preventive Medicine*, 17(1), 35–47. doi:10.1016/0091-7435(88)90070-9

Stults-Kolehmainen, M. A., Gilson, T. A., and Abolt, C. J. (2013). Feelings of acceptance and intimacy among teammates predict motivation in intercollegiate sport. *Journal of Sport Behavior*, 36(3), 306–327.

Terry-McElrath, Y. M. and O'Malley, P. M. (2011). Substance use and exercise participation among young adults: parallel trajectories in a national cohort-sequential study. *Addiction*, 106(10), 1855–1865.

Toft, D. (2013). *Fremtiden senioridræt – mellem ironman og stolemotion [Exercise for the elderly in the future – between ironman and chair based exercise]*. Copenhagen: IDAN.

Tomporowski, P. D. (2003). Effects of acute bouts of exercise on cognition. *Acta Psychologica*, 112(3), 297–324.

Wenger, E. (2000). Communities of practice and social learning systems. *Organization*, 7(2), 225–246.

Wenger, E. (2011). Communities of Practice. Retrived from http://wenger-trayner.com/introduction-to-communities-of-practice/ (accessed 18 May 2016).

Wenger, E. and Snyder, W. M. (2000). Communities of practice: the organizational frontier. *Harvard Business Review*, 78(1), 137.

Wikman, J. M., Elsborg, P., Nielsen, G., Seidelin, K., Nyberg, M., Bangsbo, J., Hellsten, Y., and Elbe, A.-M. (unpublished manuscript). Are team sport games a more motivating type of exercise than individual exercise activities for middle-aged women? A comparison of the levels of motivation associated with participating in floorball and spinning.

Willemann, M. (2004). *Motion på recept: En litteraturgennemgang med fokus på effekter og organisering [Exercise on Prescription: A Literature Review with Focus on Effects and Organisation]*. Copenhagen: Viden- og dokumentationsenheden, Sundhedsstyrelsen.

Wipfli, B. M., Rethorst, C. D., Landers, D. M., and others. (2008). The anxiolytic effects of exercise: a meta-analysis of randomized trials and dose–response analysis. *Journal of Sport & Exercise Psychology*, 30(4), 392–410.

Chapter 7

Mental health, physical activity and sport

Simon Rosenbaum, Davy Vancampfort,
Oscar Lederman and Brendon Stubbs

Why mental health?

In 1954, the first director-general of the World Health Organization, Dr Brock Chisholm, famously stated that *'without mental health there can be no true physical health'*. With a growing body of research demonstrating the interrelationship between mind and body, the significance and relevance of Dr Chisholm's statement is increasingly pertinent. Mental and substance use disorders are a global health priority and are collectively responsible for the leading cause of years lived with disability worldwide (Whiteford *et al.*, 2013). More than one in five, or an estimated 30 per cent of the population will experience a common mental disorder (depression or anxiety) throughout their lifetime (Steel *et al.*, 2014), with mental ill-health consistently listed as the primary reason for presentation to general practice/ primary care (Sauver *et al.*, 2013). Furthermore, the treatment costs of mental illness are estimated at £22.5 billion per year in the United Kingdom alone (McCrone, 2008), with this figure likely to be considerably higher if accounting for indirect costs and cost associated with disability and loss of productivity. This highlights an ongoing need for the evaluation of novel, non-pharmacological, evidence-based interventions that have the potential to improve patient outcomes.

Mental illness and mental health: two continuums

It is important to consider the distinction between *mental illness* and *mental health*, especially in the context of sport, physical activity and public health. Mental health is more than simply the absence of mental illness, and is a positive concept related to the social and emotional wellbeing of individuals and communities. Mental health is influenced by culture, but generally relates to the enjoyment of life, ability to cope with stress and sadness, the fulfilment of goals and potential, and a sense of connection to others (Hunter Institute of Mental Health, 2015). A *mental illness* is a disorder diagnosed by a medical professional that significantly interferes with an individual's cognitive, emotional or social abilities (Hunter Institute of Mental Health, 2015). Westerhof and Keyes (2010) described the two continua model of mental illness and health, stating that both mental health and mental illness are related, but distinct dimensions: one continuum indicates the presence or absence of mental health, the other the presence or absence of mental illness (Westerhof and Keyes, 2010).

Mental disorders encompass a wide variety of signs, symptoms, experiences and disorders. For example, mental illnesses can include mood disorders (e.g. major depression and bipolar disorder), anxiety disorders (e.g. generalised anxiety disorder and social anxiety disorder), psychotic disorders (e.g. schizophrenia), personality disorders (e.g. narcissistic personality disorder and borderline personality disorder) and substance use disorders (e.g. alcohol dependence or abuse) (see Figure 7.1). Mental disorders are typically classified according to the Diagnostic and Statistical Manual of Mental Disorders or other structured diagnostic classification (American Psychiatric Association, 2013). While each mental disorder may be viewed in isolation, co-morbidity with other mental disorders is common (Amerio *et al.*, 2015; Fornaro *et al.*, 2016).

Integrating mind and body: mental and physical ill-health

Poor mental health is known to be associated with adverse physical health in a bidirectional relationship. For example, people with obesity are more likely to develop depression (Luppino *et al.*, 2010), and people with pain and musculoskeletal disorders are more likely to have comorbid mental health conditions (Stubbs, Koyanagi, Thompson, *et al.*, 2016; Stubbs, Aluko, *et al.*, 2016).

Conversely, the physical health of people with established mental illness is significantly poorer than the general population culminating in a 10 to 15 years reduction in life expectancy (Olfson *et al.*, 2015). The cause of this premature mortality is multi-factorial, with high rates of cardiovascular and metabolic diseases identified as contributing factors. For example, people

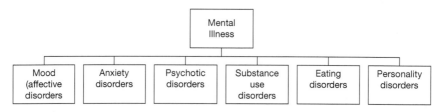

Figure 7.1 Broad classifications of mental illness (adapted from DSM-IV and ICD-10)
American Psychiatric Association, 2000

with mental illness (e.g. depression, schizophrenia or bipolar disorder) are at a significantly increased risk of developing diabetes compared to the general population (De Hert *et al.*, 2009; Vancampfort, Correll, *et al.*, 2016). Obesity, hypertension and hypercholesterolemia are all significantly more prevalent and smoking rates are approximately two to three times that seen in the general population (Newcomer and Hennekens, 2007). In addition, more than one third of all cigarettes smoked, are smoked by someone with a mental illness (Lasser *et al.*, 2000). Furthermore, there is evidence suggesting that this disparity is worsening and the mortality gap is widening (Suetani, Whiteford, and McGrath, 2015) highlighting the need for novel and effective multi-component lifestyle interventions incorporating a combination of sport, exercise and dietary components (Teasdale *et al.*, 2016; Daumit *et al.*, 2013; Schuch, Vancampfort, Richards, *et al.*, 2016). Definitive evidence exists demonstrating a significant relationship between exercise and reduced all-cause and cardiovascular mortality in the general population (Nocon *et al.*, 2008) with epidemiological evidence for the beneficial effects of physical activity dating back to a landmark study comparing active and sedentary bus and postal workers (Morris *et al.*, 1953). Exercise has since been cited in treatment guidelines and position statements for various conditions such as diabetes (Colberg *et al.*, 2010), cardiovascular disease (Thompson *et al.*, 2003), major depressive disorder (Davidson, 2010) and cancer recovery (Schmitz *et al.*, 2010). Despite this increasing recognition of the health benefits associated with being physically active, people with a mental illness are known to be less likely to be physically active compared to the general population (Vancampfort, Firth, *et al.*, 2016; Stubbs, Koyanagi, Hallgren, *et al.*, 2016; Stubbs, Firth, *et al.*, 2016). Therefore an evidence-based approach to increasing physical activity within this vulnerable population is warranted.

Figure 7.2 serves to highlight the bidirectional relationship between physical and mental health, and the co-contribution of sedentary behaviour, smoking, physical activity, dietary habits and physical fitness to the increased metabolic risk of people with mental illness. Despite medication being a necessary component of treatment for many mental disorders, substantial metabolic consequences are known to occur, in particularly with antipsychotic medication, with the most rapid deterioration of metabolic health occurring in the initial 12 months of treatment (Correll *et al.*, 2009; Perez-Iglesias *et al.*, 2008). Up to 77 per cent of previously antipsychotic naïve patients treated with antipsychotic medication will experience clinically significant (>7 per cent) weight gain within the first year of treatment (Correll *et al.*, 2009). Given that the average age of experiencing a first episode of psychosis and hence commencement of medication is between 16 and 21 years, preventing such adverse metabolic deterioration is crucial to minimising the disparity in cardiovascular related outcomes for people experiencing psychotic related mental illness (Alvarez-Jimenez *et al.*, 2008; Curtis,

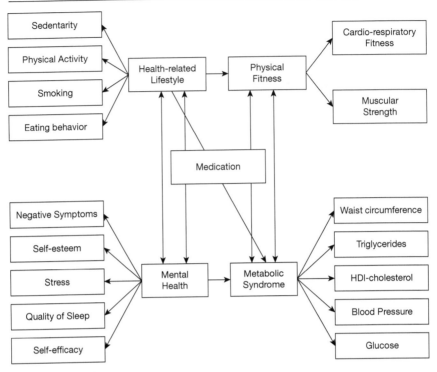

Figure 7.2 Relations between the metabolic syndrome and physical fitness, health-related lifestyle behaviour, variables of mental health and antipsychotic medication in persons with mental illness

Reproduced with permission from Vancampfort *et al.*, 2010

Newall and Samaras, 2012). A 2016 study demonstrated for the first time that a combined lifestyle and life-skills intervention comprising exercise and dietary components was effective in attenuating antipsychotic induced weight gain among young people experiencing a first episode of psychosis (Curtis *et al.*, 2016).

Physical activity, physical fitness and mental illness

People with mental illness have significantly reduced physical fitness (exercise capacity) compared to the general population, with a 2016 meta-analysis finding that people with severe mental illness have a significantly lower cardio-respiratory fitness compared to controls (n=310; Hedges' g=-1.01, 95%CI=-1.18 to -0.85, p<0.001) (Vancampfort, Rosenbaum, *et al.*, 2016). In a review of prospective cohort studies, data from 1,142,699 people found that, among both men and women, poor cardiorespiratory fitness was linked to a higher risk of developing depression, with low fitness levels associated with a 75 per cent increased risk of depression, while those with medium fitness levels had an increased risk of approximately 23 per cent (Schuch, Vancampfort, Sui, *et al.*, 2016). In a sample of 70 patients experiencing first episode schizophrenia in the United States, muscular strength and endurance, muscular flexibility and cardiorespiratory fitness were assessed using the Young Men's Christian Association standardised fitness test, with most scores below the 50th percentile compared with national norms (Gretchen-Doorly *et al.*, 2012). Furthermore patients with a higher body mass index and those who smoked had even poorer results, with a non-significant trend indicating that patients with a longer duration of illness had a further reduced exercise capacity (Gretchen-Doorly *et al.*, 2012). In another sample of 60 desired-weight and overweight patients with schizophrenia, exercise capacity and self-reported physical activity levels were assessed via the 6-minute walk test and Baecke questionnaire (Vancampfort *et al.*, 2011). Compared to healthy controls, patients with schizophrenia walked a significantly shorter distance (p<0.001) (Vancampfort *et al.*, 2011). Exercise-based interventions targeting people experiencing mental illness significantly improve cardiorespiratory fitness, typically over a relatively short period of time (typically 12 weeks) (Stubbs, Rosenbaum, *et al.*, 2016; Vancampfort, Rosenbaum, *et al.*, 2015). Improvements are greater following interventions incorporating high intensity activity, those with a higher frequency of exercise (at least three times per week), and those interventions that are supervised by qualified personnel (i.e., physiotherapists and exercise physiologists) (Stubbs, Rosenbaum, *et al.*, 2016; Vancampfort; Rosenbaum, *et al.*, 2015). In addition to improving fitness, sport, exercise and physical activity offers considerable promise as an acceptable, low-risk, accessible and efficacious component of treatment for people experiencing mental illness (Rosenbaum *et al.*, 2014). Integrating physical activity interventions as part of routine mental healthcare may also improve traditional service utilisation by reducing stigma associated with help seeking behaviour and increase engagement with treatment services to facilitate functional recovery and improve overall outcomes.

Physical activity and depression

There is evidence of a bidirectional relationship between physical activity and depression. Both physical activity (defined as any bodily movement produced by skeletal muscles that results in energy expenditure (Caspersen, Powell, and Christenson, 1985a) and exercise (i.e., a subset of physical activity that is planned, structured and repetitive (Caspersen, Powell, and Christenson, 1985b) have been identified as having prevention and treatment effects on depression (Schuch, Vancampfort, Richards, *et al.*, 2016; Mammen and Faulkner, 2013; Rebar *et al.*, 2015). Meta-analyses have demonstrated that moderate-intensity, supervised exercise programmes of at least 9 weeks duration (trials typically range from 8–16 weeks), that use a combination of aerobic and resistance-based exercise modalities, together with a group format, appear to have the greatest impact on reducing depressive symptoms (Schuch, Vancampfort, Rosenbaum, et al., 2016; Stanton and Reaburn, 2014). To date, the largest community-based trial of exercise for depression involved 946 outpatients randomised to either 12 weeks of prescribed exercise, Internet-based cognitive behavioural therapy (CBT), or usual care consisting of brief CBT-focused therapy and antidepressant treatment, found that supervised exercise three times per week resulted in significantly lower depression severity compared to usual care, and that the magnitude of the effect was equivalent to the Internet-CBT group (Hallgren et al., 2015). The results of this study are promising, especially for those groups for whom significant barriers to accessing standard clinician delivered cognitive behaviour therapy exist, including stigma and financial costs associated with seeking treatment. Nonetheless, there is ongoing debate within the scientific literature regarding the magnitude of effect of exercise on depression. Methodological differences between reviews and meta-analyses (Ekkekakis, 2015), specifically around (i) the inclusion of pragmatic interventions such as physical activity counselling and yoga, which many argue better reflect real world clinical practice and the condition-specific barriers associated with commencing and maintaining an exercise programme, and (ii) a large control group response (SMD –0.9) across exercise and depression RCTs (Stubbs et al., 2015) have resulted in an underreporting of the overall effect size. A 2016 meta-analysis of 25 RCTs including people with a diagnosis of depression and those with depressive symptoms, found a large and significant overall effect on depression after adjustment for publication bias with an SMD of –1.11, corresponding to an approximate 5-point reduction in the Hamilton Rating Scale for Depression (HAM-D), and a greater than six-point reduction in the Beck Depression Inventory (BDI), both of which are clinically significant based on the National Institute for Health and Care Excellence (NICE) guidelines (Schuch, Vancampfort, Richards, et al., 2016; NICE, 2009). Additionally, it was found that a total of 1,057 negative studies would be required to nullify the significance of the main analysis, further justifying the robustness of the analysis (Schuch, Vancampfort, Richards, et al., 2016). In a subsequent 2016 meta-analysis, Schuch et al., reviewed the literature relating to exercise for depression in older adults (60 years) and found a large, significant effect of exercise on depression across the eight included RCTs (SMD = –0.90) (Schuch, Vancampfort, Rosenbaum, et al., 2016).

The potential protective role of physical activity against poor mental health is becoming increasingly clear. A synthesis of 30 studies found that baseline physical activity was negatively associated with risk of future depression, with evidence of an effect in response to even low levels of physical activity (i.e., less that the WHO recommendation of 150 minutes per week (WHO, 2010) (Mammen and Faulkner, 2013). Evidence for the bidirectional relationship between physical activity and depression continues to increase, with a large longitudinal study demonstrating that positive lifestyle behaviours such as physical activity at baseline, were associated with a 22 per cent (RR 0.76) reduced risk of episodes of a mood disorder at 5-year follow-up (Gall et al., 2016). These data are consistent with a 2014 meta-analysis of observational studies finding that sedentary behaviour, independent of physical activity, is associated with a significantly increased risk of depression (Zhai, Zhang, and Zhang, 2015).

Physical activity as an adjunct form of medicine: mechanisms of action

The mechanisms behind the beneficial effects of physical activity on mental illness are complex and multi-factorial, including neurobiological and psychosocial adaptations that occur over both the short and long term (Schuch, Deslandes, et al., 2016). Aerobic-based exercise is the more commonly researched subtype of physical activity in both human and animal models relating to mental illness (Eyre and Baune, 2013; Rethorst and Trivedi, 2013), with a more potent effect of exercise consisting of both aerobic and resistance components generally observed (Erickson, Gildengers, and Butters, 2013). This greater effect of 'metabolic exercise' (combined aerobic and resistance exercises) is in-line with recommendations for those with type two diabetes mellitus in which a greater effect on blood glucose control have been found with combination-based exercise (Hordern et al., 2012). Among the neurochemical mechanisms associated with the benefits of physical activity for mental illness is the exercise induced increase in brain derived neurotrophic factor (BDNF) and insulin-like growth factor (IGF-1) (Cevada et al., 2013; Pajonk et al., 2010), both of which are associated with neurogenesis, angiogenesis and neuroplasticity (Erickson, Gildengers, and Butters, 2013). These trophic factors act as modulators and can be modulated by neurotransmitters such as adrenaline and noradrenaline (Dishman and O'Connor, 2009), which have an established impact on both cognition and mood (Cevada et al., 2013). BDNF is also significant for its role in supporting neural survival, growth and synaptic plasticity (Voss et al., 2013). In 2011 Erickson et al., demonstrated that aerobic exercise training increases the volume of the anterior hippocampus in older adults, and that the increased hippocampal volume was associated with greater serum levels of BDNF (Erickson et al., 2011). The hippocampal volume of people with schizophrenia(Pajonk et al., 2010), PTSD (Bremner et al., 1995) major depression (Bremner et al., 2000) and other mental disorders has repeatedly shown to be reduced compared to healthy controls with implications for memory, cognition and the progression of the conditions (DeCarolis and Eisch, 2010).

As such, hippocampal neurogenesis has been identified as a potential treatment strategy for people experiencing mental illness (DeCarolis and Eisch, 2010). Hippocampal plasticity in mental illness in response to an aerobic exercise intervention has been previously demonstrated, with Pajonk *et al.*, finding that following moderate-intensity aerobic exercise training, hippocampal volume increased significantly by an average of 12 per cent in patients with chronic schizophrenia compared with no change in a comparable, non-exercising group of patients (Pajonk *et al.*, 2010). Furthermore, the changes in hippocampal volume were strongly correlated with changes in maximal oxygen uptake (V02) (the gold standard assessment of cardio-respiratory fitness) resulting from the exercise intervention (Pajonk *et al.*, 2010). However subsequent human studies including those in people with depression and psychosis have been unable to replicate these original findings despite demonstrating improved cardio-respiratory fitness in response to an aerobic exercise intervention (Rosenbaum, Lagopoulos, *et al.*, 2015).

Several psychological theories and models have been proposed to explain the affective benefits of exercise for people experiencing mental illness (Paluska and Schwenk, 2000). For example the distraction hypothesis postulates that exercise may function as a distraction from unpleasant or stressful stimuli (Paluska and Schwenk, 2000; Daley, 2002) such as an acute period of psychiatric hospitalisation. Other popular psychological hypotheses include Bandura's theory of self-efficacy (Bandura, 1982) and Sonstroem's psychological model for physical activity (Sonstroem and Morgan, 1989). Both of these theories suggest a positive reinforcement resulting from participation in exercise (either internal or external) that subsequently increase one's drive to further participate in increasingly more activity. For example improved ability may result in higher self-esteem, and confidence to perform a specific activity (Daley, 2002; Paluska and Schwenk, 2000). The social effects of exercise participation and exercise training have also been cited as a potential mechanism (Paluska and Schwenk, 2000; Richardson *et al.*, 2005; Faulkner and Biddle, 1999), as have improved quality of life (Forsberg *et al.*, 2010; Visceglia and Lewis, 2011) and improved sleep behaviour (Youngstedt and Charton, 2005).

Delivering pragmatic physical activity and sport-based interventions

The application of physical activity as a treatment for mental illness can be traced back to the 1960s and the creation of dedicated physiotherapy training programmes in mental health (Probst, 2012), and randomised controlled trials from 1975 (Clark *et al.*, 1975) to the present day. As allied health clinicians trained in exercise prescription, physiotherapists and exercise physiologists are commonly utilised in both research and clinical settings to design and deliver exercise interventions for people with mental illness

(Probst, 2012; Lederman *et al.*, 2016). The specialty of physiotherapy in mental health gained formal recognition within the World Confederation for Physical Therapy in 2011 with the formation of the International Organization of Physical Therapists working in Mental Health (IOPTMH) (Probst, 2012). In addition, a 2016-consensus statement published in the journal *Australasian Psychiatry* outlined the unique role of exercise physiologists regarding exercise prescription in the treatment and management of mental disorders. Data relating to the effectiveness of these interventions for specific mental health conditions such as bipolar disorder (Thomson *et al.*, 2015) and posttraumatic stress disorder (Rosenbaum, Vancampfort, *et al.*, 2015) is emerging, with conditions such as schizophrenia (Vancampfort *et al.*, 2012) depression (Schuch, Vancampfort, Richards, *et al.*, 2016) and eating disorders (Vancampfort *et al.*, 2014) receiving more research attention. Despite a small number of RCTs, and significant variance in the types of interventions, there is evidence that clinical exercise interventions offer added value. Evidence to date recommends that physical therapists and exercise physiologists address barriers, and structure programmes to be informative, motivational and allow for progression while recommending adequate undergraduate training in the recognition of symptoms of severe mental illness and the side-effects of medication (Vancampfort *et al.*, 2012).

In addition to the provision of clinically focused exercise interventions, there is increasing interest in the role of professional sporting clubs who may offer an alternative or adjunct to clinical services targeting people with mental illness. Such organisations may facilitate access to traditional mental health services, particularly among young people, for whom accessing such services may be highly stigmatised and therefore offer promise as an intervention model requiring further research (Curran *et al.*, 2016). Increasing examples of sport-based programmes targeting people experiencing mental illness exist within the academic literature. The *'Imagine Your Goals'* (IYG) programme (Henderson *et al.*, 2014) developed by Everton Football Club and adopted by the Premier League in 2011, aimed to improve social inclusion and wellbeing among people with mental illnesses, as well as facilitate stigma and discrimination reduction. The success of the programme resulted in IYG being delivered by 16 English Premier League football clubs. Results of a subsequent evaluation suggested significant improvements in personal and individual skills following completion of the intervention. Other examples of sport being used to improve mental health include sport for development programmes measuring targeting mental health outcomes (Richards *et al.*, 2014; Hamilton, Foster, and Richards, 2016). Despite a lack of high quality studies, investigation into the role of sport in improving mental health outcomes in developing and post-conflict settings is clearly warranted.

Encouraging participation in sport and exercise-related activities among people with mental illness may also help to address one of the major barriers to physical activity in this population, namely amotivation. While the general population experience considerable barriers to engaging in regular physical activity including amotivation, fatigue, stress and a lack of time, these barriers are compounded for people experiencing mental illness, with motivation in particular an important consideration (Firth *et al.*, 2016). Motivation is a fundamental component of behaviour change and plays an important role in achieving long-term lifestyle modification among people experiencing mental illness (Vancampfort, Moens, *et al.*, 2016; Vancampfort, De Hert, *et al.*, 2016; Vancampfort, Madou, *et al.*, 2015). The Self-Determination Theory (SDT) describes motivation on a continuum ranging from extrinsic (or external) to intrinsic (or autonomous) motivation (Prochaska and DiClemente, 1986). Autonomous motivation is facilitated by satisfaction of the three 'psychological needs'; autonomy (freedom and choice in decisions), competency (belief in ability to achieve desired outcomes) and social relatedness (behaviour reflects previous knowledge/experience) (Deci and Ryan, 2000). Exploring methods of addressing amotivation and strategies to increase motivation to engage in physical activity among people with mental illness, such as motivational interviewing and determining 'readiness to change' according to the Transtheoretical Model of Change, are essential when considering effective physical activity interventions.

Conclusion

The impact of physical activity on mood and mental wellbeing of both the general population, and those experiencing a mental illness is becoming increasingly clear. Promoting all aspects of physical activity including sport and exercise, as an integrated component of both promoting mental wellbeing among the healthy population, and as a component of treatment among people experiencing mental illness is warranted given the overwhelming body of evidence demonstrating a significant effect on both physical and mental health outcomes.

References

Alvarez-Jimenez, M., Gonzalez-Blanch, C., Crespo-Facorro, B., Hetrick, S., Rodriguez-Sanchez, J. M., Perez-Iglesias, R., and Luis, J. (2008). Antipsychotic-induced weight gain in chronic and first-episode psychotic disorders. *CNS Drugs*, 22(7), 547–562.

American Psychiatric Association (2000). *Diagnostic and Statistical Manual of Mental Disorders (DSM-IV-TR)* text rev. Washington, DC: APA.

American Psychiatric Association (2013). *DSM 5*. American Psychiatric Association.

Amerio, A., Stubbs, B., Odone, A., Tonna, M., Marchesi, C., and Ghaemi, S. N. (2015). The prevalence and predictors of comorbid bipolar disorder and obsessive–compulsive disorder: a systematic review and meta-analysis. *Journal of Affective Disorders*, 186, 99–109.

Bandura, A. (1982). Self-efficacy mechanism in human agency. *American Psychologist*, 37(2), 122.

Bremner, J. D., Narayan, M., Anderson, E. R., Staib, L. H., Miller, H. L., and Charney, D. S. (2000). Hippocampal volume reduction in major depression. *American Journal of Psychiatry*, 157(1), 115–118.

Bremner, J. D., Randall, P., Scott, T. M., Bronen, R. A., Seibyl, J. P., Southwick, S. M., Delaney, R. C., McCarthy, G., Charney, D. S., and Innis, R. B. (1995). MRI-based measurement of hippocampal volume in patients with combat-related posttraumatic stress disorder. *The American Journal of Psychiatry*, 152(7), 973.

Caspersen, C. J., Powell, K. E., and Christenson, G. M. (1985a). Physical activity, exercise, and physical fitness: definitions and distinctions for health-related research. *Public Health Rep*, 100(2), 126–31.

Caspersen, C. J., Powell, K. E., and Christenson, G. M. (1985b). Physical activity, exercise, and physical fitness: definitions and distinctions for health-related research. *Public Health Reports*, 100, 126–131.

Cevada, T., da Cruz Rubini, E., Lattari, E., and Blois, C. (2013). Neuroscience of exercise: from neurobiology mechanisms to mental health. *Neuropsychobiology*, 68(1), 1–14.

Clark, B. A., Wade, M. G., Massey, B. H., and Van Dyke, R. (1975). Response of institutionalized geriatric mental patients to a twelve-week program of regular physical activity. *Journal of Gerontology*, 30(5), 565–73.

Colberg, S. R., Sigal, R. J., Fernhall, B., Regensteiner, J. G., Blissmer, B. J., Rubin, R. R., Chasan-Taber, L., Albright, A. L., and Braun, B. (2010). Exercise and Type 2 Diabetes The American College of Sports Medicine and the American Diabetes Association: joint position statement. *Diabetes Care*, 33(12), e147–e167.

Correll, C. U., Manu, P., Olshanskiy, V., Napolitano, B., Kane, J. M., and Malhotra, A. K. (2009). Cardiometabolic risk of second-generation antipsychotic medications during first-time use in children and adolescents. *JAMA: The Journal of the American Medical Association*, 302(16), 1765–1773.

Curran, K., Rosenbaum, S., Parnell, D., Stubbs, B., Pringle, A., and Hargreaves, J. (2016). Tackling mental health: the role of professional football clubs. *Sport in Society*, 1–11. doi:10.1080/17430437.2016.1173910

Curtis, J., Newall, H. D., and Samaras, K. (2012). The heart of the matter: cardiometabolic care in youth with psychosis. *Early Intervention in Psychiatry*, 6(3), 347–53.

Curtis, J., Watkins, A., Rosenbaum, S., Teasdale, S., Kalucy, M., Samaras, K., and Ward, P. B. (2016). Evaluating an individualized lifestyle and life skills intervention to prevent antipsychotic-induced weight gain in first-episode psychosis. *Early Intervention in Psychiatry*, 10(3), 267–276.

Daley, A. J. (2002). Exercise therapy and mental health in clinical populations: is exercise therapy a worthwhile intervention? *Advances in Psychiatric Treatment*, 8(4), 262–270.

Daumit, G. L., Dickerson, F. B., Wang, N.-Y., Dalcin, A., Jerome, G. J., Anderson, C. A., Young, D. R., Frick, K. D., Yu, A., and Gennusa, J. V III. (2013). A behavioral weight-loss intervention in persons with serious mental illness. *New England Journal of Medicine*, 368(17), 1594–1602.

Davidson, J. R. (2010). Major depressive disorder treatment guidelines in America and Europe. *Journal of Clinical Psychiatry*, 71, e04.

De Hert, M., Dekker, J. M., Wood, D., Kahl, K. G., Holt, R. I. G., and Möller, H. J. (2009). Cardiovascular disease and diabetes in people with severe mental illness position statement from the European Psychiatric Association (EPA), supported by the European Association for the Study of Diabetes (EASD) and the European Society of Cardiology (ESC). *European Psychiatry*, 24(6), 412–424. doi:10.1016/j.eurpsy.2009.01.005

DeCarolis, N. A. and Eisch, A. J. (2010). Hippocampal neurogenesis as a target for the treatment of mental illness: a critical evaluation. *Neuropharmacology*, 58(6), 884–893.

Deci, E. L. and Ryan, R. M. (2000). The 'what' and 'why' of goal pursuits: human needs and the self-determination of behavior. *Psychological inquiry*, 11(4), 227–268.

Dishman, R. K. and O'Connor, P. J. (2009). Lessons in exercise neurobiology: the case of endorphins. *Mental Health and Physical Activity*, 2(1), 4–9.

Ekkekakis, P. (2015). Honey, I shrunk the pooled SMD! Guide to critical appraisal of systematic reviews and meta-analyses using the Cochrane review on exercise for depression as example. *Mental Health and Physical Activity*, 8, 21–36.

Erickson, K. I., Gildengers, A. G., and Butters, M. A. (2013). Physical activity and brain plasticity in late adulthood. *Dialogues in Clinical Neuroscience*, 15(1), 99.

Erickson, K. I., Voss, M. W., Prakash, R. S., Basak, C., Szabo, A., Chaddock, L., Kim, J. S., Heo, S., Alves, H., and White, S. M. (2011). Exercise training increases size of hippocampus and improves memory. *Proceedings of the National Academy of Sciences*, 108(7), 3017–3022.

Eyre, H. A. and Baune, B. T. (2013). Assessing for unique immunomodulatory and neuroplastic profiles of physical activity subtypes: a focus on psychiatric disorders. *Brain, Behavior, and Immunity*, 39, 42–55.

Faulkner, G. and Biddle, S. (1999). Exercise as an adjunct treatment for schizophrenia: a review of the literature. *Journal of Mental Health*, 8(5), 441–457.

Firth, J., Rosenbaum, S., Stubbs, B., Gorczynski, P., Yung, A. R., and Vancampfort, D. (2016). Motivating factors and barriers towards exercise in severe mental illness: a systematic review and meta-analysis. *Psychological Medicine*, 1–13.

Fornaro, M., Orsolini, L., Marini, S., De Berardis, D., Perna, G., Valchera, A., Gananca, L., Solmi, M., Veronese, N., and Stubbs, B. (2016). The prevalence and predictors of bipolar and borderline personality disorders comorbidity: systematic review and meta-analysis. *Journal of Affective Disorders*, 195, 105–118.

Forsberg, K. A., Bjorkman, T., Sandman, P. O., and Sandlund, M. (2010). Influence of a lifestyle intervention among persons with a psychiatric disability: a cluster randomised controlled trail on symptoms, quality of life and sense of coherence. *Journal of Clinical Nursing*, 19(11–12), 1519–28.

Gall, S. L., Sanderson, K., Smith, K. J., Patton, G., Dwyer, T., and Venn, A. (2016). Bi-directional associations between healthy lifestyles and mood disorders in young adults: the Childhood Determinants of Adult Health Study. *Psychological Medicine* FirstView, 1–14. doi:10.1017/S0033291716000738

Gretchen-Doorly, D., Kite, R. E., Subotnik, K. L., Detore, N. R., Ventura, J., Kurtz, A. S., and Nuechterlein, K. H. (2012). Cardiorespiratory endurance, muscular flexibility and strength in first-episode schizophrenia patients: use of a standardized fitness assessment. *Early Intervention in Psychiatry*, 6(2), 185–190.

Hallgren, M., Kraepelien, M., Öjehagen, A., Lindefors, N., Zeebari, Z., Kaldo, V., and Forsell, Y. (2015). Physical exercise and Internet-based cognitive behavioural therapy in the treatment of depression: randomised controlled trial. *The British Journal of Psychiatry*, 207, 227–234. doi:10.1192/bjp.bp.114.160101

Hamilton, A., Foster, C., and Richards, J. (2016). Systematic review of the mental health impacts of sport and physical activity programmes for adolescents in post-conflict settings. *Journal of Sport for Development*, 4(6), 44–59.

Henderson, C., O'Hara, S., Thornicroft, G., and Webber, M. (2014). Corporate social responsibility and mental health: The Premier League football Imagine Your Goals programme. *International Review of Psychiatry*, 26(4), 460–466.

Hordern, M. D., Dunstan, D. W., Prins, J. B., Baker, M. K., Fiatarone Singh, M. A., and Coombes, J. S. (2012). Exercise prescription for patients with type 2 diabetes and pre-diabetes: a position statement from Exercise and Sport Science Australia. *Journal of Science and Medicine in Sport*, 15(1), 25–31.

Hunter Institute of Mental Health (2015). *Prevention First: A Prevention and Promotion Framework for Mental Health*. Newcastle, Australia: Hunter Institute of Mental Health.

Lasser, K., Boyd, J. W., Woolhandler, S., Himmelstein, D. U., McCormick, D., and Bor, D. H. (2000). Smoking and mental illness: a population-based prevalence study. *JAMA*, 284(20), 2606–2610.

Lederman, O., Grainger, K., Stanton, R., Douglas, A., Gould, K., Perram, A., Baldeo, R., Fokas, T., Nauman, F., Semaan, A., Hewavasam, J., Pontin, L., and Rosenbaum, S. (2016). Consensus statement on the role of Accredited Exercise Physiologists within the treatment of mental disorders: a guide for mental health professionals. *Australasian Psychiatry*, 24(4), 347–351. doi:10.1177/1039856621 6632400

Luppino, F. S., de Wit, L. M., Bouvy, P. F., Stijnen, T., Cuijpers, P., Penninx, B. W., and Zitman, F. G. (2010). Overweight, obesity, and depression: a systematic review and meta-analysis of longitudinal studies. *Archives of general psychiatry*, 67(3), 220–229.

Mammen, G. and Faulkner, G. (2013). Physical activity and the prevention of depression: a systematic review of prospective studies. *American Journal of Preventive Medicine*, 45, 649–657.

McCrone, P. (2008). *Paying the Price: The Cost of Mental Health Care in England to 2026*. London: The King's Fund.

Morris, J. N., Heady, J. A., Raffle, P. A. B., Roberts, C. G., and Parks, J. W. (1953). Coronary heart-disease and physical activity of work. *Lancet*, 262(6796), 1111–1120.

Newcomer, J. W. and Hennekens, C. H. (2007). Severe mental illness and risk of cardiovascular disease. *JAMA: The Journal of the American Medical Association*, 298(15), 1794–1796. doi:10.1001/jama.298.15.1794

NICE (2009). Depression: the treatment and management of depression in adults (update) NICE clinical guideline 90.

Nocon, M., Hiemann, T., Muller-Riemenschneider, F., Thalau, F., Roll, S., and Willich, S. N. (2008). Association of physical activity with all-cause and cardio-vascular mortality: a systematic review and meta-analysis. *European Journal of Cardiovascular Prevention & Rehabilitation*, 15(3), 239–246.

Olfson, M., Gerhard, T., Huang, C., Crystal, S., and Stroup, T. (2015). Premature mortality among adults with schizophrenia in the United States. *JAMA Psychiatry*, 1–10. doi:10.1001/jamapsychiatry.2015.1737

Pajonk, F.-G., Wobrock, T., Gruber, O., Scherk, H., Berner, D., Kaizl, I., Kierer, A., Muller, S., Oest, M., Meyer, T., Backens, M., Schneider-Axmann, T., Thornton, A. E., Honer, W. G., and Falkai, P. (2010). Hippocampal plasticity in response to exercise in schizophrenia. *Archives of General Psychiatry*, 67(2), 133–143.

Paluska, S. A. and Schwenk, T. L. (2000). Physical activity and mental health. *Sports Medicine*, 29(3), 167–180.

Perez-Iglesias, R., Crespo-Facorro, B., Martinez-Garcia, O., Ramirez-Bonilla, M. L., Alvarez-Jimenez, M., Pelayo-Teran, J. M., Garcia-Unzueta, M. T., Amado, J. A., and Vazquez-Barquero, J. L. (2008). Weight gain induced by haloperidol, risperidone and olanzapine after 1 year: findings of a randomized clinical trial in a drug-naive population. *Schizophrenia Research*, 99(1), 13–22.

Probst, M. (2012). The International Organization of Physical Therapists working in Mental Health (IOPTMH). *Mental Health and Physical Activity*, 5(1), 20–21. doi:http://dx.doi.org/10.1016/j.mhpa.2012.04.003

Prochaska, J. O. and DiClemente, C. C. (1986). Toward a comprehensive model of change. In W. R. Miller and N. Heather (eds), *Treating Addictive Behaviors* (pp. 3–27). New York: Springer.

Rebar, A. L., Stanton, R., Geard, D., Short, C., Duncan, M. J., and Vandelanotte, C. (2015). A meta-meta-analysis of the effect of physical activity on depression and anxiety in non-clinical adult populations. *Health Psychology Review*, 9, 1–78. doi:10.1080/17437199.2015.1022901

Rethorst, C. D. and Trivedi, M. H. (2013). Evidence-based recommendations for the prescription of exercise for major depressive disorder. *Journal of Psychiatric Practice*, 19(3), 204–212.

Richards, J., Foster, C., Townsend, N., and Bauman, A. (2014). Physical fitness and mental health impact of a sport-for-development intervention in a post-conflict setting: randomised controlled trial nested within an observational study of adolescents in Gulu, Uganda. *BMC Public Health*, 14(1), 619.

Richardson, C. R., Faulkner, G., McDevitt, J., Skrinar, G. S., Hutchinson, D. S., and Piette, J. D. (2005). Integrating physical activity into mental health services for persons with serious mental illness. *Psychiatric Services*, 56(3), 324–31.

Rosenbaum, S., Lagopoulos, J., Curtis, J., Barry, B., Taylor, L., Watkins, A., and Ward, P. B. (2015). Aerobic exercise intervention in young people with schizophrenia spectrum disorders; improved fitness with no change in hippocampal volume. *Psychiatry Research: Neuroimaging*, 232, 200–201.

Rosenbaum, S., Tiedemann, A., Sherrington, C., Curtis, J., and Ward, P. B. (2014). Physical activity interventions for people with mental illness: a systematic review and meta-analysis. *J Clin Psychiatry*, 75(9), 964–74. doi:10.4088/JCP.13r08765

Rosenbaum, S., Vancampfort, D., Steel, Z., Newby, J. M., Ward, P. B., and Stubbs, B. (2015). Physical activity in the treatment of posttraumatic stress disorder: a systematic review and meta-analysis. *Psychiatry Res*, 230, 130–136.

Sauver, J. L., St., Warner, D. O., Yawn, B. P., Jacobson, D. J., McGree, M. E., Pankratz, J. J., Melton, L. J., Roger, V. L., Ebbert, J. O., and Rocca, W. A. (2013). Why patients visit their doctors: assessing the most prevalent conditions in a defined american population. *Mayo Clinic Proceedings*, 88(1), 56–67.

Schmitz, K. H., Courneya, K. S., Matthews, C., Demark-Wahnefried, W., Galva, D. A., Pinto, B. M., Irwin, M. L., Wolin, K. Y., Segal, R. J., Lucia, A., Schneider, C. M., von Gruenigen, V. E., and Schwartz, A. L. (2010). American College of

Sports Medicine roundtable on exercise guidelines for cancer survivors. *Medicine & Science in Sports & Exercise*, 10, 1409–1426.

Schuch, F. B., Vancampfort, D., Rosenbaum, S., Richards, J., Wards, P. B., and Stubbs, B. (2016). Exercise for depression in older adults: a meta-analysis of randomised trials adjusting for publication bias. *Revista Brasileira de Psiquiatria*, 1–8. doi:10.1590/1516-4446-2016-1915

Schuch, F. B., Deslandes, A. C., Stubbs, B., Gosmann, N. P., Silva, C. T., and Fleck, M. P. (2016). Neurobiological effects of exercise on major depressive disorder: a systematic review. *Neurosci Biobehav Rev*, 61, 1–11. doi:10.1016/j.neubiorev.2015.11.012

Schuch, F. B., Vancampfort, D., Richards, J., Rosenbaum, S., Ward, P. B., and Stubbs, B. (2016). Exercise as a treatment for depression: a meta-analysis adjusting for publication bias. *Journal of Psychiatric Research*, 77, 42–51. doi:10.1016/j.jpsychires.2016.02.023

Schuch, F. B., Vancampfort, D., Sui, X., Rosenbaum, S., Firth, J., Richards, J., Ward, P. B., and Stubbs, B. (2016). Are lower levels of cardiorespiratory fitness associated with incident depression? A systematic review of prospective cohort studies. *Preventive Medicine*, 93, 159–165.

Sonstroem, R. J. and Morgan, W. P. (1989). Exercise and self-esteem: rationale and model. *Medicine & Science in Sports & Exercise*, 21(3), 329–337.

Stanton, R. and Reaburn, P. (2014). Exercise and the treatment of depression: a review of the exercise program variables. *Journal of Science and Medicine in Sport*, 17(2), 177–182.

Steel, Z., Marnane, C., Iranpour, C., Chey, T., Jackson, J. W., Patel, V., and Silove, D. (2014). The global prevalence of common mental disorders: a systematic review and meta-analysis 1980–2013. *International Journal of Epidemiology*, 43(2), 476–493.

Stubbs, B., Rosenbaum, S., Vancampfort, D., Ward, P. B., and Schuch, F. B. (2016). Exercise improves cardiorespiratory fitness in people with depression: a meta-analysis of randomized control trials. *J Affect Disord*, 190, 249–53. doi:10.1016/j.jad.2015.10.010

Stubbs, B., Aluko, Y., Myint, P. K., and Smith, T. O. (2016). Prevalence of depressive symptoms and anxiety in osteoarthritis: a systematic review and meta-analysis. *Age and Ageing*, 45(2), 228–235.

Stubbs, B., Firth, J., Berry, A., Schuch, F. B., Rosenbaum, S., Gaughran, F., Veronesse, N., Williams, J., Craig, T., and Yung, A. R. (2016). How much physical activity do people with schizophrenia engage in? A systematic review, comparative meta-analysis and meta-regression. *Schizophrenia Research*, 171(1–3), 103–109.

Stubbs, B., Koyanagi, A., Hallgren, M., Firth, J., Richards, J., Schuch, F., Rosenbaum, S., Mugisha, J., Veronese, N., Lahti, J., and Vancampfort, D. (2016). Physical activity and anxiety: a perspective from the World Health Survey. *Journal of Affective Disorders*. doi:http://dx.doi.org/10.1016/j.jad.2016.10.028

Stubbs, B., Koyanagi, A., Thompson, T., Veronese, N., Carvalho, A. F., Solomi, M., Mugisha, J., Schofield, P., Cosco, T., and Wilson, N. (2016). The epidemiology of back pain and its relationship with depression, psychosis, anxiety, sleep disturbances, and stress sensitivity: data from 43 low-and middle-income countries. *General Hospital Psychiatry*, 43, 63–70.

Stubbs, B., Vancampfort, D., Rosenbaum, S., Ward, P. B., Richards, J., Ussher, M., and Schuch, F. B. (2015). Challenges establishing the efficacy of exercise as an antidepressant treatment: a systematic review and meta-analysis of control group responses in exercise randomised controlled trials. *Sports Medicine*, 46, 699–713. doi:10.1007/s40279-015-0441-5

Suetani, S., Whiteford, H. A., and McGrath, J. J. (2015). An Urgent Call to Address the Deadly Consequences of Serious Mental Disorders. *JAMA Psychiatry*, 1–2.

Teasdale, S. B., Ward, P. B., Rosenbaum, S., Samaras, K., and Stubbs, B. (2016). Solving a weighty problem: systematic review and meta-analysis of nutrition interventions in severe mental illness. *The British Journal of Psychiatry*, 209(5).

Thompson, P. D., Buchner, D., Piña, I. L., Balady, G. J., Williams, M. A., Marcus, B. H., Berra, K., Blair, S. N., Costa, F., and Franklin, B. (2003). Exercise and physical activity in the prevention and treatment of atherosclerotic cardiovascular disease a statement from the Council on Clinical Cardiology (Subcommittee on Exercise, Rehabilitation, and Prevention) and the Council on Nutrition, Physical Activity, and Metabolism (Subcommittee on Physical Activity). *Circulation*, 107(24), 3109–3116.

Thomson, D., Turner, A., Lauder, S., Gigler, M. E., Berk, L., Singh, A. B., Pasco, J., Berk, M., and Sylvia, L. (2015). A brief review of exercise, bipolar disorder and mechanistic pathways. *Name: Frontiers in Psychology*, 6, 147.

Vancampfort, D., Madou, T., Moens, H., De Backer, T., Vanhalst, P., Helon, C., Naert, P., Rosenbaum, S., Stubbs, B., and Probst, M. (2015). Could autonomous motivation hold the key to successfully implementing lifestyle changes in affective disorders? A multicentre cross sectional study. *Psychiatry Research*, 228(1), 100–106.

Vancampfort, D., Moens, H., Madou, T., De Backer, T., Vallons, V., Bruyninx, P., Vanheuverzwijn, S., Mota, C. T., Soundy, A., and Probst, M. (2016). Autonomous motivation is associated with the maintenance stage of behaviour change in people with affective disorders. *Psychiatry Research*, 240, 267–271. doi:10.1016/j. psychres.2016.04.005

Vancampfort, D., Rosenbaum, S., Ward, P. B., and Stubbs, B. (2015). Exercise improves cardiorespiratory fitness in people with schizophrenia: a systematic review and meta-analysis. *Schizophr Res*, 169(1–3), 453–457. doi:10.1016/j.schres. 2015.09.029

Vancampfort, D., Correll, C. U., Galling, B., Probst, M., De Hert, M., Ward, P. B., Rosenbaum, S., Gaughran, F., Lally, J., and Stubbs, B. (2016). Diabetes mellitus in people with schizophrenia, bipolar disorder and major depressive disorder: a systematic review and large scale meta-analysis. *World Psychiatry*, 15(2), 166–174.

Vancampfort, D., De Hert, M., Broderick, J., Lederman, O., Firth, J., Rosenbaum, S., and Probst, M. (2016). Is autonomous motivation the key to maintaining an active lifestyle in first-episode psychosis? *Early Intervention in Psychiatry*.

Vancampfort, D., Firth, J., Schuch, F., Rosenbaum, S., De Hert, M., Mugisha, J., Probst, M., and Stubbs, B. (2016). Physical activity and sedentary behavior in people with bipolar disorder: a systematic review and meta-analysis. *Journal of Affective Disorders*, 201, 145–152.

Vancampfort, D., Knapen, J., Probst, M., van Winkel, R., Deckx, S., Maurissen, K., Peuskens, J., and De Hert, M. (2010). Considering a frame of reference for physical activity research related to the cardiometabolic risk profile in schizophrenia. *Psychiatry Research*, 177(3), 271.

Vancampfort, D., Probst, M., Skjaerven, L. H., Catalán-Matamoros, D., Lundvik-Gyllensten, A., Gómez-Conesa, A., Ijntema, R., and De Hert, M. (2012). Systematic review of the benefits of physical therapy within a multidisciplinary care approach for people with schizophrenia. *Physical Therapy*, 92(1), 11–23.

Vancampfort, D., Probst, M., Sweers, K., Maurissen, K., Knapen, J., and De Hert, M. (2011). Relationships between obesity, functional exercise capacity, physical activity participation and physical self-perception in people with schizophrenia. *Acta Psychiatrica Scandinavica*, 123(6), 423–430.

Vancampfort, D., Rosenbaum, S., Schuch, F., Ward, P. B., Richards, J., Mugisha, J., Probst, M., and Stubbs, B. (2016). Cardiorespiratory fitness in severe mental illness: a systematic review and meta-analysis. *Sports Medicine*, 1–10.

Vancampfort, D., Vanderlinden, J., De Hert, M., Soundy, A., Adámkova, M., Skjaerven, L. H., Catalán-Matamoros, D., Lundvik Gyllensten, A., Gómez-Conesa, A., and Probst, M. (2014). A systematic review of physical therapy interventions for patients with anorexia and bulimia nervosa. *Disability and Rehabilitation*, 36(8), 628–634.

Visceglia, E. and Lewis, S. (2011). Yoga therapy as an adjunctive treatment for schizophrenia: a randomized, controlled pilot study. *Journal of Alternative and Complementary Medicine*, 17(7), 601–607.

Voss, M. W., Vivar, C., Kramer, A. F., and van Praag, H. (2013). Bridging animal and human models of exercise-induced brain plasticity. *Trends in Cognitive Sciences*, 17(10), 525–544.

Westerhof, G. J. and Keyes, C. L. (2010). Mental illness and mental health: the two continua model across the lifespan. *Journal of Adult Development*, 17(2), 110–119.

Whiteford, H. A., Degenhardt, L., Rehm, J., Baxter, A. J., Ferrari, A. J., Erskine, H. E., Charlson, F. J., Norman, R. E., Flaxman, A. D., and Johns, N. (2013). Global burden of disease attributable to mental and substance use disorders: findings from the Global Burden of Disease Study 2010. *The Lancet*, 382(9904), 1575–1586. doi:http://dx.doi.org/10.1016/ S0140-6736(13)61611-6

WHO (2010). Global recommendations on physical activity for health. *Geneva: World Health Organization*, 8–10.

Youngstedt, S. D. and Charton, J. (2005). Exercise and sleep. In G. E. J. Faulkner and A. H. Taylor (eds), *Exercise, Health and Mental Health: Emerging Relationships*. London: Routledge.

Zhai, L., Zhang, Y., and Zhang, D. (2015). Sedentary behaviour and the risk of depression: a meta-analysis. *British Journal of Sports Medicine*, 49, 705–709. doi:10.1136/bjsports-2014-093613

Chapter 8

Sport, physical activity and public health policy

Bob Snape and Kathryn Curran

Introduction

Declining levels of participation in physical activity has become of pan-European concern with over 65 per cent of the population estimated not to take sufficient physical exercise (Rind and Jones, 2014; Hunter *et al.*, 2015). Low levels of physical activity are associated with a number of health risks, notably obesity, coronary heart disease, diabetes and some forms of cancer (Booth, Roberts and Laye, 2012). The importance of physical activity to health is such that its promotion is a key strategic aim of the World Health Organization which has identified physical inactivity as the fourth leading risk factor for global mortality and published recommendations of appropriate levels of activity (World Health Organization, 2010). The potential benefits to public health of increased physical activity and the economic savings to be gained in avoiding the medical treatment of these sicknesses have been noted by politicians, and in the United Kingdom physical activity has become part of government policy in health, sport and education. There is, however, little cohesion between these disparate policy fields. Sport policy, by definition, prioritises sport but has, over recent decades, incorporated objectives related to increased participation in physical activity as a means of preventing obesity, dementia and mental health problems, and seems set to continue to do so (Department of Culture, Media and Sport, 2015; Sport England, 2015). The implication in much sport policy documentation however, is that physical activity is ancillary rather than integral to sport. Health policy, on the other hand, focuses primarily on physical activity in the wider and usually non-sporting sense, with clearly articulated guidelines for practice and explicit statements on its potential health benefits for both young and older people. Unlike sport policy, for which an established framework is available for implementation among governmental and non-profit sector organisations, there is, in the United Kingdom, very little state machinery for the active promotion and engagement of people in physical activity at the level of the local communities. The policy relationships between sport and physical activity are potentially problematic in several western countries, with the distinctions between them becoming blurred and displaying a lack of joined-up thinking between the health and sport sectors (Christiansen, Kahlmeier and Racioppi, 2014; Stuji and Stovkis, 2015). This chapter provides a critical evaluation of both sport and health policy. It draws from the historical development of these policy fields, offers evidence to explain governmental failure to increase participation to any significant degree and advocates the need for a new policy approach to physical activity for public health.

Sport policy and physical activity

With increasing concern about the health risks associated with physical inactivity, various governments have looked to sport as a means of delivering health policy. This reached its zenith in London's bid for the 2012 Olympic Games which would, it was proclaimed, create a more inclusive, more active community, leading to a fitter society and reducing health inequalities (London Organising Committee of the Olympic Games and the Paralympic Games Limited, n.d.). The perceived ability of sport to improve public health was highlighted by Sebastian Coe, the Prime Minister's Olympic Ambassador, as the legacy strand with the potential to have the biggest long-term impact for the nation's health as, inspired by the Olympics, people would seize opportunities to participate in sport or physical activity more often (Mayor of London, 2013). The importance attached to health benefits was embodied within the Games' legacy under a Sport and Healthy Living Strand and by 2013 it was claimed that this had led to 1.4 million more people playing sport once a week since the winning of the bid in 2005. As Coe noted, although as a sportsman physical activity came as second nature to him, for many it did not; however, as the report noted, £1 billion had been invested over 4 years into youth and community sport (Mayor of London, 2013). Who these new participants were or precisely what additional health benefits had been gained was not made clear. The optimistic claims of the Olympic bid were consistent with a trend towards grandiose governmental claims for sport since the turn of the last century, expressed not only in terms of improved health but through assumptions that spending on sport would automatically increase participation and improve public health, the evidence usually being clear in terms of funding and virtually non-existent in terms of health improvement (Department for Culture, Media and Sport, 2003; Sport England, 2004a). Even Tracey Crouch, newly appointed as minister for sport following the general election of 2015, accepted Sport England's culpability in stating that

> Government is in part to blame in that we have got a sport strategy that is very much out of date and that is the strategy that Sport England is

designed to deliver. I'm saying that I'm going to rip up that strategy and start again.

(Daily Telegraph, 2015)

As with other sport events legacies, policy objectives in health and physical activity were not achieved (Feng and Hong, 2013; Bauman, Bellew and Craig, 2015; Misener *et al.*, 2015; Ramchandani *et al.*, 2015).

Like other fields of social policy, that of sport suffers from political short-termism and unanticipated events. Both have been instrumental in determining the policy relationships between sport, physical activity and health in England since the early twentieth century. Within the last decade the change from a New Labour to a Conservative administration and the winning of the bid to host the London 2012 Olympics have arguably been detrimental to policy on physical activity. In 2004, Sport England's strategic plan was innovatory in adopting the Council of Europe's definition of sport as:

> '*all forms of physical activity which, through casual participation, aim at expressing or improving physical fitness and mental well-being, forming social relationships or obtaining results in competition at all levels.*'

(Sport England, 2004a)

Its principal strategic aim was to increase participation in sport and physical activity across all social classes and age groups in ways which reflected people's motivations, their lifestyle preferences and the realities of their day-to-day life circumstances. Based upon empirical evidence and cited research (Sport England, 2004b) it laid out a long-term plan to implement the government's strategic aims for physical activity and sport as identified in *Game Plan* which set a target of 70 per cent of the population in England being reasonably active (30 minutes of moderate exercise five times per week) active by 2020 (Great Britain Prime Minister's Strategy Unit, 2002). While stating a commitment to support elite sport and international success in sporting competitions, the emphasis of the strategy was firmly on increasing participation in sport, as understood in the above definition, among all age groups and to create a 'culture of lifelong participation'. Importantly, it also laid out the details of a well-funded machinery of sport and physical activity provision and development with clearly stated roles for local authorities and third sector organisations.

In 2008, approximately 4 years into its projected 20-year life, this strategy was replaced by a new one which radically curtailed the emphasis on physical activity in noting that Sport England's future role would be to focus exclusively on sport and to maintain a clear distinction from the physical activity agenda which would be driven by other departments, including the

Department of Health and Department of Transport (Sport England, 2008). The rationale for this abrupt change of policy direction was the winning of the bid to host the London 2012 Olympics which had provided a focal point for developing a 'world-leading community sport system' and 'maximising English sporting success in all its forms' (Sport England, 2008). A key plank of the new strategy was an emphasis on the role of the sports club with its coaching, facilities and competitions. By working with National Governing Bodies of sport, Sport England's intent was now to place the sports club at the centre of a bid to increase participation, not in physical activity but specifically in sport.

The replacement of the New Labour government in 2010 by a Conservative–Liberal Democrat coalition was followed by severe funding cuts to the local authorities and voluntary organisations that had formed the structure through which participation in sport and physical activity was to have been increased (Parnell, Millward and Spracklen, 2015). These included the abolition of the School Sports Partnerships (Phillpots, 2013; Phillpots and Grix, 2014) which had created links between education institutions and sports clubs to encourage extra-curricular sport among young people, which was particularly controversial as the principal strategic policy aim in sport became to fulfil the 2012 Olympic legacy aim by creating a community sport legacy through increased participation in sport at a grassroots level. Local authorities could bid for funding but the principal agents of change remained the National Governing Bodies which were required to set out details of their plans to increase participation in their respective sport as a condition of funding (Sport England, 2012). The latest Sport England strategy, *A Sporting Future*, published in 2015, returns to a definition of sport which accommodates physical activity but depends largely for its implementation upon local authorities which are simultaneously undergoing far-reaching and substantial reductions in government funding and the strategy does in fact concede that there will be limited public funding available to support it (Sport England, 2015; Parnell, Cope, Bailey and Widdop, 2016). In a final gesture that many would see as beyond ironic, the government announced in its spring budget of 2016 a tax on sugary drinks to raise money to support school sports that would be limited and only available through competitive bidding.

There is, accordingly, little evidence to indicate that sport policy has had or indeed will have for the foreseeable future, any significant effect on increasing participation in physical activity. Indeed, in June 2015 Sport England reported that the number of people playing sport at least once a week had declined by 222,000 in 6 months, while the percentage of those on the lowest incomes participating in sport was at the lowest level since records began in 2005–2006 (Gibson, 2015). While the explanations of sport's failure to increase participation in physical activity and thus contribute to public health are complex, there is a body of evidence to suggest why this became the case. It would seem incontrovertible that recurrent shifts in policy objectives outlined above, together with fundamental changes in public and voluntary were in part responsible; however other contributory factors have been identified. Research on the 2010 Olympic Games in Vancouver, for example, found that a flawed policy design meant that interventions and programmes to increase participation did not address the identified target populations, and this resonates with the generality of policy in England which exhibited very little indication of how inactive adult groups might be engaged (Derom and Lee, 2014). Policy failure can thus be partly attributed a failure to distinguish clearly between the general community and specific demographic groups in which addressing physical non-activity was a health priority (Bauman, Murphy and Matsudo, 2013). Furthermore, international research has shown that the support of sports clubs in sport-based health-enhancing physical activity cannot be assumed; their primary aim is not to provide physical activity opportunities for non-active people and their involvement has to be negotiated (Ooms, Veenhof, Schipper-van Veldhoven and de Bakker, 2015).

Implementing policy on physical activity

The World Health Organization's Global Strategy on Diet, Physical Activity and Health (World Health Organization, 2004) highlighted the importance of scaling up national policy action to address physical activity (Milton and Bauman, 2015). The UK governments' Department of Health and Department of Transport have attempted to address this call through physical activity and public health policy. Policy on physical activity is produced primarily by the Department of Health, where it is integrated within a more general set of policies around healthy living and lifestyle which include diet, reduced alcohol consumption and smoking cessation (Department of Health, 2011). However, while policy on physical activity is clear on recommended guidelines, there remains a lack of awareness of these (Hunter *et al.*, 2014). The National Health Service publishes advice on the benefits of physical activity but does not provide facilities. Engagement and active support for physical activity for health thus fall within the remit of public health. In theory this should not be problematic, but instability and change in health policy has militated against a long-term holistic approach through which health needs in terms of physical activity can be addressed through the provision of facilities and, more importantly, the active engagement and support of those who would most benefit from participation in physical activity (Big Lottery Fund, 2007).

From policy to practice

The dysfunctional nature of policy on physical activity in terms of health is reflected in practice. However it is also the case that excellent practice exists despite this. We move now to a brief analysis of health-orientated intervention in physical activity. Interventions have increasingly been informed by the collection of data specific to non-sport-based physical activity is important to public health. In 1991 the Department of Health established the Health Survey for England (HSE), an annual interview-based survey which examines the changes in the health and physical activity behaviours of people living in England. The data collected by the HSE provides vital information which is used by central government (e.g. the Department of Health and Public Health England) and local government for a range of purposes, including: monitoring changes in health and lifestyles, monitoring the prevalence of specific health conditions, planning services, policy development, monitoring and evaluating policy.

In October 2005, Sport England launched a population telephone-based survey capturing data on the sport and recreation behaviours of people in England. The Active People Survey (APS) tracks the number of people playing sport on an annual basis (with the exception of 2006–2007). The findings of the APS have become a valuable resource for the sports sector. The APS provides information on the national picture of who is taking part in sport and how are they participating. This can be broken down by demographics such as age, gender ethnicity, as well as by the way people are engaging (i.e., participation by volunteering or club membership). The APS also provides a local picture of who plays sport and how. This includes information about different geographical areas, including local authorities, county sport partnerships and regions; a picture of the participation by individual sports (i.e., who plays sport and how they participate). Rowe (2009) argues that the APS has given Sport England, the Department for Culture, Media and Sport and the 354 local authorities the strongest data for sport policy making in the world. It cannot, however, be argued to provide reliable data on non-sporting physical activity. Both the HSE and the APS have been criticised for their methodological limitations; given the self-report nature of both surveillance systems, the validity of answers offered has often come under question. Furthermore, while both are repeated measure surveys, they are not longitudinal on an individual level and changes in the questions related to physical activity have led to criticism due to inability to differentiate the true changes in physical activity (Stamatakis, Ekelund and Wareham, 2007; Milton and Bauman, 2015). The adequacy of Sport England's Active People Survey as a tool for evidence-based practice is thus deeply flawed and ultimately costly in terms of the misdistribution of funding.

Exercise referral

A common physical activity intervention in health policy is the Exercise Referral Scheme programme which is widely adopted within public health as a means of encouraging physical activity and normally offered as a non-clinical corollary of public health provision. However as a means of policy implementation these schemes have a chequered reputation and quantitative evaluations have revealed concerns about their effectiveness in enabling significant weight loss (Williams, Hendry, France and Lewis, 2007; Forster, Veerman, Barendregt and Vos, 2011; Pavey, Anokye, Taylor, Trueman, Moxham et al., 2011). A principal challenge to their effectiveness has been the non-retention of clients (Dudgill, Graham, and McNair, 2005; Morton, Biddle and Beauchamp, 2008). Programmes designed with strategies to improve adherence may thus have a higher chance of improving retention and gaining better overall results (Taylor, Doust and Webborn, 1998). Research also suggests that clients who self-refer may already be internally motivated and therefore more likely to adhere (Moore, Moore and Murphy, 2011). The short-term nature of exercise referral schemes has also been identified as a potential flaw, even where the scheme itself has shown short-term behavioural change (Moore, Moore and Murphy, 2011). Nevertheless, despite their potential shortcomings, exercise referral schemes remain one of the few means of encouraging physically inactive people, especially those suffering from conditions which make participation difficult, to participate in exercise.

There are, however, examples of successful engagement in physical activity within public health provision, notably through the Healthy Living Centres established under the New Labour government which integrated expertise in public health with community engagement interventions. Where promoted to non-active and unhealthy people as part of a change of lifestyle for health, participation in physical activity can be increased (Big Lottery Fund, 2007). A recent programme delivered by Blackburn with Darwen Healthy Living, a third sector organisation established from the former Blackburn with Darwen Healthy Living Centre. 'Aspire' was a programme established in 2012 to help acutely obese people to lose weight through dietary change and participation in physical activity. The design of the programme placed an emphasis on personal support and the client group was thus restricted to twelve adults. The 6-month duration of the programme was adopted to allow sufficient time to enable clients to adopt changed patterns of eating and levels of physical activity and to achieve significant loss of weight.

Aspire was a self-referral scheme and its success corresponds with evidence to suggest that successful long-term participation in daily movement requires the matching of exercise regimens and physical activity outlets to individual preferences and environmental conditions; in other words, referral schemes must take into account the personal and social circumstances of their clients (Deusinger, 2012). The programme was successful in retaining clients over a 6-month programme with high levels of personal support and individual counselling which were considered crucial to its success. The emphatic view of its clients that the social networks formed through participation would lead to a longer-term maintenance of the levels of physical activity achieved during the scheme also reflect evidence that policy sustainability is aided where long-term social networks of support are formed which enable post-scheme continuity (Moore, Moore and Murphy, 2011).

It appears that public health is better equipped that the sport sector in understanding the relationships between physical activity and, being undistracted by competition and elite performance, is better able to engage physically inactive communities. However, Sport England (associated with the Department for Culture, Media and Sport) has also adopted a role in addressing physical activity participation. For example, Sport England's 2012–2017 Youth and Community Sport Strategy (Sport England, 2012) outlined how £1billion of National Lottery and Exchequer funding was to be invested in Youth and Community Sport over a 5-year period. As part of this strategy, Sport England invested £17 million to create 153 full-time sports development professionals – College Sport Makers – within the Further Education sector. The College Sport Makers' role was to link colleges with community sport and physical activity opportunities in order to widen the offer for students; raising student participation in sport and physical activity and reducing the drop out of young people from sport and physical activity, especially at 16 and 18 years old.

In 2014 Sport England launched 'This Girl Can', a national campaign which aimed to empower and encourage more women to participate in sport and physical activity. Females are under-represented in sport and physical activity participation (Deaner, Balish and Lombardo, 2016). The campaign aimed to tell the 'real' story of women who play sport and participate in physical activity by using images that challenge the idealised and stylised images that are commonly portrayed in the media. The campaign website provided guidance for women to find an approach of being physically active in a way which is best suited to their activity preferences and abilities. Detail on the opportunities and facilities available to them were also accessible via the campaign website.

However, it remains unclear what impact (if any) the College Sport Makers have had on participation and drop out, and indeed, if their roles will be re-funded or not. Similarly, to date, little evidence exists on the effectiveness of the 'This Girl Can' campaign, however through a 'snapshot' investigation, Sport England report that 2.8 million 14–40-year-old women say they have done some, or more, activity as a result of our campaign (Sport England, 2016). Furthermore, neither of these policies dis-aggregates physical activity from sport. This is problematic as sport and physical activity represent inherently different behaviours and distinctive challenges, incentives and meanings for every potential recruit (McKenna et al., 2016).

Community asset approach

In 2013 public health spending was transferred from Primary Care Trusts to Clinical Commissioning Groups. This shift has been argued to be one of the most significant extensions of local government powers and duties in a generation (Carrier and Kendall, 2015). Alongside this change in power however, local government and health services faced significant cuts to funding. As a result, there has been an increasing dependence on community-centred approaches for health promotion and reduction in health inequalities (Public Health England, 2015). Utilising everyday environments as a 'setting' to promote health and reduce health inequalities has therefore become increasingly popular with public health agencies in the United Kingdom. This approach has been used by public health agencies to deliver interventions aimed at tackling lifestyle issues such as smoking, poor diets and physical inactivity and has been adopted in schools, workplaces, hospitals and prisons (Department of Health, 2010).

Over the last 10 years, professional sport clubs have been subject to pressure from the government, national governing bodies and stakeholders towards the need for a greater contribution to public health (Drygas *et al.*, 2013). As a result, a growing number of Community Trusts (financially independent charities that harness the brand of the sports club) have been established within professional sports clubs (Parnell, Curran and Philpott, 2016). Through their Community Trusts, professional sports stadia have been utilised as settings to deliver on a range of public health outcomes including physical inactivity, smoking cessation, poor diets, cancer awareness and mental health (Curran, Drust and Richardson, 2014). This has been achieved by engaging fans, visitors, workforces and local communities in interventions delivered both on match days and non-match days (Curran, Bingham, Richardson and Parnell, 2014; Hunt *et al.*, 2014; Parnell and Pringle, 2016).

Evidence suggests that professional sports clubs provide an acceptable setting and communications vehicle to positively influence health-related behaviour of their communities (Curran *et al.*, 2015). However, sports stadia based health interventions have often been coordinated and delivered by community sport coaches and practitioners who are not qualified or trained in public health and have therefore received criticism related to their delivery and evaluation (Parnell, Stratton, Drust and Richardson, 2013). If public health outcomes are going to continue to be delivered through professional sport clubs (and/or other community settings), appropriate resources and training (human and financial) for effective delivery and evaluation are essential (Curran *et al.*, 2016).

Public education

National Campaigns are considered a cornerstone of physical activity and public health promotion (Milton and Bauman, 2015). Mass media campaigns are widely used to expose high proportions of large populations to public health messages through routine uses of existing media, such as television, radio and newspapers (Wakefield, Loken, and Hornik, 2010). Change4Life was launched in January 2009 by the Department of Health. Change4Life is a national campaign that uses a range of communication channels (i.e., TV advertisement, newspaper advertising, posters, website and social media) to encourage people to 'Eat well, Move more and Live longer'. Initially, the government invested £75 million to run the campaign for a 3-year period. In its first year Change4Life reported to have been a success with more than 1 million mothers claiming to have made changes to their children's behaviours as a direct result of the campaign (Department of Health, 2011). However, during the same period, the Health Survey for England reported a reduction in the proportion of children aged 5–15 years meeting the physical activity guidelines (Health Survey for England, 2012). This, therefore, questioned the success of the campaign on improving children's physical activity behaviours.

Following the change in government in England in 2010, the financial support for campaign from the government was reduced to £10.9 million per annum and the commercial sector and local authorities were called upon to 'fill the gap'. As a result, numerous harmful food organisations from the commercial sector partnered with the campaign including Pepsico and Britvic, producers of sugary drinks including Pepsi, Tango and 7-UP (Milton and Bauman, 2015) an outcome which now seems ironic given the governments Spring 2016 Budget which outlined a tax sugary drinks tax to improve health and tackle obesity.

In 2016 Public Health England launched 'One You' – a national campaign to help adults aged 40–60 years to avoid future diseases caused by modern day life. It has been suggested that everyday habits and behaviours such as poor diets, drinking more alcohol than is recommended, smoking, physical inactivity and sedentary behaviour, are responsible for around 40 per cent of all deaths in England and cost the NHS more than £11 billion a year (Weiler and Stamatakis, 2010). The One You campaign provides resources, support and encouragement which aim to encourage middle aged adults to take control of their health. Through public relations, social media and a 60-second TV advertisement, One You encourages adults to reappraise their lifestyle choices. Evidence suggests that public health mass media campaigns such as 'Change4Life' and 'One You' can produce positive changes and/or prevent negative changes in health-related behaviours across large populations. However it is argued that continued investment in these campaigns is essential in order to achieve adequate population exposure to media messages (Wakefield, Loken and Hornik, 2010). Many lifestyle changes are generational in implementation – the 50-year campaign on the dangers of cigarette smoking, for example – and sustained promotion rather than short-term and under-funded policy would seem essential to progress.

Conclusions

This chapter has argued that the policy framework for sport, physical activity and health in the United Kingdom is dysfunctional, with insufficient strategic coordination between the public sectors of sport and health. The claim that the London 2012 Olympics would lead to wider participation in physical activity has not been fulfilled and the evidence presented here lends support to previous research which has suggested the policy disaggregation of sport and physical activity (Bauman, Murphy and Matsudo, 2013). The question remains, however, of where responsibility for policy on physical activity might reside. Sport England, as we have argued, has proved unable to deliver a measurable national physical activity policy nor to become integrated with public health. It remains for the government to determine how to raise the status of physical activity policy and, equally importantly, construct a public health-based framework in which it can be promoted and sustained at a national level for the whole population.

References

Bauman, A., Bellew, B., and Craig, C. (2015). Did the 2000 Sydney Olympics increase physical activity among adult Australians? *British Journal of Sports Medicine*, 49(4), 243–247.

Bauman, A., Murphy, N., and Matsudo, V. (2013). Is a population-level physical activity legacy of the London 2012 Olympics likely? *Journal of Physical Activity and Health*, 10(1), 1–3.

Big Lottery Fund (2007). *Learning from Healthy Living Centres: The Changing Policy Context*. Available at: www.biglotteryfund.org.uk/er_eval_hlc_final_eval_summ.pdf (last accessed 28/04/16).

Booth, F., Roberts, C., and Laye, M. (2012). Lack of exercise is a major cause of chronic diseases. *Comprehensive Biology*, 2(2), 1143–1211.

Carrier, J. and Kendall, I. (2015). *Health and the National Health Service*. London: Routledge.

Christiansen, N., Kahlmeier, S., and Racioppi, F. (2014). Sport promotion policies in the European Union: results of a contents analysis. *Scandinavian Journal of Medicine and Science in Sports*, 24(2), 428–439.

Curran, K., Bingham, D. D., Richardson, D., and Parnell, D. (2014). Ethnographic engagement from within a Football in the Community programme at an English Premier League football club. *Soccer and Society*, 15(6), 934–950.

Curran, K., Drust, B., and Richardson, D. (2014). 'I just want to watch the match!' A practitioner's reflective account of men's health themed match day events at an English Premier League Football Club. *Soccer and Society*, 15(6), 919–933.

Curran, K., Drust, B., Murphy, R., Pringle, A., and Richardson. D. (2015). The challenge and impact of engaging hard-to-reach populations in regular physical activity and health behaviours: an examination of an English Premier League 'Football in the Community' men's health programme. *Public Health*, 135, 14–22.

Curran, K., Rosenbaum, S., Parnell, D., Stubbs, B., Pringle, A., and Hargreaves, J. (2016). Tackling mental health: the role of professional football clubs. *Sport in Society*. doi:10.1080/17430437.2016.1173910

Daily Telegraph (11 June 2015) Sports Minister blasts failing strategy. Available at http://telegraph.co.uk/sport/olympics/swimming/11669313/Sports-Minister-blasts-failing-strategy-as-participation-numbers-drop-and-swimming-shows-the-worst-decline.html (last accessed 28/04/16).

Deaner, R., Balish, S., and Lombardo, M. (2016). Sex differences in sports interest and motivation: an evolutionary perspective. *Evolutionary Behavioral Sciences*, 10(2), 73.

Department of Culture, Media and Sport (2003). *Olympics. Government Response to 'A London Olympic Bid for 2012'* (HC 268) Report of the Culture, Media and Sport Select Committee Session 2002–2003. http://webarchive.nationalarchives.gov.uk/+/http:/www.culture.gov.uk/NR/rdonlyres/ezywinmeztnlirwxkpb66tfbonr6oxcgqheqxhcknvenozjjapyzwl4vxkty3yx73wtjkbktbfbovpzm2pcnapa4s4c/OlympicsCm5867.pdf

Department of Culture, Media and Sport (2015). *A New Strategy for Sport: Consultation Paper*. Available at https://gov.uk/government/consultations/a-new-strategy-for-sport-consultation (last accessed 28/04//16).

Department of Health (2010). Healthy lives, healthy people. Available at https://gov.uk/government/uploads/system/uploads/attachment_data/file/216096/dh_127424.pdf (last accessed 28/04/16).

Department of Health (2011). Change4Life three year social marketing strategy. Available at https://gov.uk/government/uploads/system/uploads/attachment_data/file/213719/dh_130488.pdf (last accessed 28/04/16).

Department of Health (2011). Start active, stay active. Available at https://gov.uk/government/publications/start-active-stay-active-a-report-on-physical-activity-from-the-four-home-countries-chief-medical-officers (last accessed 28/04/16).

Derom, I. and Lee, D. (2014). Vancouver and the 2010 Olympic games: physical activity for all? *Journal of Physical Activity and Health*, 11, 1556–1564.

Deusinger, S. (2012). Exercise intervention for management of obesity. *Pediatric Blood and Cancer*, 58, 135–139.

Drygas, W., Ruszkowska, J., Philpott, M., Björkström, O., Parker, M., Ireland, R., and Tenconi, M. (2013). Good practices and health policy analysis in european sports stadia: results from the 'Healthy Stadia' project. *Health Promotion International*, 28(2), 157–65.

Dudgill, L., Graham, R., and McNair, F. (2005). Exercise referral: the public health panacea for physical activity promotion? A critical perspective of exercise referral schemes; their development and evaluation. *Ergonomics*, 48, 1390–1410.

Feng, J. and Hong, F. (2013). The legacy: did the Beijing olympic games have a long-term impact on grassroots sport participation in Chinese townships? *International Journal of the History of Sport*, 30(4), 407–422.

Forster, M., Veerman, J., Barendregt, J., and Vos, T. (2011). Cost-effectiveness of diet and exercise interventions to reduce overweight and obesity. *International Journal of Obesity*, 35(8), 1071–1078.

Gibson, O. (2015). How the Olympics failed. *Guardian Sports Section*. Available at https://theguardian.com/sport/blog/2015/jul/05/olympic-legacy-failure-london-2012-message-millstone (last accessed 28/04/16).

Great Britain. Prime Minister's Strategy Unit (2002). *Game Plan, a strategy for delivering Government's sport and physical activity objectives*. London: Cabinet Office.

Hunt, K., Wyke, S., Gray, C., Anderson, A., Brady, A., Bunn, C., Donnan, P., *et al.* (2014). A gender-sensitised weight loss and healthy living programme for overweight and obese men delivered by scottish premier league football clubs (Ffit): a pragmatic randomised controlled trial. *The Lancet*, 383(9924), 1211–21.

Hunter, R., Boeri, M., Tully, M., Donnelly, P., and Kee, F. (2015). Addressing inequalities in physical activity participation: implications for public health policy and practice. *Preventive Medicine*, 72, 64–9.

Hunter, R., Tully, M., Donnelly, P., Stevenson, M., and Kee, F. (2014). Knowledge of UK physical activity guidelines: implications for better targeted health promotion. *Preventive Medicine*, 65, 33–9.

London Organising Committee of the Olympic Games and the Paralympic Games Ltd (n.d.). *Olympic Games Official Report*, Volume One. Available at https://publications.parliament.uk/pa/cm200607/cmselect/cmcumeds/69/69ii.pdf (last accessed 28/04/16).

Mayor of London (2013). *Inspired by 2012: The Legacy from the London 2012 Olympic and Paralympic Games. A Joint UK Government and Mayor of London Report*, Cabinet Office. Available at https://gov.uk/government/uploads/system/uploads/attachment_data/file/224148/2901179_OlympicLegacy_acc.pdf (last accessed 28/04/16).

McKenna, J., Quarmby, T., Kime, N., Parnell, D., and Zwolinsky, S. (2016). Lessons from the field for working with Healthy Stadia: physical activity practitioners reflect on sport. *Sport in Society*. doi:10.1080/17430437.2016.1173913.

Milton, K. and Bauman, A. (2015). A critical analysis of the cycles of physical activity policy in England. *International Journal of Behavioural Nutrition and Physical Activity*, 12(1), 8.

Misener, L., Taks, M., Chalip, L., and Green, C. (2015). The elusive 'trickle-down effect' of sport events: assumptions and missed opportunities. *Managing Leisure*, 20(2), 135–147.

Moore, G., Moore, L., and Murphy, S. (2011). Facilitating adherence to physical activity: exercise professionals' experiences of the National Exercise Referral Scheme in Wales: a qualitative study. *BMC Public Health*, 11, 935.

Morton, K., Biddle, S., and Beauchamp, S. (2008). Changes in self-determination during an exercise referral scheme. *Public Health*, 11, 1257–1260.

NHS Digital (2012). *Health Survey for England (2012)*. Available at http://hscic.gov.uk/catalogue/PUB13218 (last accessed 28/04/16).

Ooms, L., Veenhof, C., Schipper-van Veldhove, N., and de Bakker, D. (2015). Sporting programs for inactive population groups: factors influencing implementation in the organized sports setting. *BMC Sports Science, Medicine and Rehabilitation*, 7(1), 1.

Parnell, D. and Pringle, A. (2016). Football and health improvement: an emerging field. *Soccer and Society*, 17(2), 171–174.

Parnell, D., Cope, E., Bailey, R., and Widdop, P. (2016). Sport policy and English primary physical education: the role of professional football clubs in outsourcing. *Sport in Society*, doi:10.1080/17430437.2016.1173911

Parnell, D., Curran, K., and Philpott, M. (2016). Healthy stadia: an insight from policy to practice. *Sport in Society*, doi:10.1080/17430437.2016.1173914

Parnell, D., Millward, P., and Spracklen, K. (2015). Sport and austerity in the UK: an insight into Liverpool 2014. *Journal of Policy Research in Tourism, Leisure and Events*, 7(2), 200–203.

Parnell, D., Stratton, G., Drust, B., and Richardson, D. (2013). Football in the community schemes: exploring the effectiveness of an intervention in promoting healthful behaviour change. *Soccer and Society*, 14, 35–51.

Pavey, T., Anokye, N., Taylor, A., Trueman, P., and Moxham, T. (2011). The clinical effectiveness and cost-effectiveness of exercise referral schemes: a systematic review and economic evaluation. *FalseHealth Technology Assessment*, 15, 1–254.

Phillpots, L. (2013) An analysis of the policy process for physical education and school sport: the rise and demise of school sport partnerships. *International Journal of Sports Policy*, 5(2), 193–211.

Phillpots, L. and Grix, J. (2014). New governance and physical education and school sport policy: a case study of school to club links. *Physical Education and Sport Pedagogy*, 19(1), 76–96.

Public Health England (2015). A guide to community centred approaches for health and wellbeing. Available at https://gov.uk/government/uploads/system/uploads/attachment_data/file/402889/A_guide_to_community-centred_approaches_for_health_and_wellbeing__briefi___.pdf (last accessed 28/04/16).

Ramchandani, G., Davies, L., Coleman, R., Shibli, S., and Bingham, J. (2015). Limited or lasting legacy? The effect of non-mega sport event attendance on participation. *European Sport Management Quarterly*, 15(1), 93–111.

Rind, E. and Jones, A. (2014). Declining physical activity and the socio-cultural context of the geography of industrial restructuring: a novel conceptual framework. *Journal of Physical Activity and Health*, 11, 683–692.

Rowe, N. (2009). The active people survey: a catalyst for transforming evidence-based sport policy in England. *International Journal of Sport Policy*, 1(1), 89–98.

Sport England (2004a). *The Framework for Sport in England*. London: Sport England.

Sport England (2004b). *Driving Up Participation: the Challenge for Sport*. London: Sport England.

Sport England (2008). *Sport England Strategy 2008–2011*. London: Sport England.

Sport England (2012). *A Sporting Habit for Life: 2012–2017*. London: Sport England.

Sport England (2012). Youth and community sport strategy. Available at: www.sportengland.org/media/3662/a-sporting-habit-for-life-a4-1.pdf. (last accessed 28/04/16).

Sport England (2015). *Sporting Future. A New Strategy for an Active Nation*. Available at https://gov.uk/government/publications/sporting-future-a-new-strategy-for-an-active-nation (last accessed 28/04/16).

Sport England (2016). 'This Girl Can' delivers results one year on. Available at https://sportengland.org/news-and-features/news/2016/january/12/thisgirlcanbirthday/ (last accessed 28/04/16).

Stamatakis, E., Ekelund, U., and Wareham, N. (2007). Temporal trends in physical activity in England: the Health Survey for England 1991 to 2004. *Preventive Medicine*, 45(6), 416–423.

Stuji, M. and Stovkis, R. (2015). Sport, health and the genesis of a physical activity policy in the Netherlands. *International Journal of Sport Policy*, 7(2), 217–233.

Taylor, A., Doust, J., and Webborn, N. (1998). Randomised controlled trial to examine the effects of a GP exercise referral programme in Hailsham, East Sussex, on modifiable coronary heart disease risk factors. *Journal of Epidemiology and Community Health*, 52(9), 595–601.

Wakefield, M., Loken, B., and Hornik, R. (2010). Use of mass media campaigns to change health behaviour. *The Lancet*, 376(9748), 1261–1271.

Weiler, R. and Stamatakis, E. (2010). Physical activity in the UK: a unique crossroad? *British journal of sports medicine*, 44(13), 912–914.

Williams, N., Hendry, M., France, B., and Lewis, R. (2007). Effectiveness of exercise-referral schemes to promote physical activity in adults: systematic review. *The British Journal of General Practice: the Journal of the Royal College of General Practitioners*, 57(545), 979–986

World Health Organization (2004). Global strategy on diet, physical activity and health. Available at http://who.int/dietphysicalactivity/strategy/eb11344/strategy_english_web.pdf (last accessed 28/04/16).

World Health Organization (2010). *Global Recommendations on Physical Activity for Health*. Available at http://apps.who.int/iris/bitstream/10665/44399/1/978924 1599979_eng.pdf (last accessed 28/04/16).

Chapter 9

Sport and health
The unique challenge of elite sport

Shawn M. Arent and Alan J. Walker

Introduction

Citius, Altius, Fortius. Three simple Latin words that form the Olympic motto. They also capture the mindset of high-level and elite athletes as they push the limits of their physical abilities. The pursuit of excellence embodies much of what we value about sport. At the highest levels of competition, athletes almost take on a mythical quality for the fans. We see them through a skewed lens of invincibility and superhuman capabilities. We watch as records fall, trophies and medals are won, and our concepts of human limits are challenged. Elite athletes do not train to be average. They train to demonstrate superiority. They train to be better. In many ways, this is exactly what they accomplish. Whether it is enhanced aerobic capacity, greater speed, or higher power output, athletes at the highest levels certainly possess traits that exemplify a healthy ideal. There is inherent value in sport socially, culturally, financially, psychologically, and, certainly, physically (Bailey *et al.*, 2012, 2013). Despite these benefits, however, elite sport may present a very different reality for some. In their efforts to run faster, jump higher and become stronger, athletes are often willing to jeopardise their health and wellbeing in order to accomplish their goals or reap an economic windfall. The inherent mindset of an elite athlete is not necessarily one of optimising health. Instead, a 'win-at-all-costs' mentality may drive their decisions and actions in order to take advantage of a narrowing window of opportunity.

Elite athletes may be willing to resort to doping and PEDs, play through injury and pain, cause permanent damage to their bodies and risk damage to their brains through concussion in order to win. They may even risk addiction to painkillers and recreational drugs to dull the pain and allow them to continue to play. Efforts to become lighter in order to run faster or in the pursuit of a perceived 'ideal' image for some sports may result in the development of eating disorders or disordered eating. This chapter will examine this conundrum and explore the impacts of participation in elite sport on long-term health. For the purpose of this chapter, 'elite athletes' will be defined as those competing at the highest level of national championships, international championships, or at the professional level (de Hon, Kuipers, and van Bottenburg, 2015). Given the differences in organisational constructs between countries, we will also at times consider Division I college athletes in the United States as part of the relevant discussion as they are often competing at a similar level to second and third division professional teams in other regions.

Doping and PEDs

Ben Johnson. Lance Armstrong. Alberto Contador. Diego Maradona. Barry Bonds. Marion Jones. Maria Sharapova. The list could go on and on, but these are just some of the more high-profile examples of athletes who have been suspended or had careers ended because of doping or PEDs. Given the media attention these cases received, along with the news just before the 2016 Rio Olympics about the discovery of the prolific and systematic doping programme that Russia had been employing, it would clearly seem that there is a PED epidemic. However, being able to substantiate this is difficult. If doping control tests are any indication, it would seem that there are no more than 1–2 per cent of elite athletes doping (de Hon, *et al.*, 2015). On the other hand, some anecdotal evidence or research utilising questionnaires and often asking athletes about their own use as well as their opinion on overall use has rates as high as 70 to 90 per cent (de Hon *et al.*, 2015; Berning, Adams, and Stamford, 2004). Both of these methods of assessment are clearly not without their problems, however. The first method (positive tests) assumes – incorrectly – that all doping athletes are caught. The second method (questionnaires and anecdotes) assumes that athletes are being honest. Given the illegality and potential repercussions of PED use, it is highly unlikely that this is the case, even if the assessment is anonymous. Additionally, asking about *competitors'* use will likely result in questions being answered driven by ego and perception that he or she could not possibly be beaten unless everyone else was on drugs. A potentially more accurate method utilising randomised response technique would put use rates somewhere between 14 and 39 per cent (de Hon, *et al.*, 2015), though even this may not fully capture the dynamics and prevalence of doping.

The increasing concern about PED use in sports would make it seem as if this is somehow a new or novel issue. In fact, Greek athletes in the third century BC were said to have ingested stimulants in order to improve their performance (Verroken, 2001). Attempts to gain a competitive edge through substances believed to be ergogenic have a long history in elite sport. Though we will touch on some of the ethical issues surrounding PEDs and doping, that is not the main purpose of this chapter. Instead, the question that needs to be asked is whether or not athletes are putting themselves at risk from a health standpoint rather than just from a legal one. In truth, many of the ethical arguments against drug use in sport are not entirely useful for understanding this behaviour. For example, the notion of doping being inconsistent with the idea of 'fair play' is problematic because athletes do not train to provide a *fair* playing field, they train so that they have an advantage.

The search for an advantage, or even to level the playing field if they believe everyone else is doping, is certainly a driving motivation behind PED use (Donahue *et al.*, 2006). The potential health risks and moral dilemma take a distant secondary consideration to winning and financial gain (Verroken, 2001). Admittedly, once the decision is made to violate doping rules and cross a perceived ethical boundary, any health risks may seem quite minor. Much of what is reported regarding these risks primarily pertains to andro-genic-anabolic steroids (AAS). Some of the potential adverse effects include hypertension, myocardial hypertrophy, gynecomastia, acne, testicular atrophy, increased triglycerides, reduced HDL, polycythemia and decreased endogenous testosterone production (Pärssinen and Seppälä, 2002; van Amsterdam, Opperhuizen, and Hartgens, 2010). In females, increased clitoral enlargement, hirsutism, and irregular menstruation are also possible (van Amsterdam *et al.*, 2010). It is important to note that many of these side-effects tend to acute in nature and reverse upon cessation of AAS, unless use was excessively prolonged. The impacts on cardiovascular disease cannot be readily dismissed and may ultimately represent the more severe and chronic of the problems with AAS use (van Amsterdam *et al.*, 2010). It has also been suggested that AAS may lead to enhanced aggression, depression, psychotic episodes, and mood swings (Pärssinen and Seppälä, 2002). Though these effects should not be trivialised, the evidence (particularly for their likelihood) is not particularly strong. Likewise, attempts have been made to link AAS use to enhanced risk for certain cancers (namely hepatic and prostate), but most of this is based on very few cases where other etiology cannot be discounted.

In an athlete's perspective, it would be easy to see how some of these health risks could be easily dismissed. Furthermore, the medical community did itself a disservice by contesting the fact that AAS enhance performance for so many years (Hoberman, 2002). By doing so, a great degree of credibility was lost and athletes are less likely to believe the stated medical risks of taking the drugs. Furthermore, elite athletes may have an air of invincibility and a 'superman' complex (Arent and Lutz, 2015). In other words, though these side-effects may occur in others, they will not occur in *them*. For every negative example a physician may provide about damage from AAS use, the athlete can think of dozens and dozens more where no long-term effects were seen. Coupled with the intense desire to win, this makes the discussion about health risks quite complicated. While more rigorous testing program-mes may serve as an enhanced deterrent, simultaneous inclusion of better prevention programmes would seem warranted. There is also an incredible irony at work here in that the health risks of AAS could be greatly diminished if used under medical supervision (Berning, Adams, and Stamfords, 2004). However, the current rule structure and doping policies make this extremely unlikely.

When evaluating the health risks associated with AAS use in particular, one must keep in mind that they are rarely used in isolation. Ancillary drugs taken to combat side effects, stimulants taken to enhance endurance or focus, benzodiazepines taken to counteract the effects of the stimulants so the athlete can sleep, and diuretics used to try to mask AAS or to try to make weight for weight-category sports can all be much more dangerous than the AAS themselves. Additionally, there is increasing use of peptides such as growth hormone (GH) and insulin-like growth factor 1 (IGF-1), which have been implicated in cell proliferation and tumour growth, particularly in supraphysiological doses (Tentori and Graziani, 2007). Blood doping and recombinant human erythropoietin (rhEPO) have the potential to not only benefit endurance by increasing oxygen carrying capacity and cardiac output, but can also increase blood viscosity (Corrigan, 2002). In turn, this can increase coagulation and increase demand on the cardio-vascular system, particularly when losing plasma volume due to sweating. All of the above represent significant health risks to which the elite athlete may expose themselves in an effort to gain a competitive edge.

When it comes to drugs in sport, there is a remarkable hypocrisy on the part of the governing bodies, organisations, and physicians as it relates to the health of the athlete. While doping and PEDs are demonised and placed in a position that all but eliminates the likelihood of medical super-vision, painkillers and NSAIDs are dispensed at an alarming rate (Tscholl and Dvorak, 2012). For example, during the 2010 World Cup, physician-reported use of medication by athletes during the tournament was over 70 per cent, while 60 per cent took painkillers at least once (Tscholl and Dvorak, 2012). Almost 40 per cent of the players took a painkiller *before every game*. This included 32 injections into a joint and 20 intramuscular injections of glucocorticoids. Use of these drugs are not without risk, including impaired healing of both tendon and bone (Vuolteenaho, Moilanen, and Moilanen, 2008; Virchenko, Skoglund, and Aspenberg, 2004), impaired muscular regeneration (Mikkelsen *et al.*, 2009), and systemic problems (Alaranta *et al.*, 2006), including kidney and heart failure. This was all done in an attempt to keep athletes on the field, yet the use of AAS in recovery and repair from injury is considered 'cheating'. Furthermore, there are numerous stories of athletes who have succumbed to addiction to painkillers and recreational drugs in an attempt to deal with the pain inflicted by their sport. Whether elite athletes are looking for a competitive edge, to prolong a career, to keep up with other doping athletes, or simply to remain on the field because it is expected that they play through injury, it is clear that drug use in sport, and not just PED use in sport, presents a notable challenge to their health and wellbeing.

Playing through pain and injury

One of the greatest compliments you can give an athlete is to refer to them as 'tough'. For most, this suggests that they will play through anything and put their bodies on the line. The term carries with it a perceived connotation of valour. Elite athletes, particularly in team and combat sports, are often seen as modern-day gladiators willing to sacrifice and display 'courage' to achieve the elusive victory.

Playing through pain and injury is often perceived as part of the elite sport culture (Roderick, Waddington, and Parker, 2000) and is not only accepted, but it is often celebrated. Athletes may even be elevated to 'legend' status after displaying extreme tolerance for pain and seemingly overcoming something that should sideline the mere mortal. There was Kerri Strug, US gymnast, successfully landing the gold-medal winning vault on a badly damaged ankle in the 1996 Olympics only to have to be carried to the medal podium by her coach. Ronnie Lott, Hall of Fame safety of the San Francisco 49ers of the NFL, had part of his mangled finger amputated during a game so that he could go back in and play. Franz Beckenbauer, vaunted German footballer, finished the semifinal of the 1970 World Cup with a broken collarbone. Bert Trautmann, goalkeeper for Manchester City, finished a match in 1956 after injuring his neck making a save. It was later discovered that he had played the match with several dislocated vertebrae and two *broken* ones. Finally, Hall of Fame NFL Quarterback Brett Favre set the record for consecutive starts with 297 (a record unlikely to ever be broken) despite various injuries including a broken thumb, concussions, and a badly damaged ankle that required surgery in the off-season. He later revealed that he had become addicted to the painkillers that had allowed him to continue to play. These have become the standards by which we now judge 'toughness' of an athlete.

Pain and injury are related, yet conceptually distinct terms. Injury is more objective and can be considered a structural breakdown that can affect physical function (Howe, 2001). Pain, on the other hand, is a subjective experience as it may not 'mean' the same thing to everyone. It is an indicator of injury and is generally considered unpleasant both physically and emotionally (Howe, 2001). Furthermore, pain can be classified as either acute or chronic. Of the two, the persistent effects of chronic pain tend to place emotional, social, physical, and even financial stress on the athlete (Howe, 2001). Injuries are an inherent part of athletics. Rather than this being a silent issue, they are often celebrated as a badge of honour in a way and freely discussed – unless the injury could cost the player a spot on the field, in which case they are readily covered up by the athletes (Howe, 2001). There are certainly risks involved, particularly in contact sports. Even in non-contact sports like cycling, crashes and overuse injuries are a reality. A study in English professional football (Hawkins and Fuller, 1998) found that there was over a 12 per cent chance of a player needing medical treatment during the course of a match, with almost 15 per cent of those incidents resulting in the player missing at least one subsequent match. Furthermore, over 800 players out of approximately 2,600 in English and Welsh football clubs incurred an injury during a game that required them to miss at least one additional game (Hawkins and Fuller, 1998). This says nothing, however, of the number who were injured but still managed to play through the pain. As noted previously, over half of the athletes in the 2010 World Cup took painkillers to get through a match (Tscholl and Dvorak, 2012).

The 'culture of risk' in sport (Nixon, 1993) has created an environment where athletes are now often expected to play when hurt or injured. The pressure to do so comes from management, other players, and even themselves (Roderick et al., 2000). At the professional level, the pressure to win and the monetary stakes have exceeded the concern for the athletes' health and wellbeing (Howe, 2001). From a management and ownership standpoint, a highly paid athlete sitting on the bench due to injury is a poor investment and often seen as worthless (Murphy and Waddington, 2007). It is not uncommon for players who are injured to be isolated and 'inconvenienced' so that they try to return to play more quickly (Nelson, 1996; Roderick et al., 2000). This includes things like reducing their normal benefits, making them come in extremely early for treatment, having them stay late for treatment so that they are purposely caught in rush-hour traffic, and not letting them participate in organisational activities with their 'healthy' teammates (Roderick et al., 2000). Ironically, these actions place even more stress on the athlete and could easily contribute to a delayed healing and recovery process. However, at that level of competition, the reality is that being healed and being ready to return to play are not necessarily the same thing.

Just as elite athletes see playing through pain and injury as 'part of the job' (Hammond, Lilley, Pope et al., 2014), team physicians and physiotherapists have adopted this same perspective (Roderick et al., 2000; Murphy and Waddington, 2007). Rather than focusing on getting players back to a state of health and cured following an injury, the medical staff is tasked with getting them back on the field as expeditiously as possible. This is an important distinction. As noted by Roderick et al. (2000), at least one physiotherapist acknowledged that patients in his private practice receive better treatment than the players, despite access to better equipment and treatment options. By playing through an injury, the athlete may never have the chance to fully and properly heal. This may be one critical reason that previous injury drastically increases the risk of future injury (Hägglund, Waldén, and Ekstrand, 2006). In a prospective study of 12 elite male Swedish football teams, researchers found that injury in the previous season produced an increased hazard ratio of 2.7 for injuries in the subsequent season (Hägglund et al., 2006). Hamstring, groin, and knee injuries were particularly problematic, with players being two to three times more likely to suffer the same injury in the next season (Hägglund *et al.*, 2006). Additionally, playing while in pain or injured may cause the athlete to compensate with modified biomechanics, thereby making them more susceptible to other injuries.

Many athletes believe that the sports medicine team works in the best interests of the owners and organisation rather than in the players' best interests, which has led to an increasing distrust of the motives and qualifications of team doctors and medical staff (Murphy and Waddington, 2007). This further complicates the pain/injury continuum because athletes may be reluctant to disclose certain things to the medical staff, which impacts treatment options and decision making processes. Additionally, there may be information withheld from the athletes which would be important for them to consider when making *their* decision about whether to play through pain or injury (Murphy and Waddington, 2007; Roderick *et al.*, 2000).

Pain plays an important role in the diagnosis and treatment of an injury, and, in some cases may be a more revealing indicator of damage than diagnostic equipment (Howe, 2001). One of the challenges this presents is that different athletes may have very different pain thresholds, thereby impacting the degree of attention and treatment by sports medicine. A second challenge is the over-reliance on painkillers, NSAIDs and cortisone injections to reduce the pain to a level that allows the athlete to play. This approach to 'medical management' places the athlete at greater risk because of the minimisation of cues and signals crucial to injury assessment. There is a remarkable irony in the fact that painkillers are systematically used to allow return to play while likely still injured, yet AAS or GH use is banned despite the fact that these substances can help an athlete actually heal faster. Further compounding the issue is the notion that coaches and managers often decide whether an athlete is fit to play, thus overstepping their expertise and overriding sports medicine staff recommendations (Murphy and Waddington, 2007). This is both a cultural and ethical problem and represents a failure on the part of the physicians and trainers.

Regardless of the potentially enabling behaviour by the medical staff, athletes have a variety of reasons for being willing to play through pain and injury. To say that this is due solely to the culture of sport or the pressure from ownership or sponsors would be an oversimplification. For example, older athletes nearing the end of their career, those with contract bonuses in sight, or those in the last year of their contracts may be more likely to play while injured (Hammond *et al.*, 2014). The perceived importance of upcoming games is also a factor, with athletes reporting more pressure to play in critical matches, particularly when team size is limited and there may not be enough other players to cover their absence (Hammond *et al.*, 2014). They may also be so tightly tied to the identity of 'elite athlete' that they will do whatever they can to remain on the field and part of the team in order to maintain their self-identity (Hammond *et al.*, 2014). Despite claims of the 'masculinity' of this behaviour, it does not appear that there are major gender differences in the willingness to play while hurt (Malcom, 2006; Young, 1997; Weinberg, Vernau, and Horn, 2013), though there may be differences in the degree to which males and females are willing to tolerate pain and injury (Nixon, 1996). In order to justify sacrificing their bodies, as well as their brains when it comes to concussion, elite athletes minimise or even deny the long-term consequences of playing through injury (Weinberg et al., 2013; Walk, 1997). Unfortunately, there are consequences.

There are both psychological and physiological repercussions stemming from injury, and trying to play through the injury may only serve to compound these. After an injury, elite athletes tend to have increased anger, greater symptoms of depression, and suicidal thoughts (Quackenbush and Crossman, 1994; Baum, 2005). The challenge that an injury can present to their identity as an athlete, particularly if it threatens their career, can have a major emotional impact (O'Connell and Manschreck, 2012). When they feel isolated following an injury or with an increased pressure to return from teammates, coaches and management, athletes often resort to alcohol or drug use to cope unless they have developed alternative strategies or have a well-established social support network (O'Connell and Manschreck, 2012). The impacts of playing hurt are felt long after the athlete leaves the field. Data collected on former professional football players from England indicated that 49 per cent of the 284 surveyed athletes had developed osteoarthritis, a rate five times greater than that of age-matched males in the general population (Roderick et al., 2000). Additionally, 15 per cent of the former players were considered disabled. In a large-scale survey of 1,617 retired American football players from the NFL, approximately 15 per cent reported moderate-to-severe depression and almost 50 per cent reported that they commonly or very commonly experienced pain (Schwenk, Gorenflo, Dopp, and Hipple, 2007). Pain and depression were associated with difficulties with sleep, relationships, exercise and fitness (Schwenk et al., 2007). Though the authors speculate that the decrease in functional ability limited exercise and fitness, which then contributed to the depression (Schwenk et al., 2007), it is also possible that the mental health problems were at least in part due to head trauma suffered while playing. Given the increasing understanding of concussion and long-term consequences, particularly in the NFL, this possibility cannot be dismissed and represents an area of elite athlete health that deserves its own consideration beyond simply playing with pain and injury.

Concussions

'Concussions are part of the profession, an occupational risk' was a conclusion reached in 1994 by the NFL's Mild Traumatic Brain Injury (MTBI) Committee. Since then, the premature deaths of Mike Webster, Justin Strzelczyk, Terry Long, Andre Waters, Dave Duersons, Ray Easterling,

Junior Seau, and college player Owen Thomas have all been a resounding acknowledgement of that apparent 'occupational risk'. The ground-breaking work of Dr. Bennet Omalu sent shockwaves through the sports world when he published findings linking repeated blows to the head to a condition he called Chronic Traumatic Encephalopathy (CTE), signs of which were found in the brain tissues of the aforementioned American football players (Omalu et al., 2005). These players exhibited outward signs of confusion and Alzheimer's like symptoms that have since been attributed to CTE developed while playing (Omalu et al., 2005). Since Dr. Omalu's findings were first published, public opinion and overall understanding of the dangers of repeated head blows and concussions has, fortunately, changed. Unfortunately, the willingness of athletes to play through injury coupled with the individuality of MTBI severity and duration of effects make concussions one of the more dangerous threat to elite athlete health.

Sports medicine professionals began to track the number of concussions sustained during play beginning in the early 1990s. Since that time, there has been a steady increase in the number of recorded concussions (Harmon et al., 2013). This leads to an important question, though: are more concussions actually occurring or are we just better at detecting them? There are several possible explanations for these findings, including bigger and stronger athletes, new techniques in detecting the signs and symptoms, and willingness to self-report. Concussions are non-discriminatory; they affect athletes in any sport and occur in both men and women. In fact, in a study of 25 NCAA sports, there was at least one concussion during the competitive season for every sport with the exception of men's cross-country (Zuckerman et al., 2015). Furthermore, the rate of having a repeat concussion was 13.9 per cent in men and 10.3 per cent in women (Zuckerman et al., 2015). While concussions are possible in any sport, there is an increased likelihood in sports with a higher degree of contact such as ice hockey, rugby, American football, boxing and football (soccer). For example, rugby players experience 8–17.1 concussion per 1,000 playing hours (Gardner et al., 2015). Due to the competitive nature and 'gladiator' mentality of elite athletes, many concussive episodes likely go unreported and undiagnosed which could underestimate the true frequency. In order to better protect athletes, medical and coaching staffs need to prevent them from 'pushing through' head injuries, as well as to ensure that they are fully recovered before returning to play.

With the increase in media attention, return to play policies has been scrutinised and questions have arisen regarding the risk for subsequent injuries. Current procedures for a suspected MTBI include on-field diagnosis of somatic, cognitive, or neuropsychiatric signs and symptoms and may result in immediate removal from competition (Okonkwo, Tempel, and Maroon, 2014). The initial assessment is then followed by a series of cognition, balance, and memory tests which are compared to previously established baselines. The outcomes of the various evaluations should inform the medical decision on overall readiness for return to play (Cancelliere *et al.*, 2014; Okonkwo *et al.*, 2014). Premature clearance and return may exacerbate the inherent risk for future injury tied to concussive episodes. Current research shows that players who sustain concussions are 2.2 times more likely to incur a subsequent injury in the following year (Nordström, Nordström, and Ekstrand, 2014), perhaps suggesting that concussed athletes may become more susceptible to future injuries, the mechanism for which remains unknown (Nordström *et al.*, 2014; Okonkwo *et al.*, 2014). It is worth noting that players who sustain concussions have also been found to be more 'injury-prone' even prior to the concussion (Burman, Lysholm, Shahim, Malm, and Tegner, 2016). This could simply be due to their style of play or positional demands leading to an increased relative risk of injury (Burman *et al.*, 2016). Though not all research is in agreement, it has also been shown that most athletes recover and return to baseline testing values within days to a few weeks depending on the severity and number of previous concussions (Cancelliere *et al.*, 2014). Unfortunately, as noted previously, these on- and off-field decisions can be greatly influenced by the coaches, team owners, players, and the game situation/schedule (Roderick *et al.*, 2000). These external pressures along with an internal drive to play and win can put athletes at an increased risk and severely compromise health.

Despite the recently increased attention to the implications of repeated blows to the head and concussions, the effects have actually been recognised and documented for almost a century. An article titled 'Punch Drunk' was published in 1928 which described an altered conscious state in professional boxers after repeated blows to the head (Martland, 1928). These immediate effects of severe concussions are readily recognisable and can include confusion, amnesia, headaches, loss of consciousness, and deficits in orientation and concentration (McCrea, Kelly, Randolph, Cisler, and Berger, 2002). However, it is common for these to go undetected in more mild cases, especially if the athlete attempts to hide symptoms in order to continue to play (McCrea *et al.*, 2002). As an athlete sustains more concussions, the effects increase in severity and duration (Harmon *et al.*, 2013). Recent research in this area has resulted in athletes being put through a more stringent evaluation. This also serves to discourage them to play through these symptoms and almost serves as a means to protect them from themselves.

Knowledge of the long-term effects of sustaining multiple concussions is very limited at this point and primarily focuses on the cognitive function and mental health of retired American football players. Twenty years post-injury, former athletes who sustained multiple concussions show cognitive changes that demonstrate deficits in fine dexterity, visuomotor reaction time and intracortical inhibition when compared to non-concussion controls (Pearce *et al.*, 2014). Three decades after retirement, cognitive and motor system alterations consisting of decreases in episodic memory, deteriorated frontal lobe functions, motor execution slowness and early onset of Alzheimer's were evident (De Beaumont *et al.*, 2009). Even in younger athletes at 9 months post-concussion, decreased motor control functions and increased intercortical inhibition have been seen. Particularly alarming, the severity of these changes increased with the number of concussions experienced (De Beaumont *et al.*, 2011). The delayed impact on motor execution slowness, which was observed only in the older population, suggests a possible aging effect (De Beaumont *et al.*, 2011). This may indicate that certain effects of concussions can go undetected until later in life. Along with alterations in cognitive function and memory impairment, there is evidence suggesting a link between multiple concussions and dementia-related symptoms as well as an increased risk of depression (Guskiewicz *et al.*, 2005; Guskiewicz *et al.*, 2007). The silent threat of cognitive dysfunction, depression and possibly even early onset of diseases such as Alzheimer's and dementia poses serious threats to elite athletes later in life (Guskiewicz *et al.*, 2005; Guskiewicz *et al.*, 2007; De Beaumont *et al.*, 2009).

While the short-term consequences of concussions can be concerning for athletes, it is the fear of long-term disability and even early death that has caused some players to decide to retire early. Until recently, there was no direct evidence linking concussions and long-term effects. This resulted in speculation and doubt about the likelihood, plausibility, or severity of such an association. The autopsy reports published by Omalu *et al.* in 2005 and 2006 were the first to show direct evidence of physical changes in brain matter due to repeated concussions. These case studies exhibited a change in brain matter and morphology and evidence of CTE resulting from multiple concussions and repeated sub-concussive blows to the head (Omalu *et al.*, 2005, 2006). In the latter part of their lives, the individuals Omalu autopsied exhibited altered mood and conscious state. They experienced feelings of, among other things, being dazed, mental fogginess, headaches, and vertigo, as well as early onset of Alzheimer's symptoms (Omalu *et al.*, 2005, 2006). Though this was the first diagnosis of CTE, earlier research had found significantly altered brain matter and structure in former professional boxers (Corsellis, Bruton, and Freeman-Browne, 1973). The findings of Omalu *et al.* have resulted in the development of new ways to detect these alterations in the brain prior to autopsy. Recently, new positron emission tomography (PET) scan techniques revealed significant morphological changes and atrophy of brain matter in former NFL players showing signs of CTE (Coughlin *et al.*, 2015). The new and developing techniques to identify the life altering effects of CTE are a step in the right direction for elite athletes, but the deadly consequences of multiple concussions remain.

Concussions may be hidden depending on their severity and may go unreported by players in big game situations for fear of looking weak or losing their spot. Coaches may also encourage them to 'shake it off' and continue to play because they do not appreciate the ramifications or consequences of even a minor concussion. This misunderstanding by both players and coaches alike can exacerbate the problem and result in effects that the players will have to endure for the rest of their lives. Athletes who play contact sports are certainly the most prone to experience concussions, though all athletes need to be aware of the dangers they pose. Through better monitoring, assessment, and continued research this condition can be better understood and improve the quality of life in elite athletes who have suffered from multiple concussions. Sports organisations have begun to implement rules that they hope will lessen the incidence of concussion and reduce the exposure to sub-concussive contact. Equipment manufacturers are trying to find ways to improve the safety of headgear and helmets to lessen the forces that may lead to cortical damage. Despite the medical, technical, technological, rule, and safety advances, concussions remain a very serious threat to the health of athletes and must not be considered an acceptable 'occupational risk' any longer.

Eating disorders

When milliseconds separate immortalised Olympic champions from forgotten fourth place finishers, elite athletes must often have everything perfect in order to win. The pursuit of perfection is often accompanied by an elevated need for a sense of control and harsh self-assessment. Coaches and significant others may further exacerbate these feelings, which can lead to even greater pressure and feelings of inadequacy. While this may have positive outcomes in some cases, for example increasing adherence to a training programme or diet, it can also lead athletes to go to extremes to compensate. For some this may mean use of PEDs or playing through pain and injury. For others it may be reflected in their rigid adherence to body image or bodyweight standards or expectations. In the latter case, disordered eating (DE) or diagnosed eating disorders (ED) may be the end result. This may seem counterintuitive to the general public and leave them wondering how athletes performing at such a high level could suffer from these issues. However, the pressure to win, perform, and maintain peak physical appearance leads to an increased rate of both DE and ED in elite athletes (Bratland-Sanda and Sundgot-Borgen, 2013; Joy, Kussman, and Nattiv, 2016; Sundgot-Borgen and Torstveit, 2004).

Athletes from a number of different sports can be affected by DE, which is an alteration in the diet ranging from restrictive eating to abnormal eating habits including over consumption of food (McArdle, Meade, and Moore, 2015; Sundgot-Borgen and Torstveit, 2004). If DE tendencies are left untreated they can progress to ED, which include such conditions as anorexia nervosa and bulimia nervosa (Lebrun and Rumball, 2002). Due to the mentality of elite athletes and the complexity of their unique lifestyle, Sundgot-Brogen *et al.* coined the term 'anorexia athletica' to describe athletes with symptoms of EDs who do not meet the full criteria of anorexia nervosa and bulimia nervosa (Lebrun and Rumball, 2002; Sundgot-Borgen and Torstveit, 2004). This specific condition for athletes is recognised due to the prevalence of DE in this population.

Elite athletes have been found to be at a greater risk of DE and ED when compared to the general population, with varying degrees of severity depending on the specific sporting population being evaluated (Bratland-Sanda and Sundgot-Borgen, 2013; Joy et al., 2015; Sundgot-Borgen and Torstveit, 2004). Individuals who participate in weight class sports, aesthetic sports, and sports that put an emphasis on leanness are all at elevated risk, and females tend to be at greater risk than males (Joy et al., 2015). The incidence of ED in aesthetic sports has been found to range between 18 and 42 per cent across both male and female athletes, and has been shown to be as high as 24 per cent in endurance sports (Joy et al., 2015; Sundgot-Borgen and Torstveit, 2004). This is in comparison to 5 per cent in non-athlete counterparts (Sundgot-Borgen and Torstveit, 2004). Those effected by an ED are also at an increased risk for depression, anxiety, obsessive compulsive disorder, and substance abuse (Joy et al., 2015). Along with possible nutrient/vitamin deficiencies due to dietary imbalances and reduced energy availability, ED can have detrimental effects on both performance and health (Joy et al., 2015).

Unique to female athletes is the added element of the Female Athlete Triad, which results from the combined effects of DE, amenorrhea and osteoporosis (Lebrun and Rumball, 2002). DE is often the precipitating factor of development of the Female Athlete Triad. The decrease in energy availability due to DE may be the underlying cause of menstrual disturbances, which are further exacerbated by excessive energy expenditure through training. The state of chronic energy deficiency can lead to hormonal dysregulation and amenorrhea (Loucks, 2003; Lebrun and Rumball, 2002; Stand, 2007), which may ultimately result in the development of osteoporosis. Young female athletes may be at particular risk of long-term health consequences from the triad because attainment of peak bone mass during the late teenage years is compromised, thus resulting in increased likelihood of developing osteoporosis (Lebrun and Rumball, 2002; Stand, 2007).

While male athletes are at a relatively lower risk for experiencing DE and ED, this should not be construed as inferring immunity from the disorders. Certain groups of male athletes, such as rowers, wrestlers, martial artists, and jockeys have demonstrated greater risk for DE and ED (Baum, 2006; Bratland-Sanda and Sundgot-Borgen, 2013). While the overall risk is lower in males, 10 per cent of endurance athletes, 17 per cent of weight class athletes and 42 per cent of antigravity sport athletes are effected by EDs (Joy et al., 2015). Of these populations, weight-restricted athletes such as jockeys and wrestlers have a higher tendency to skip meals, reduce fluid and caloric intake, and use drugs (e.g. amphetamines and laxatives) to reduce hunger, inhibit weight gain, and aid in weight loss in an effort to improve performance (Baum, 2006). Unfortunately, due to the pressures and sport-specific acceptance of many of these tactics, these practices can easily go unreported (Baum, 2006).

While extreme eating methods or restriction in order to reduce weight or maintain 'ideal' aesthetics garners considerable attention, the opposite behaviour of over consumption may play an equally detrimental role in long-term health. This stems from a form of body dysmorphia in which athletes feel the need to constantly become bigger and stronger in order to be successful, a condition more commonly referred to as *The Adonis Complex* (Arent and Lutz, 2015; Pope, Phillips, and Olivardia, 2000). This mindset can result in large increases in body weight after athletes retire due to a drastic reduction in energy expenditure while maintaining an inappropriately high caloric intake (Stephan, Torregrosa, and Sanchez, 2007). In line with these observations, American football, basketball, and ice hockey players are at risk of increased weight-related complications after retirement, particularly in comparison to endurance athletes (Baron, Hein, Lehman, and Gersic, 2012; Stephan *et al.*, 2007). Educating these athletes on healthy eating behaviours may be a critical, but often underutilised, step for helping them successfully transition into retirement and positively impacting their health.

To athletes, DE and ED may seem to be an acceptable part of a willingness to do anything to be great, much like playing through injury or pain. In fact, many athletes, coaches, team owners and trainers deny that EDs are a problem (McArdle *et al.*, 2015; Sundgot-Borgen and Torstveit, 2004). The combined expectations of the coaching staff, public perspective, and the athletes themselves may be creating pressuring to strive for a certain 'look' for the sport (Hammond *et al.*, 2014; Bratland-Sanda and Sundgot-Borgen 2013; McArdle *et al.*, 2015), even when this may be at the expense of optimal performance. The intense nature of elite athletics causes ED and DE to often be overlooked despite the serious health and performance conse-quences that are created.

The studies performed on elite athletes suggest that those in certain types of sports are at a higher risk for DE and ED than the general population (McArdle *et al.*, 2015). Similar to doping and PEDs, injuries, and concus-sions, one is left to wonder whether these data are actually under-repre-sentations of the magnitude of the problem because of self-report bias in most cases. To further confound the issue, the vast majority of the studies evaluating DE and ED are primarily based on Norwegian athletes. While this work has given the subject unparalleled insight, the significant reliance on this population could be a misrepresentation of elite athletes worldwide who may participate in a more diverse sport range, perform at different levels, and have different ideologies. Regardless, it is clear the issue of DE and ED involves aspects of performance, health, and both internal and external pressures that shape elite athletes' decisions and habits.

Conclusions

Sport is an enduring and important part of our culture and society. Besides numerous developmental, psychological, and physical benefits resulting from participation, it also has critical social and economic implications. However, *elite* sport presents a very unique situation. Despite the physical prowess of athletes at this level and the fact that athletes in some sports (i.e. endurance-based) have better health and longer life expectancy than the general public (Garatachea *et al.*, 2014; Baum, 2006), there are some very real, very impact-ful ramifications that accompany participation on the elite stage. These athletes knowingly and unknowingly put themselves at risk. While certain aspects may be a 'part of sport culture', this does not mean that these have to be accepted at face value. By working to change the culture and holding leagues, organisations, teams, management, and medical staff accountable, we can at least strive to make a *safer* environment, even if it is not entirely risk-free.

As technology and rule changes develop to try to make sport safer, parti-cularly with respect to injuries and concussions, there also needs to be a systematic and concerted effort to properly educate and assist players and coaches to help them make better decisions themselves. A trend towards increased involvement of qualified sport scientists and sport nutritionists is a positive step. These individuals possess the capability and knowledge to help properly monitor athletes, assess deficiencies and risk factors, and apply training, recovery, and nutritional strategies to help them reach full potential without unnecessarily jeopardising health. It is both unrealistic and unfair to expect athletes and coaches to be fully knowledgeable in these areas. In fact, most of them simply do 'what has always been done'. Unfortunately, this mindset contributes to the elevated risk and it is imperative that we move away from it.

The battlefield triage mentality of patching up the athletes so that they can keep going has to be tempered. While the health impacts of PEDs may be slightly overstated in an effort to justify ethical arguments, the consideration of the reliance on pain killers and their health impacts seems to be remarkably understated. The issue of concussions also needs to remain in the spotlight. Education on both identifying the signs and symptoms as well as long-term ramifications to dissuade premature return-to-play must be emphasised. It is time for medical ethics to play a larger role. In what other profession would the current level of risk and injury-rate be considered acceptable?

Even with advances in understanding, educational programmes, medicine and technology, we must realise that there will continue to be at least some elevated level of risk to health in elite sport. Whether the issue is doping and PEDs, playing through injury and pain, sustaining concussions, or developing disordered eating or eating disorders, elite athletes are willing to risk their health and bodies to get that added advantage, that last step, that .01 second difference that makes them the best in the world. They willingly play the role of modern-day gladiator for the fans. And as Maximus asked the crowd in the movie *Gladiator*: 'Are you not entertained?'

References

Alaranta, A., Alaranta, H., Holmila, J., Palmu, P., Pietilä, K., and Helenius, I. (2006). Self-reported attitudes of elite athletes towards doping: differences between type of sport. *International Journal of Sports Medicine*, 27(10), 842–846.

Arent, S. M. and Lutz, R. S. (2015). The psychology of supplementation in sport and exercise: motivational antecedents and biobehavioral outcomes. In *Nutritional Supplements in Sports and Exercise* (pp. 23–48). New York: Springer.

Bailey, R., Hillman, C., Arent, S., and Petitpas, A. (2012). Physical activity as an investment in personal and social change: the human capital model. *Journal of Physical Activity and Health*, 9(8), 1053–1055.

Bailey, R., Hillman, C., Arent, S., and Petitpas, A. (2013). Physical activity: an underestimated investment in human capital. *Journal of Physical Activity and Health*, 10(3), 289–308.

Baron, S. L., Hein, M. J., Lehman, E., and Gersic, C. M. (2012). Body mass index, playing position, race, and the cardiovascular mortality of retired professional football players. *The American Journal of Cardiology*, 109(6), 889–896.

Baum, A.L. (2005). Suicide in athletes: a review and commentary. *Clinics in Sports Medicine*, 24(4), 853–859.

Baum, A.L. (2006). Eating disorders in the male athlete. *Sports Medicine*, 36(1), 1–6.

Berning, J. M., Adams, K. J., and Stamford, B. A. (2004). Anabolic steroid usage in athletics: facts, fiction, and public relations. *The Journal of Strength & Conditioning Research*, 18(4), 908–917.

Bratland-Sanda, S. and Sundgot-Borgen, J. (2013). Eating disorders in athletes: overview of prevalence, risk factors and recommendations for prevention and treatment. *European Journal of Sport Science*, 13(5), 499–508.

Burman, E., Lysholm, J., Shahim, P., Malm, C., and Tegner, Y. (2016). Concussed athletes are more prone to injury both before and after their index concussion: a data base analysis of 699 concussed contact sports athletes. *BMJ Open Sport & Exercise Medicine*, 2(1), e000092.

Cancelliere, C., Hincapié, C. A., Keightley, M., Godbolt, A. K., Côté, P., Kristman, V. L., Stålnacke, B.M., Carroll, L.J., Hung, R., Borg, J., and Nygren-de Boussard, C. (2014). Systematic review of prognosis and return to play after sport concussion: results of the International Collaboration on Mild Traumatic Brain Injury Prognosis. *Archives of Physical Medicine and Rehabilitation*, 95(3), S210-S229.

Corrigan, B. (2002). Beyond EPO. *Clinical Journal of Sport Medicine*, 12(4), 242–244.

Corsellis, J. A. N., Bruton, C. J., and Freeman-Browne, D. (1973). The aftermath of boxing. *Psychological Medicine*, 3(3), 270–303.

Coughlin, J. M., Wang, Y., Munro, C. A., Ma, S., Yue, C., Chen, S., Airan, R., Kim, P. K., Adams, A. V., Garcia, C., Sair, H. I., Sawa, A., Smith, G., Lyketsos, C. G., Caffo, B., Kassiou, M., Guilarte, T. R., Pomper, M. G., and Higgs, C. (2015).

Neuroinflammation and brain atrophy in former NFL players: an in vivo multi-modal imaging pilot study. *Neurobiology of Disease*, 74, 58–65.

De Beaumont, L., Mongeon, D., Tremblay, S., Messier, J., Prince, F., Leclerc, S., Lassonde, M., and Théoret, H. (2011). Persistent motor system abnormalities in formerly concussed athletes. *Journal of Athletic Training*, 46(3), 234–240.

De Beaumont, L., Theoret, H., Mongeon, D., Messier, J., Leclerc, S., Tremblay, S., Ellemberg, D., and Lassonde, M. (2009). Brain function decline in healthy retired athletes who sustained their last sports concussion in early adulthood. *Brain*, 132(3), 695–708.

de Hon, O., Kuipers, H., and van Bottenburg, M. (2015). Prevalence of doping use in elite sports: a review of numbers and methods. *Sports Medicine*, 45(1), 57–69.

Donahue, E. G., Miquelon, P., Valois, P., Goulet, C., Buist, A., and Vallerand, R. J. (2006). A motivational model of performance-enhancing substance use in elite athletes. *Journal of Sport & Exercise Psychology*, 28(4), 511–520.

Garatachea, N., Santos-Lozano, A., Sanchis-Gomar, F., Fiuza-Luces, C., Pareja-Galeano, H., Emanuele, E., and Lucia, A. (2014). Elite athletes live longer than the general population: a meta-analysis. *Mayo Clinic Proceedings*, 89(9), 1195–1200.

Gardner, A., Iverson, G. L., Levi, C. R., Schofield, P. W., Kay-Lambkin, F., Kohler, R. M., and Stanwell, P. (2015). A systematic review of concussion in rugby league. *British Journal of Sports Medicine*, 49(8), 495–498.

Guskiewicz, K. M., Marshall, S. W., Bailes, J., McCrea, M., Cantu, R. C., Randolph, C., and Jordan, B. D. (2005). Association between recurrent concussion and late-life cognitive impairment in retired professional football players. *Neurosurgery*, 57(4), 719–726.

Guskiewicz, K. M., Marshall, S. W., Bailes, J., McCrea, M., Harding, H. P., Matthews, A., Mihalik, J. R., and Cantu, R. C. (2007). Recurrent concussion and risk of depression in retired professional football players. *Medicine & Science in Sports & Exercise*, 39(6), 903.

Hägglund, M., Waldén, M., and Ekstrand, J. (2006). Previous injury as a risk factor for injury in elite football: a prospective study over two consecutive seasons. *British Journal of Sports Medicine*, 40(9), 767–772.

Hammond, L. E., Lilley, J. M., Pope, G. D., Ribbans, W. J., and Walker, N. C. (2014). 'We've just learnt to put up with it': an exploration of attitudes and decision-making surrounding playing with injury in English professional football. *Qualitative Research in Sport, Exercise and Health*, 6(2), 161–181.

Harmon, K. G., Drezner, J. A., Gammons, M., Guskiewicz, K. M., Halstead, M., Herring, S. A., Kutcher, J. S., Pana, A., Putukian, M., and Roberts, W. O. (2013). American Medical Society for Sports Medicine position statement: concussion in sport. *British Journal of Sports Medicine*, 47(1), 15–26.

Hawkins, R. D. and Fuller, C. W. (1998). A preliminary assessment of professional footballers' awareness of injury prevention strategies. *British Journal of Sports Medicine*, 32(2), 140–143.

Hoberman, J. (2002). Sports physicians and the doping crisis in elite sport. *Clinical Journal of Sport Medicine*, 12(4), 203–208.

Howe, P. D. (2001). An ethnography of pain and injury in professional rugby union: the case of Pontypridd RFC. *International Review for the Sociology of Sport*, 36(3), 289–303.

Joy, E., Kussman, A., and Nattiv, A. (2016). 2016 update on eating disorders in athletes: a comprehensive narrative review with a focus on clinical assessment and management. *British Journal of Sports Medicine*, *50*(3), 154–162.

Lebrun, C. M. and Rumball, J. S. (2002). Female athlete triad. *Sports Medicine and Arthroscopy Review*, *10*(1), 23–32.

Loucks, A. B. (2003). Energy availability, not body fatness, regulates reproductive function in women. *Exercise and Sport Sciences Reviews*, *31*(3), 144–148.

Malcom, N. L. (2006). 'Shaking It Off' and 'Toughing It Out': socialization to pain and Injury in girls' softball. *Journal of Contemporary Ethnography*, *35*(5), 495–525.

Martland, H. S. (1928). Punch drunk. *Journal of the American Medical Association*, *91*(15), 1103–1107.

McArdle, S., Meade, M. M., and Moore, P. (2015). Exploring attitudes toward eating disorders among elite athlete support personnel. *Scandinavian Journal of Medicine & Science in Sports*, *26*(9), 1117–1127.

McCrea, M., Kelly, J. P., Randolph, C., Cisler, R., and Berger, L. (2002). Immediate neurocognitive effects of concussion. *Neurosurgery*, *50*(5), 1032–1042.

Mikkelsen, U. R., Langberg, H., Helmark, I. C., Skovgaard, D., Andersen, L. L., Kjaer, M., and Mackey, A. L. (2009). Local NSAID infusion inhibits satellite cell proliferation in human skeletal muscle after eccentric exercise. *Journal of Applied Physiology*, *107*(5), 1600–1611.

Murphy, P. and Waddington, I. (2007). Are elite athletes exploited? *Sport in Society*, *10*(2), 239–255.

Nelson, G. (1996). *Left Foot Forward. A Year in the Life of a Journeyman Footballer*. London: Headline.

Nixon, H. L. (1993). Accepting the risks of pain and injury in sport: mediated cultural influences on playing hurt. *Sociology of Sport Journal*, *10*(2), 183–196.

Nixon, H. L. (1996). Explaining pain and injury attitudes and experiences in sport in terms of gender, race, and sports status factors. *Journal of Sport and Social Issues*, *20*, 33–44.

Nordström, A., Nordström, P., and Ekstrand, J. (2014). Sports-related concussion increases the risk of subsequent injury by about 50% in elite male football players. *British Journal of Sports Medicine*, *48*(19), 1447–1450.

O'Connell, S. and Manschreck, T. C. (2012). Playing through the pain: psychiatric risks among athletes. *Current Psychiatry*, *11*(7), 16–20.

Okonkwo, D. O., Tempel, Z. J., and Maroon, J. (2014). Sideline assessment tools for the evaluation of concussion in athletes: a review. *Neurosurgery*, *75*, S82–S95.

Omalu, B. I., DeKosky, S. T., Hamilton, R. L., Minster, R. L., Kamboh, M. I., Shakir, A. M., and Wecht, C. H. (2006). Chronic traumatic encephalopathy in a national football league player: part II. *Neurosurgery*, *59*(5), 1086–1093.

Omalu, B. I., DeKosky, S. T., Minster, R. L., Kamboh, M. I., Hamilton, R. L., and Wecht, C. H. (2005). Chronic traumatic encephalopathy in a National Football League player. *Neurosurgery*, *57*(1), 128–134.

Pärssinen, M. and Seppälä, T. (2002). Steroid use and long-term health risks in former athletes. *Sports Medicine*, *32*(2), 83–94.

Pearce, A. J., Hoy, K., Rogers, M. A., Corp, D. T., Maller, J. J., Drury, H. G., and Fitzgerald, P. B. (2014). The long-term effects of sports concussion on retired

Australian football players: a study using transcranial magnetic stimulation. *Journal of Neurotrauma*, *31(13)*, 1139–1145.

Pope, H., Phillips, K. A., and Olivardia, R. (2000). *The Adonis Complex: The Secret Crisis of Male Body Obsession*. Simon and Schuster.

Quackenbush, N. and Crossman, J. (1994). Injured athletes: a study of emotional responses. *Journal of Sport Behavior*, *17(3)*, 178–187.

Roderick, M., Waddington, I., and Parker, G. (2000). Playing hurt: managing injuries in English professional football. *International Review for the Sociology of Sport*, *35(2)*, 165–180.

Schwenk, T. L., Gorenflo, D. W., Dopp, R. R., and Hipple, E. (2007). Depression and pain in retired professional football players. *Medicine & Science in Sports & Exercise*, *39(4)*, 599–605.

Stand, P. (2007). The female athlete triad. *Medicine & Science in Sports & Exercise*, *39(10)*, 1867–82.

Stephan, Y., Torregrosa, M., and Sanchez, X. (2007). The body matters: psychophysical impact of retiring from elite sport. *Psychology of Sport and Exercise*, *8(1)*, 73–83.

Sundgot-Borgen, J. and Torstveit, M. K. (2004). Prevalence of eating disorders in elite athletes is higher than in the general population. *Clinical Journal of Sport Medicine*, *14(1)*, 25–32.

Tentori, L. and Graziani, G. (2007). Doping with growth hormone/IGF-1, anabolic steroids or erythropoietin: is there a cancer risk? *Pharmacological Research*, *55(5)*, 359–369.

Tscholl, P. M. and Dvorak, J. (2012). Abuse of medication during international football competition in 2010–lesson not learned. *British Journal of Sports Medicine*, *46(16)*, 1140–1141.

van Amsterdam, J., Opperhuizen, A., and Hartgens, F. (2010). Adverse health effects of anabolic–androgenic steroids. *Regulatory Toxicology and Pharmacology*, *57(1)*, 117–123.

Verroken, M. (2001). Ethical aspects and the prevalence of hormone abuse in sport. *Journal of Endocrinology*, *170(1)*, 49–54.

Virchenko, O., Skoglund, B., and Aspenberg, P. (2004). Parecoxib impairs early tendon repair but improves later remodeling. *The American Journal of Sports Medicine*, *32(7)*, 1743–1747.

Vuolteenaho, K., Moilanen, T., and Moilanen, E. (2008). Non-steroidal anti-inflammatory drugs, cyclooxygenase-2 and the bone healing process. *Basic & Clinical Pharmacology & Toxicology*, *102(1)*, 10–14.

Walk, S. R. (1997). Peers in pain: the experiences of student athletic trainers. *Sociology of Sport Journal*, *14(1)*, 22–56.

Weinberg, R., Vernau, D., and Horn, T. (2013). Playing through pain and injury: psychosocial considerations. *Journal of Clinical Sport Psychology*, *7(1)*, 41–59.

Young, K. (1997). Women, sport and physicality: preliminary findings from a Canadian study. *International Review for the Sociology of Sport*, *32(3)*, 297–305.

Zuckerman, S. L., Kerr, Z. Y., Yengo-Kahn, A., Wasserman, E., Covassin, T., and Solomon, G. S. (2015). Epidemiology of sports-related concussion in NCAA athletes from 2009–2010 to 2013–2014 incidence, recurrence, and mechanisms. *The American Journal of Sports Medicine*, *43(11)*, 2654–2662.

Chapter 10

Sport and health

The prevention and treatment of non-communicable diseases

Peter Krustrup and Morten Bredsgaard Randers

Introduction

According to WHO, non-communicable diseases are by far the leading cause of death in the world, representing more than 60 per cent of all annual deaths. Physical inactivity is the primary cause of most non-communicable diseases (Booth *et al.*, 2012), and it is well established that physical activity is a cornerstone in the prevention and treatment of non-communicable diseases (Booth *et al.*, 2012; Pedersen and Saltin, 2015). Evidence has even suggested that, in certain cases, exercise therapy is as effective as medical treatment and, in some cases, even more effective (Pedersen and Saltin, 2015).

The terms physical activity and exercise are often used interchangeably, but they are not synonymous. Physical activity, defined as '*any bodily movement produced by skeletal muscles that results in energy expenditure*', which is distinguished from exercise, defined as '*planned, structured, and repetitive bodily movement done to improve or maintain one or more components of physical fitness*' (Caspersen *et al.*, 1985). Thus, exercise is part of a person's total physical activity, which also includes household tasks, transportation, occupational, leisure-time activities and so on. Sport is another term often used interchangeably with exercise, but sport has a set of rules, a defined goal and is often competitive. Competing in a marathon would thus be sport, whereas training for the event is exercise.

The strong relationship between physical inactivity and morbidity and mortality emphasises that considerable attention must be given to increasing physical activity in a population (Pedersen and Saltin, 2006). This could include increases in occupational physical activities, transportation and leisure-time activities. High occupational physical activity has, however, been negatively related to health profile and mortality, probably due to the relationship between high occupational and low leisure-time physical activity (Korshøj *et al.*, 2016). Some types of physical activity must be performed on a regular basis due to the fact that a short period of inactivity leads to major negative changes in health profile (Pedersen and Saltin, 2006). Taken together, leisure-time activities such as exercise and sport participation seem important for public health, and a recent paper in *The Lancet* concluded that exercise and sport have the potential to '*improve the health of a nation*' (Khan *et al.*, 2012). But what type of sport or exercise should be suggested for preventing lifestyle-related diseases and to improving health profile? Traditionally, prolonged low-to-moderate-intensity aerobic exercise training such as brisk walking, continuous running or cycling has been recommended for the prevention and treatment of cardiovascular and metabolic diseases (Cornelissen and Fagard, 2005; Pedersen and Saltin, 2015). Newer research has now shown that brief but very intense exercise has a significant impact on cardiorespiratory fitness, skeletal muscle oxidative capacity and insulin action (Babraj *et al.*, 2009; Burgomaster *et al.*, 2008; Gibala, 2007), and studies have shown that high intensity interval training is superior to prolonged moderate intensity exercise and strength training in improving cardiorespiratory fitness (Helgerud *et al.*, 2007; Nybo *et al.*, 2010; Schjerve *et al.*, 2008; Pattyn *et al.*, 2014; Weston *et al.*, 2014).

In 2011, the American College of Sports Medicine (ACSM) made an important update to its 1998-version position stand '*The recommended quantity and quality of exercise for developing and maintaining cardiorespiratory and muscular fitness, and flexibility in healthy adults*' (ACSM position stand, 1998; 2011). The update related directly to the intensity and type of physical activity. The 2011-version emphasises the importance of vigorous-intensity cardiorespiratory exercise. Hence, the newest recommendations include moderate-intensity cardiorespiratory exercise training for at least 30 minutes 5 days a week to accumulate at least 150 minutes a week, 20 minutes vigorous training 3 days a week to accumulate at least 75 minutes a week, or a combination of moderate and vigorous exercise. Moreover, strength training 2–3 times a week for major muscle groups and neuromotor exercise including agility, balance, and coordination are recommended. To prevent the development of lifestyle diseases adults should engage in sport and/or exercise training that covers several training types.

Figure 10.1 gives an overview of the impact of different types of exercise on various fitness capacities and their relationship to the risk of certain lifestyle diseases. This model can be used to analyse different exercise modes and sports disciplines. Traditional exercise, such as brisk walking, continuous running and cycling, falls in the training categories of aerobic low intensity and aerobic moderate intensity. As shown in the model, these training categories have suboptimal yet positive effects on metabolic and cardiovascular fitness. The high intensity interval training used in several recent studies has a marked positive effect on metabolic and cardiovascular fitness (Burgomaster *et al.*, 2008; Gibala *et al.*, 2007; Nybo *et al.*, 2010) and, to some extent, also musculoskeletal fitness (Figure 10.1). This model can also be applied to more complex exercise modes and sports, for example, racket sports such as squash and badminton, and team sports such as football, team

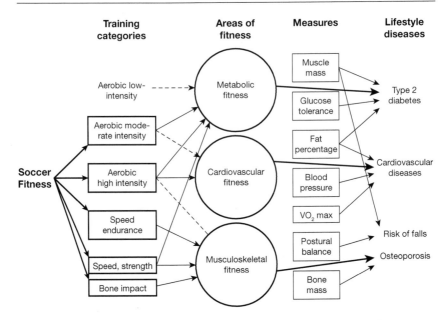

Figure 10.1 Holistic model on how various types of training can prevent and treat lifestyle diseases

Adapted from Krustrup *et al.*, 2010a

handball, basketball, floorball and volleyball. An increasing number of studies have used tracking systems and physiological measurements to describe activity profile and physiological demands during recreational sporting activities (Krustrup *et al.*, 2017; Fernandez-Fernandez, 2009; Smekal *et al.*, 2001; Sheppard *et al.*, 2009; Povoas *et al.*, 2017), whereas strong scientific evidence through a substantial number of randomised controlled trials has only been obtained for a few selected sports disciplines.

A recent review and meta-analysis (Oja *et al.*, 2015) aimed at assessing '*the quality and strength of evidence for the health benefits of specific sport disciplines*'. In that review, it was concluded that the '*best evidence was found for recreational football and running*'. For recreational cycling and swimming, some inconclusive evidence of health benefits was found, but no solid evidence was found for any other sport (Oja *et al.*, 2015).

The potential of a given sport to promote public health does not depend solely on the health benefits of that sport but also on its prevalence in a given society. Football is the most popular sport in the world with more than 270 million registered players, so football has the potential to make a global impact on health (Blatter and Dvorak, 2014). The knowledge base for the health effects of football, comprising more than 120 scientific papers published from 2009 to 2017, reveals that recreational football training conducted as small-sided games (4v4 to 7v7) has substantial and broad-spectrum fitness and health benefits for participants across the lifespan and for a number of patient groups, including patients with Type 2 diabetes, hypertension, obesity and osteoporosis.

Activity profile and physiological response to recreational football

The average heart rate in small-sided recreational football games of 3v3 to 9v9 has been shown to be 80–90 per cent of individual maximal heart rate (HRmax) in untrained men, women, children and elderly (Krustrup et al., 2009; 2010; Randers et al., 2010a; 2014). This is observed irrespective of social status, skill level and prior experience of football (Randers et al., 2012). It is also observed that heart rate reaches near maximal values and fluctuates up and down between 70 and 100 per cent HRmax during training sessions, with 10–50 per cent of the time in the highest HR zone above 90 per cent HRmax in school children and untrained healthy women and men aged 18–80 (Bendiksen et al., 2014; Krustrup et al., 2009; Randers et al., 2010a, 2014; Andersen et al., 2014b). These observations are similar for groups of patients with hypertension, Type 2 diabetes and prostate cancer (Krustrup et al., 2013; Andersen et al., 2014c; Uth et al., 2014; De Sousa et al., 2014).

Average blood lactate values in untrained men and women, as well as men with type 2 diabetes, reach 5–7 mmol/L, and individual values fluctuate between 2 and 14 mmol/L (Andersen et al., 2014c; Krustrup et al., 2010d; Randers et al., 2010a; 2014). Plasma ammonia has also been shown to increase 55–103 per cent above rest during training sessions (Randers et al., 2014; 2017), which is another sign of very intense periods during small-sided recreational football games. Although intensity is high, the intermittent nature of football allows significant blood flow to adipose tissue, which promotes the release of fatty acids. Marked increases in FFA in the blood have been observed during training sessions, even with high lactate concentration, which is known as a suppressor of lipolysis (Randers et al., 2010a; 2014; 2017). Thus, all the metabolic energy systems are used during small-sided football games for participant groups across the lifespan, which is supported by muscle biopsy analysis showing increases in muscle lactate and creatine phosphate utilisation (Krustrup et al., 2010d; Randers et al., 2010a). It is also evident that most muscle groups are active during football training due to the highly diverse movement pattern and the fact that all striated muscle fibre types are recruited, as revealed by high glycogen utilisation in red slow-twitch fibres (Type I) and white fast-twitch fibres (Type IIa and IIx) (Krustrup et al., 2010d; Randers et al., 2010a). Thus, it is clear from these observations that small-sided recreational football games combinine endurance training with high intensity interval training for basically everyone.

Motion analysis using video recordings and GPS tracking in various groups has clearly shown that small-sided recreational football games constitute intense, versatile interval training with multiple repetitions of orthodox and unorthodox movements including sprints, accelerations, decelerations, turns, shots and tackles (Pedersen *et al.*, 2009; Randers *et al.*, 2010a; Krustrup *et al.*, 2010d). The mean running intensity is ~50–90 m/min, giving totals for distance covered per session of ~2.5–5.5. Although mean running speed is rather low, the nemerous activity changes, brief intense actions and involvements with the ball impose high cardiovascular and metabolic demands, as explained above. Moreover, these many actions impose a high and multi-faceted stimulus to muscles and bones (Jackman *et al.*, 2013; Krustrup *et al.*, 2010c; Randers *et al.*, 2010b; Helge *et al.*, 2010; 2014). A 1-hour session of 7v7 for untrained men involved 886 activity changes at various speeds, of which 98 were high intensity runs, 16 were sprints and 59 were backwards and sideways runs (Krustrup *et al.*, 2010d), with corresponding values for untrained women with no prior football experience of 954, 101, 15 and 46, respectively (Randers *et al.*, 2010a). Additionally, multiple specific intense actions are performed, totalling an average of 192 for the untrained women during a 1-hour 7v7 session, with 66 turns, 28 stops, 40 shots and passes, 17 dribbles, 21 shoulder contacts and 17 foot tackles (Pedersen *et al.*, 2009). Interestingly, similar movement patterns were observed during 1v1, 2v2, 3v3 and 4v4 for untrained women and men (Randers *et al.*, 2010a), for homeless men playing 4v4 football on asphalt (Helge *et al.*, 2014b) and for untrained young men playing 5v5 on sand, asphalt and artificial turf (Brito *et al.*, 2012), with the only difference being more sideways and backwards running and short intense running bouts as the number of players decreases due to higher game involvement.

A recent study using GPS tracking of a 45-min Football Fitness session for elderly men with prostate cancer has also shown that, despite a total distance (2.65 km) of about half that observed in young men, the players performed as many as 194 accelerations, 296 decelerations and 100 running bouts (Uth *et al.*, 2015a). Thus, there are extensive and multi-faceted musculoskeletal demands during small-sided recreational football games for participants across the lifespan. When applying these studies of activity profile and acute physiological demands to the model in Figure 10.1, it is clear that recreational football played as small-sided games combines all training categories and affects all fitness categories, and therefore has the potential to be a broad-spectrum health-enhancing activity.

In the following sections of this chapter, we will provide some of the many studies – mostly RTCs – that led to the conclusion by Oja *et al.* (2015) that the '*best evidence* [for the health benefits of sports disciplines] *was found for recreational football and running*', and to recreational football being mentioned as a contributor to the health of nations in *The Lancet* (Khan *et al.*, 2012).

Cardiorespiratory fitness

A central component of health profile seems to be cardiorespiratory fitness, as low cardiorespiratory fitness is associated with several non-communicable diseases (Pedersen and Saltin, 2015). Relative risk of all-cause mortality is more strongly related to cardiorespiratory fitness than to physical activity (Lee *et al.*, 2010), which is why more attention must be paid to enhancing the cardiorespiratory fitness in the fight against morbidity and mortality from cardiovascular diseases (Pattyn *et al.*, 2014; Weston *et al.*, 2014). Thus, increasing cardiorespiratory fitness is of high importance and recreational football, with the many brief intense actions and periods with very high heart rate, is effective in this matter.

After 3–6 months of recreational football training VO$_2$max increased in untrained men from 39.6 to 44.6 ml/min/kg (Krustup *et al.*, 2009) and in type 2 diabetes patients from 30.5 to 34.1 ml/min/kg (Schmidt *et al.*, 2013). A recent systematic review and meta-analysis of recreational football concluded that the average increase in maximal oxygen uptake after 3–4 months of Football Fitness training was 3.5 ml/min/kg (Milanovic *et al.*, 2015). This equates to an increment of 1 MET, which has been associated with a decrement of 10–25 per cent in mortality risk (Kokkinos *et al.*, 2011).

Obesity – visceral adipose tissue

Obesity has long been considered a major risk factor for a number of non-communicable diseases. Obesity is not only linked to coronary heart diseases but also a risk factor indirectly through its adverse effect on hypertension and insulin resistance (Kokkinos and Myers, 2010). However, it has been discussed whether obesity per se is a risk factor, as there is increasing evidence to show that mortality risk is not associated with fatness when adjusting for fitness (Barry *et al.*, 2014). It has been shown that obese men have a 2.6 times higher mortality risk of cardiovascular diseases than normal-weight men (Wei *et al.*, 1999), but leanness does not increase health benefits in fit men and being fit reduces the risks of being obese (Lee *et al.*, 1999). In adults >60 years, waist circumference has been associated with mortality, but this association was not significant when adjusted for fitness (Sui *et al.*, 2007). These findings are supported by several studies, showing lower risk of all-cause and/or CVD mortality in fit but obese compared to unfit but lean men and women (Katzmarzyk *et al.*, 2004; Lee *et al.*, 2010; Farrell *et al.*, 2010; Church *et al.*, 2005). Moreover, a newer meta-analysis concluded that unfit individuals had twice the mortality risk, regardless of BMI, and that fit overweight and fit obese individuals had similar risk to fit normal-weight individuals (Barry *et al.*, 2014). Nevertheless, losing body fat has a positive effect on risk of developing osteoschlerosis, not only in the weight-bearing joints, but also as a result of joint damage caused by adipokines (Pottie *et al.*, 2006).

Several studies have shown that 12–16 weeks of small-sided football training leads to positive changes in body composition in healthy untrained men and women, with 1–3 kg less fat and 1–2.5 kg more muscle mass (Krustrup *et al.*, 2009; Randers *et al.*, 2012; Connolly *et al.* 2014). Similar reductions in fat mass have been observed in middle-aged men with T2DM (Andersen *et al.*, 2014c) and women with hypertension (Mohr *et al.*, 2014), and the fat loss was as high as 3.4 kg for 48–68-year-old Brazilian women and men with Type 2 diabetes when using a 12-week intervention combining football training and a calorie-restricted diet (de Sousa *et al.*, 2014). Weight loss of 4.9 kg was accompanied by a loss in waist circumference in Scottish men after a 12-week football intervention, with no further change at 12-month follow-up (Hunt *et al.*, 2014). It has been proposed that body fat distribution is more strongly linked to cardiovascular diseases than total body fat, with increased risk of CVD with increasing abdominal fat (Wu *et al.*, 1998; Wirklund *et al.*, 2008).

Few studies have measured waist circumference as an indirect measure of abdominal fat, and a reduction of 5.4 cm in Type 2 diabetic men and women was found after a 12-week intervention involving diet restriction and small-sided football training (de Sousa *et al.*, 2014). However, the diet-only group had similar changes in waist circumference, making the effect of football-only difficult to evaluate. A 3.3-cm reduction has been found after 12 weeks of training in hypertensive men (Knoepfli-Lenzin *et al.*, 2010), and several studies have found changes in android fat percentage using whole-body DXA-scans and 5–11 per cent decrements in android fat percentage in hypertensive men, Type 2 diabetics and homeless men (Andersen *et al.*, 2010; Andersen *et al.*, 2014c; Randers *et al.*, 2012). Thus, recreational small-sided football leads not only to decrements in total fat mass but also to a more favourable body fat composition.

Insulin sensitivity/resistance – Type 2 diabetes (DM2)

Insulin secretion rises as insulin sensitivity falls due to lack of physical activity. As inactivity continues insulin sensitivity declines further and, at a certain point insulin secretion cannot compensate for the decreased insulin sensitivity, indicating pre-diabetes. A continued decline in insulin sensitivity and insulin secretion leads to Type 2 diabetes and hyperglycaemia. It is well established that exercise is a central component in the prevention and treatment of Type 2 diabetes and the different pre-states (Pedersen and Saltin, 2015).

Few studies have investigated the effect of recreational football on glucose tolerance and insulin sensitivity in Type 2 diabetics. After 24 weeks of recreational football training for Type 2 diabetic men, fasting blood glucose was decreased compared to inactive controls (Andersen *et al.*, 2014c). Moreover, HbA1c was lowered after 12 weeks, with no further change in the following 12 weeks (Schmidt *et al.*, 2013). Similar changes were observed in Brazilian men and women diagnosed with Type 2 diabetes after a combined intervention comprising football training and diet restriction, but the changes did not differ from the group that only had diet restriction (de Sousa *et al.*, 2014). However, favourable changes in HOMA-IR, proinsulin, proinsulin:insulin ratio and glucagon were only observed in the combined football and diet group (de Sousa *et al.*, 2014).

Lipids and lipoproteins

Dyslipidaemia entails an elevated risk of atherosclerosis and is related to the risk of cardiovascular diseases and, in particular, coronary artery disease (Durstine *et al.*, 2002). Thus, lowering LDL cholesterol and triglycerides and increasing HDL cholesterol is important for health. For every 1 per cent that LDL cholesterol is lowered, it is suggested that the relative risk of coronary artery disease and major coronary heart disease events decreases by 1–3 per cent (Leon and Sanchez, 2001; Booth *et al.*, 2012).

In several studies, but not all, short-term training has also resulted in positive alterations in blood lipid profile, exemplified by 0.2–0.5 mM reductions in LDL cholesterol values in untrained young men, homeless men, hypertensive women and Type 2 diabetics as well as 0.2–0.4 mM reductions in triglycerides in the two latter studies (Krustrup *et al.*, 2009; Randers *et al.*, 2012; Mohr *et al.*, 2014; de Sousa *et al.*, 2014). The risk of coronary artery disease increases progressively with increasing LDL cholesterol above 2.6 mmol/L (Leon-Sanchez *et al.*, 2001), so the 12–15 per cent reduction observed in untrained men, homeless men and Type 2 diabetic men and women, who all had elevated LDL cholesterol (2.7–3.2 mmol/L) prior to the football training intervention, is of great importance (Krustrup *et al.*, 2009; de Sousa *et al.*, 2014; Randers *et al.*, 2012).

Increasing HDL cholesterol has a protective effect, but increases in HDL cholesterol have not been observed after football training interventions. One explanation for this may be that the intervention period (12–16 weeks) is too short to cause changes in HDL cholesterol (Durstine *et al.*, 2002), but changes were not observed in long-term studies (Randers *et al.*, 2010b; Krustrup *et al.*, 2010c). However, HDL cholesterol changes in a dose-dependent manner with increased energy expenditure and it has been proposed that extra energy expenditure of at least 5000 kJ per week is needed to increase HDL cholesterol (Durstine *et al.*, 2002; Kokkinos and Fernhall, 1999). The energy expended during a 1-hour football training session has been estimated at approximately 3,000 kJ in men and 2,100 kJ in women (Krustrup *et al.*, 2010b). Thus, in the two long-term studies the extra weekly energy expenditure would be ~4,000 kJ in both men and women due to the difference in training frequency (Randers *et al.*, 2010b; Krustrup *et al.*, 2010c).

Hypertension and cardiovascular disease risk

Hypertension is a major risk factor for cardiovascular diseases and the most common risk factor present in individuals suffering stroke, heart failure and sudden death (Kokkinos and Myers, 2010). Although hypertension is defined as systolic blood pressure (SBP) >140 mmHg or diastolic blood pressure (DBP) >90 mmHg in otherwise healthy individuals, with corresponding values of 130/80 mmHg in diabetics, the risk of cardiovascular death decreases log-linearly with decreasing blood pressure until at least 115/75 mmHg. An increase of 20 mmHg in SBP and 10 mmHg in DBP doubles the risk of cardiovascular mortality (Lewington et al., 2002).

After 12–16 weeks of recreational small-sided football games, SBP and DBP were lowered by 7–9 and 3–5 mmHg in normotensive men and women (Krustrup et al., 2009; 2010), which was maintained after 1 year with reduced training frequency (2.4 to 1.3 training sessions per week) (Randers et al., 2010b). No significant changes were found in SBP and DBP in a long-term study in premenopausal women (Krustrup et al., 2010c), a 12-week street football intervention for homeless men (Randers et al., 2012), and in ~70-year-old healthy elderly men following 1-year football training (Schmidt et al., 2015). However, in all three studies pre-values were rather low (women: 114/74 mmHg; homeless: 116/73 mmHg; elderly: 125/74 mmHg), and in the long-term studies on premenopausal women and the elderly comprehensive transthoracic echocardiography revealed marked changes in myocardial structure and systolic and diastolic function (Krustrup et al., 2010c; Schmidt et al., 2014). Such significant changes in structural and functional myocardial alterations were also observed in 8–10-year-old school children after 10 weeks of football training, whereas SBP and DBP were unaltered (Krustrup et al., 2014). In 526 10–12-year-old Danish school children, an 11-week school-based 'FIFA 11 for Health'-football training intervention led to 4.4 and 2.3 mmHg decreases in SBP and DBP, respectively (Orntoft et al., 2017). Interestingly, the effects were even greater (6/3 mmHg) in the 29 per cent of the children, who did not participate in sports-club activities in their leisure time. These changes were greater than reported in a meta-analysis of physical activity intervention studies in 6–12-year-old children (Cesa et al., 2014).

A reduction in SBP of 7–9 mmHg and in DBP of 3–5 mmHg in normotensive adults is considered to have significant health effects at least down to 115/75 mmHg (Lewington et al., 2002), and these training-induced changes are greater than typically observed in normotensive adults (Cornelissen and Fagard, 2005; Whelton et al., 2002). A Norwegian study (Molmen-Hansen et al., 2011) found aerobic high intensity interval training to be superior to isocaloric moderate intensity continuous training for lowering SBP and DBP, so it may be speculated that the high intensity bouts during football games have a favourable influence on blood pressure. However, changes similar to those observed in recreational football were seen also in continuous running (Krustrup *et al.*, 2009; 2010), which is in line with meta-analyses reporting no relationship between training intensity and changes in blood pressure (Fagard, 2001; Whelton *et al.*, 2002). Nevertheless, recreational football is very effective at preventing the development of hypertension.

Several studies have also investigated small-sided football games as treatment for hypertension in already diagnosed hypertensive men and women (Andersen *et al.*, 2010; 2014a; Krustrup *et al.*, 2013; Knoepfli-Lenzin *et al.*, 2010; Mohr *et al.*, 2014a). Decrements in blood pressure in the hypertensive participants were observed to be larger than in normotensive, with an average decrement in mean arterial pressure of almost 10 mmHg (SBP: 10–13 mmHg; DBP: 6–9 mmHg). Meta-analyses have shown net reductions in SBP and DBP averaged 7 and 5 mmHg, respectively (Fagard, 2001), hence recreational football can be considered a very effective type of exercise for reducing blood pressure and a potent non-pharmaceutical intervention tool for treating hypertension. As seen in normotensive men, recreational football also led to alterations in myocardial structure and systolic and diastolic function in hypertensive men (Andersen *et al.*, 2014a).

The lowered blood pressure was accompanied by a drop in resting heart rate of 4–7 bpm in untrained men and women as well as homeless participants (Krustrup *et al.*, 2009; 2010; Randers *et al.*, 2012). Resting heart rate has been suggested as a non-invasive independent predictor of cardiovascular diseases (Hsia *et al.*, 2009; Thayer and Lane, 2007), since the risk of cardiovascular diseases increases with increasing resting heart rate above at least 60 bpm (Fox *et al.*, 2007).

The lower resting heart rate may reflect a reduction in sympathetic outflow and thereby reduced systemic vascular resistance. In the study by Knoepfli-Lenzin *et al.* (2010), heart rate variability was measured in supine and standing positions and, based on their findings, they suggested an increase in parasympathetic rather than sympathetic activity and therefore an improved vagal modulation, which is linked to a reduction in cardiovascular mortality (Malik, 1996). Studies have also shown increases in muscular capillarisation after an intervention involving recreational small-sided football games in untrained men (23 per cent), women (18 per cent) and Type 2 diabetics (7 per cent) (Krustrup *et al.*, 2009; 2010; Andersen *et al.*, 2014c), which also is likely to decrease peripheral vascular resistance and thereby contribute to lowered blood pressure.

Osteoporosis

Osteoporosis is characterised by a decrease in bone mineral density (BMD) and bone mineral content (BMC), and hence reduced bone strength leading to higher risk of bone fracture. Within the last 2–3 decades vertebra and hip fractures have increased by a factor of 2–4 in men and women (Pedersen and Saltin, 2015), so the health costs of osteoporosis are rising. Immobilisation due to fractures increases several risk factors of CVD and mortality, so prevention is of major importance. Weight-bearing activities during childhood and adolescence play a major role and BMD in youth and early adulthood is related to BMD in later adulthood (Kemper *et al.*, 2000). Moreover, a meta-analysis has shown that weight-bearing activities increase bone strength in children, whereas there was insufficient evidence for such an effect in adults (Nikander *et al.*, 2010), so increasing weight-bearing physical activity in childhood seems important.

Cross-sectional studies have shown that children and adolescents participating in football and basketball had higher BMC and BMD than inactive and comparable individuals participating in low-impact sports such as swimming (Ferry *et al.*, 2011; Zribi *et al.*, 2014; Vicente-Rodriguez *et al.*, 2003). A recent RCT (Larsen *et al.*, 2016) using football as the major component of a ball-game intervention found increased BMD and BMC after a 10-month school-based intervention comprising 3 × 40 minutes of training per week. Another school-based RCT (Larsen *et al.*, 2017) investigated 3v3 small-sided games, predominantly football, but also basketball, floorball and team handball, and interval running 5 × 12 minutes per week in 8–10-year-olds, but found no significant changes in BMD or BMC, although the mechanical strain in the 5 × 12-min intervention was similar to that in 3 × 40-min intervention. Thus, the weekly loading may be of significant importance, though another explanation might be that the duration of each session was longer and consequently imposed more pronounced fatigue development towards the end of the session, reducing the muscles ability to absorb shocks and increasing strain on the bone (Larsen *et al.*, 2017).

A number of recent investigations in adults have shown that periods of recreational small-sided football games incduce a marked osteogenic response, as evidenced by training-induced increases in circulating levels of the bone formation marker osteocalcin in untrained young women (37 per cent, 16 weeks, Jackman *et al.*, 2013), 25–65-year-old female hospital workers (21 per cent, 12 weeks, Barene *et al.*, 2014), hypertensive women (37 per cent, 15 weeks, Mohr *et al.*, 2015), homeless men (27 per cent, 12 weeks, Helge *et al.*, 2014a), elderly untrained men (45 per cent, 16 weeks, Helge *et al.*, 2014b) and elderly prostate cancer patients undergoing anti-androgen treatment (34 per cent, 12 weeks, Uth *et al.*, 2015a). Similarly, football interventions have caused improvements in BMC and BMD in young, middle-aged and elderly participants, with greater effects from recreational football than from swimming, continuous running and interval running (Krustrup *et al.*, 2010c; Helge *et al.*, 2010; Mohr *et al.*, 2015). Thus, tibia BMD and leg BMC increased by 2–3 per cent in untrained healthy women and men as well as hypertensive women after 12–16 weeks of 2–3 × 1-hour football sessions per week (Krustrup *et al.*, 2010a; Helge *et al.*, 2010; Mohr *et al.*, 2015). Furthermore, several studies have shown that BMD increases in clinically important sites such as the femoral shaft, femoral neck and hip, by 1–2 per cent over 12–16 weeks in hypertensive women and elderly men (Mohr *et al.*, 2015; Helge *et al.*, 2014b; Uth *et al.*, 2015a), but even more with medium-term and long-term football interventions, with increases of 2–5 per cent in elderly healthy men (52 weeks, Helge *et al.*, 2014a) and elderly prostate cancer patients (32 weeks, Uth *et al.*, 2015b). Interestingly, the study by Uth *et al.* (2015a) revealed a significant correlation (r=0.65) between the number of decelerations during training and the 12-week increase in leg BMC, supporting a link between the movement pattern and the training-induced skeletal effects.

When it comes to preventing fractures, an important aspect of training, besides the improvements in BMC and BMD, is the improvement in rapid muscle force and postural balance, which prevented falls, especially in elderly individuals. Studies involving recreational football have also shown marked effects on muscular function, including postural balance, muscle strength and functional capacity. A cross-sectional study (Sundstrup *et al.*, 2010) showed that 70-year-old lifelong trained male football players had similar balance and rapid muscle force to 30-year-old untrained men. Improvements in postural balance have been observed after 12–16 weeks of small-sided football training in untrained young men (Krustrup *et al.*, 2009; Jakobsen *et al.*, 2011), untrained young women (Krustrup *et al.*, 2010b) and homeless men (Helge *et al.*, 2014b), but not in elderly healthy men and elderly prostate cancer patients over 12–52-week intervention periods (Andersen *et al.*, 2014b; Uth *et al.*, 2015a, b), which may be due to a lack of sensitivity of the applied balance test given that elderly men had several other measurable improvements in functional capacity. Thus, despite a lack of testosterone due to the antiandrogen treatment, the elderly men with prostate cancer had an increase in muscle mass of 0.7 kg and an increase in leg muscle strength of 15 per cent compared to controls after 12 weeks of small-sided football training. Moreover, 8–15 per cent improvements in jump performance, sit-to-stand performance and stair climbing were observed after 32 weeks, and the healthy elderly men had a 29 per cent increase in sit-to-stand performance after 16 weeks of football training (Andersen *et al.*, 2014b).

It is thus clear that participation in small-sided football training leads to several improvements, including increased BMD, BMC, and rapid muscle force, and improved muscular functionality and postural balance, which together reduce the risk of fractures.

Implementation of Football Fitness

Football Fitness is a new type of football that can attract new participant groups, as it focuses on 3v3 to 7v7 football training among friends rather than on 11v11 competitive matches (Bennike *et al.*, 2014). Apart from its broad-spectrum fitness and health effects, investigations of Football Fitness have also shown that it is considered fun, enjoyable and motivating, and that it develops social capital, networking and general wellbeing (Ottesen *et al.*, 2010; Bruun *et al.*, 2014; Nielsen *et al.*, 2014). The focus on team-mates, opponents and on the small-sided football game itself has also been shown to increase flow and to lower perceived exertion, despite the high physical demands (Krustrup *et al.*, 2010a; Elbe *et al.*, 2010). These elements, including flow during training, motivational factors and the development of social capital, are very important for regular participation in and long-term adherence to sport (Elbe *et al.*, 2016).

The concept of Football Fitness was developed between 2007 and 2010 in a close collaboration between the Danish FA and a group of researchers led by Professor Peter Krustrup, and the concept was introduced across Denmark in 2011. The concept has now been implemented in as many as 275 Danish football clubs (15–20 per cent) and the vision is to reach a total of 600 clubs (35 per cent) over the next 5-year period. A majority of the participants are untrained women aged 30–50, but there are also middle-aged and elderly men and women, along with different types of teams, including patient groups with hypertension and prostate cancer and teams of unemployed men and women in job training programmes (Bennike *et al.*, 2014). In spring 2015, the Football Fitness concept was introduced with great success nationwide in the small country of the Faroe Islands. Indeed, as many as 1.5 per cent of the population started up before the summer, including 6 per cent of all Faroese women aged 30–50, with the number of female members of the Faroese FA doubling in 9 months. In 2015, the FC Prostate study was expanded into the FC Prostate Community project, where patients are recruited from six hospitals across Denmark to play football in football clubs in close proximity to the hospitals (Bruun *et al.*, 2014). There are also ongoing projects in the Prevention Centres in the Municipality of Copenhagen, where ball games are now used as part of a 12-week training regime offered to 40–80-year-old patients with lifestyle diseases and many of these participants are encouraged to continue physical activity by playing Football Fitness in local football clubs. Together these projects clearly emphasises that football is an interesting model for worldwide health promotion through sport. Football is already by far the most popular sport in the world and there are already 400–500 million people playing regularly in sports club or on an unorganised basis. Nevertheless, using a concept like Football Fitness with new groups of untrained participants for the prevention and treatment of lifestyle diseases offers a huge potential for an increased participation and for a considerable contribution to worldwide health through sports.

References

Andersen, L. J., Randers, M. B., Hansen, P. R., Hornstrup, T., Schmidt, J. F., Dvorak, J., Søgaard, P., Krustrup, P., and Bangsbo, J. (2014a). Structural and functional cardiac adaptations to 6 months of football training in untrained hypertensive men. *Scand J Med Sci Sports*, 24 (Suppl. 1), 27–35.

Andersen, L. J., Randers, M. B., Westh, K., Martone, D., Hansen, P. R., Junge, A., Dvorak, J., Bangsbo, J., and Krustrup, P. (2010). Soccer as a treatment for hypertension in untrained 30–55-year-old men: a prospective randomized study. *Scand J Med Sci Sports*, 20 (Suppl. 1), 98–102.

Andersen, T. R., Schmidt, J. F., Nielsen, J. J., Randers, M. B., Sundstrup, E., Jakobsen, M. D., Andersen, L. L., Suetta, C., Aagaard, P., Bangsbo, J., and Krustrup, P. (2014b). The effect of football or strength training on functional ability and physical performance in elderly untrained men. *Scandinavian Journal of Medicine & Science in Sports*, 24(S1), 76–85.

Andersen, T. R., Schmidt, J. F., Thomassen, M., Hornstrup, T., Frandsen, U., Randers, M. B., Hansen, P. R., Krustrup, P., and Bangsbo, J. (2014c). A preliminary study: effects of football training on glucose control, body composition, and performance in men with type 2 diabetes. *Scandinavian Journal of Medicine & Science in Sports*, 24(S1), 43–56.

Babraj, J. A., Vollaard, N. B., Keast, C., Guppy, F. M., Cottrell, G., and Timmons, J. A. (2009). Extremely short duration high intensity interval training substantially improves insulin action in young healthy males. *BMC Endocr Disord*, 9, 3.

Barene, S., Krustrup, P., Jackman, S. R., Brekke, O. L., and Holtermann, A. (2014). Do soccer and Zumba exercise improve fitness and indicators of health among female hospital employees? A 12-week RCT. *Scandinavian Journal of Medicine & Science in Sports*, 24(6), 990–999.

Barry, V. W., Baruth, M., Beets, M. W., Durstine, J. L., Liu, J., and Blair, S. N. (2014). Fitness vs. fatness on all-cause mortality: a meta-analysis. *Progress in Cardiovascular Diseases*, 56(4), 382–390.

Bendiksen, M., Williams, C. A., Hornstrup, T., Clausen, H., Kloppenborg, J., Shumikhin, D., Brito, J., Horton, J., Barene, S., Jackman, S. R., and Krustrup, P. (2014). Heart rate response and fitness effects of various types of physical education for 8- to 9-year-old schoolchildren. *European Journal of Sport Science*, 14(8), 861–869.

Bennike, S., Wikman, J. M., and Ottesen, L. S. (2014). Football Fitness – a new version of football? A concept for adult players in Danish football clubs. *Scandinavian Journal of Medicine & Science in Sports*, 24(S1), 138–146.

Blatter, J. S. and Dvorak, J. (2014). Football for Health–Science proves that playing football on a regular basis contributes to the improvement of public health. *Scandinavian Journal of Medicine & Science in Sports*, 24(S1), 2–3.

Booth, F. W., Roberts, C. K., and Laye, M. J. (2012). Lack of exercise is a major cause of chronic diseases. *Comprehensive Physiology* 2(2), 1143–1211.

Brito, J., Krustrup, P., and Rebelo, A. (2012). The influence of the playing surface on the exercise intensity of small-sided recreational soccer games. *Human Movement Science*, 31(4), 946–956.

Bruun, D. M., Krustrup, P., Hornstrup, T., Uth, J., Brasso, K., Rørth, M., Christensen, J. F., and Midtgaard, J. (2014). 'All boys and men can play football': a qualitative investigation of recreational football in prostate cancer patients. *Scandinavian Journal of Medicine and Science Sports*, 24(S1), 113–121.

Burgomaster, K. A., Howarth, K. R., Phillips, S. M., Rakobowchuk, M., MacDonald, M. J., McGee, S. L., and Gibala, M. J. (2008). Similar metabolic adaptations during exercise after low volume sprint interval and traditional endurance training in humans. *J Physiol*, 586, 151–160.

Caspersen, C. J., Powell, K. E., and Christenson, G. M. (1985). Physical activity, exercise, and physical fitness: definitions and distinctions for health-related research. *Public Health Reports*, 100(2), 126.

Cesa, C. C., Sbruzzi, G., Ribeiro, R. A., Barbiero, S. M., de Oliveira Petkowicz, R., Eibel, B., Machado, N. B., das Virgens Marques, R., Tortato, G., dos Santos, T. J., and Leiria, C. (2014). Physical activity and cardiovascular risk factors in children: meta-analysis of randomized clinical trials. *Preventive Medicine*, 69, 54–62.

Church, T. S., LaMonte, M. J., Barlow, C. E., and Blair, S. N. (2005). Cardiorespiratory fitness and body mass index as predictors of cardiovascular disease mortality among men with diabetes. *Archives of Internal Medicine*, 165(18), 2114–2120.

Connolly, L. J., Scott, S., Mohr, M., Ermidis, G., Julian, R., Bangsbo, J., Jackman, S. R., Bowtell, J. L., Davies, R. C., Hopkins, S. J., and Fulford, J. (2014). Effects of small-volume soccer and vibration training on body composition, aerobic fitness, and muscular PCr kinetics for inactive women aged 20–45. *Journal of Sport & Health Science*, 3(4), 284–292.

Cornelissen, V. A. and Fagard, R. H. (2005). Effects of endurance training on blood pressure, blood pressure-regulating mechanisms, and cardiovascular risk factors. *Hypertension*, 46, 667–675.

de Sousa, M. V., Fukui, R., Krustrup, P., Pereira, R. M., Silva, P. R., Rodrigues, A. C., Andrade, J. L., Hernandez, A. J., and da Silva, M. E. (2014). Positive effects of football on fitness, lipid profile, and insulin resistance in Brazilian patients with type 2 diabetes. *Scandinavian Journal of Medicine & Science in Sports*, 24(S1), 57–65.

Durstine, J. L., Grandjean, P. W., Cox, C. A., and Thompson, P. D. (2002). Lipids, lipoproteins, and exercise. *J Cardiopulm Rehabil*, 22, 385–398.

Elbe, A. M., Strahler, K., Krustrup, P., Wikman, J., and Stelter, R. (2010). Experiencing flow in different types of physical activity intervention programs: three randomized studies. *Scandinavian Journal of Medicine and Science in Sports*, 20 (Suppl. 1), 111–117.

Fagard, R. H. (2001). Exercise characteristics and the blood pressure response to dynamic physical training. *Med Sci Sports Exerc*, 33, S484–S492.

Farrell, S. W., Fitzgerald, S. J., McAuley, P. A., and Barlow, C. E. (2010). Cardiorespiratory fitness, adiposity, and all-cause mortality in women. *Medicine and science in sports and exercise*, 42(11), 2006–2012.

Fernandez-Fernandez, J., Sanz-Rivas, D., and Mendez-Villanueva, A. (2009). A review of the activity profile and physiological demands of tennis match play. *Strength & Conditioning Journal*, 31(4), 15–26.

Ferry, B., Duclos, M., Burt, L., Therre, P., Le Gall, F., Jaffré, C., and Courteix, D. (2011). Bone geometry and strength adaptations to physical constraints inherent in different sports: comparison between elite female soccer players and swimmers. *Journal of Bone and Mineral Metabolism*, 29(3), 342–351.

Fox, K., Borer, J. S., Camm, A. J., Danchin, N., Ferrari, R., Sendon, J. L. L., Steg, P. G., Tardif, J. C., Tavazzi, L., Tendera, M., and Heart Rate Working Group. (2007). Resting heart rate in cardiovascular disease. *Journal of the American College of Cardiology*, 50(9), 823–830.

Garber, C. E., Blissmer, B., Deschenes, M. R., Franklin, B. A., Lamonte, M. J., Lee, I. M., and Swain, D. P. (2011). American College of Sports Medicine position stand. Quantity and quality of exercise for developing and maintaining cardiorespiratory, musculoskeletal, and neuromotor fitness in apparently healthy adults: guidance for prescribing exercise. *Medicine and Science in Sports and Exercise*, 43(7), 1334–1359

Gibala, M. J. (2007). High-intensity interval training: a time-efficient strategy for health promotion? *Curr Sports Med Rep 6*, 211–213.

Helge, E. W., Andersen, T. R., Schmidt, J. F., Jørgensen, N. R., Hornstrup, T., Krustrup, P., and Bangsbo, J. (2014b). Recreational football improves bone mineral density and bone turnover marker profile in elderly men. *Scandinavian Journal of Medicine and Science in Sports*, 24(S1), 98–104.

Helge, E. W., Aagaard, P., Jakobsen, M. D., Sundstrup, E., Randers, M. B., Karlsson, M. K., and Krustrup, P. (2010). Recreational football training decreases risk factors for bone fractures in untrained premenopausal women. *Scandinavian Journal of Medicine & Science in Sports*, 20(suppl 1), 31–39.

Helge, E. W., Randers, M. B., Hornstrup, T., Nielsen, J. J., Blackwell, J., Jackman, S. R., and Krustrup, P. (2014a). Street football is a feasible health-enhancing activity for homeless men: biochemical bone marker profile and balance improved. *Scand J Med Sci Sports*, 24(Suppl 1), 122–129.

Helgerud, J., Høydal, K., Wang, E., Karlsen, T., Berg, P., Bjerkaas, M., Simonsen, T., Helgesen, C., Hjorth, N., Bach, R., and Hoff, J. (2007). Aerobic high-intensity intervals improve VO$_2$max more than moderate training. *Medicine & Science in Sports & Exercise*, 39(4), 665–771.

Hsia, J., Larson, J. C., Ockene, J. K., Sarto, G. E., Allison, M. A., Hendrix, S. L., Robinson, J. G., LaCroix, A. Z., and Manson, J. E. (2009). Resting heart rate as a low tech predictor of coronary events in women: prospective cohort study. *BMJ*, 338, b219.

Hunt, K., Wyke, S., Gray, C. M., Anderson, A. S., Brady, A., Bunn, C., Donnan, P. T., Fenwick, E., Grieve, E., Leishman, J., and Miller, E. (2014). A gender-sensitised weight loss and healthy living programme for overweight and obese men delivered by Scottish Premier League football clubs (FFIT): a pragmatic randomised controlled trial. *The Lancet*, 383(9924), 1211–1221.

Jackman, S. R., Scott, S., Randers, M. B., Orntoft, C., Blackwell, J., Zar, A., Helge, E. W., Mohr, M., and Krustrup, P. (2013). Musculoskeletal health profile for elite female footballers versus untrained young women before and after 16 weeks of football training. *Journal of Sports Sciences*, 31(13), 1468–1474.

Jakobsen, M. D., Sundstrup, E., Krustrup, P., and Aagaard, P. (2011). The effect of recreational soccer training and running on postural balance in untrained men. *European Journal of Applied Physiology*, 111(3), 521–530.

Katzmarzyk, P. T., Church, T. S., and Blair, S. N. (2004). Cardiorespiratory fitness attenuates the effects of the metabolic syndrome on all-cause and cardiovascular disease mortality in men. *Arch Intern Med*, 164, 1092–1097.

Kemper, H. C. G., Twisk, J. W. R., Van Mechelen, W., Post, G. B., Roos, J. C., and Lips, P. T. A. M. (2000). A fifteen-year longitudinal study in young adults on the relation of physical activity and fitness with the development of the bone mass: The Amsterdam Growth And Health Longitudinal Study. *Bone, 27*(6), 847–853.

Khan, K. M., Thompson, A. M., Blair, S. N., Sallis, J. F., Powell, K. E., Bull, F. C., and Bauman, A. E. (2012). Sport and exercise as contributors to the health of nations. *Lancet, 380*(9836), 59–64.

Knoepfli-Lenzin, C., Sennhauser, C., Toigo, M., Boutellier, U., Bangsbo, J., Krustrup, P., Junge, A., and Dvorak, J. (2010). Effects of a 12-week intervention period with football and running for habitually active men with mild hypertension. *Scandinavian Journal of Medicine & Science in Sports, 20*(suppl 1), 72–79.

Kokkinos, P. F. and Fernhall, B. (1999). Physical activity and high density lipoprotein cholesterol levels: what is the relationship? *Sports Med, 28*, 307–314.

Kokkinos, P. and Myers, J. (2010). Exercise and physical activity. *Circulation, 122*(16), 1637–1648.

Kokkinos, P., Sheriff, H., and Kheirbek, R. (2011). Physical inactivity and mortality risk. *Cardiology Research and Practice, 211*, 924–945.

Korshøj, M., Ravn, M. H., Holtermann, A., Hansen, Å. M., and Krustrup, P. (2016). Aerobic exercise reduces biomarkers related to cardiovascular risk among cleaners: effects of a worksite intervention RCT. *International Archives of Occupational and Environmental Health, 89*(2), 239–249.

Krustrup, P. (2017). Soccer fitness: prevention and treatment of lifestyle diseases. In J. Bangsbo, P. Krustrup, P. R. Hansen, L. Ottesen, G. Pfister, and A.-M. Elbe (eds), *Science and Football VIII: The Proceedings of the Eighth World Congress on Science and Football* (pp. 61–70). London: Routledge.

Krustrup, P., Aagaard, P., Nybo, L., Petersen, J., Mohr, M., and Bangsbo, J. (2010a). Recreational football as a health promoting activity: a topical review. *Scandinavian Journal of Medicine & Science in Sports, 20*(suppl. 1), 1–13.

Krustrup, P., Christensen, J. F., Randers, M. B., Pedersen, H., Sundstrup, E., Jakobsen, M. D., Krustrup, B. R., Nielsen, J. J., Suetta, C., Nybo, L., and Bangsbo, J. (2010d). Muscle adaptations and performance enhancements of soccer training in untrained men. *European Journal of Applied Physiology, 108*, 1248–1257.

Krustrup, P., Hansen, P. R., Andersen, L. J., Jakobsen, M. D., Sundstrup, E., Randers, M. B., Christiansen, L., Helge, E. W., Pedersen, M. T., Søgaard, P., and Bangsbo, J. (2010c). Long-term musculoskeletal and cardiac health effects of recreational football and running for premenopausal women. *Scandinavian Journal of Medicine & Science in Sports, 20*(suppl 1), 58–65.

Krustrup, P., Hansen, P. R., Randers, M. B., Nybo, L., Martone, D., Andersen, L. J., Bune, L. T., Junge, A., and Bangsbo, J. (2010b). Beneficial effects of recreational football on the cardiovascular risk profile in untrained premenopausal women. *Scand J Med Sci Sports, 20*(Suppl 1), 40–49.

Krustrup, P., Nielsen, J. J., Krustrup, B. R., Christensen, J. F., Pedersen, H., Randers, M. B., Aagaard, P., Petersen, A. M., Nybo, L., and Bangsbo, J. (2009). Recreational soccer is an effective health-promoting activity for untrained men. *British Journal of Sports Medicine, 43*, 825–831.

Krustrup, P., Skoradal, M. B., Randers, M. B., Weihe, P., Uth, J., Mortensen, J., Mohr, M. (2017). Broad-spectrum health improvements with one year of soccer training in inactive mildly hypertensive middle-aged women. *Scand J Med Sci Sports*. Jan 25. doi:10.1111/sms.12829

Krustrup, P., Randers, M. B., Andersen, L. J., Jackman, S. R., Bangsbo, J., and Hansen, P. R. (2013). Soccer improves fitness and attenuates cardiovascular risk factors in hypertensive men. *Med Sci Sports Exerc*, 45, 553–560.

Larsen, M. N., Nielsen, C. M., Helge, E. W., Madsen, M., Manniche, V., Hansen, L., Hansen, P. R., Bangsbo, J., and Krustrup, P. (2016). Positive effects on bone mineralisation and muscular fitness after 10 months of intense school-based physical training for children aged 8–10 years: FIT FIRST randomised controlled trial. *British Journal of Sports Medicine*.

Larsen, M. N., Nielsen, C. M., Orntoft, C., Randers, M. B., Helge, E. W., Madsen, M., Manniche, V., Hansen, L., Hansen, P. R., Bangsbo, J., and Krustrup, P. (2016). Fitness effects of 10-month frequent low-volume ball game training or interval running for 8–10-year-old school children. *BioMed Res Int*.

Lee, C. D., Blair, S. N., and Jackson, A. S. (1999). Cardiorespiratory fitness, body composition, and all-cause and cardiovascular disease mortality in men. *Am J Clin Nutr*, 69, 373–380.

Lee, D. C., Sui, X., Ortega, F. B., Kim, Y. S., Church, T. S., Winett, R. A., Ekelund, U., Katzmarzyk, P. T., and Blair, S. N. (2010). Comparisons of leisure-time physical activity and cardiorespiratory fitness as predictors of all-cause mortality in men and women. *Br J Sports Med*, 45(6), 504–510.

Leon, A. S. and Sanchez, O. A. (2001). Response of blood lipids to exercise training alone or combined with dietary intervention. *Med Sci Sports Exerc*, 33, S502–S515.

Lewington, S., Clarke, R., Qizilbash, N., Peto, R., and Collins, R. (2002). Age-specific relevance of usual blood pressure to vascular mortality: a meta-analysis of individual data for one million adults in 61 prospective studies. *The Lancet*, 360, 1903–1913.

Malik, M. (1996). Heart rate variability. *Annals of Noninvasive Electrocardiology*, 1(2), 151–181.

Milanović, Z, Pantelić, S, Čović, N., Sporiš, G., and Krustrup, P. (2015). Is Recreational Soccer Effective for Improving VO2max A Systematic Review and Meta-Analysis. *Sports Med*, 45, 1339–1353.

Mohr, M., Helge, E. W., Petersen, L. F., Lindenskov, A., Weihe, P., Mortensen, J., Jørgensen, N. R., and Krustrup, P. (2015). Effects of soccer vs swim training on bone formation in sedentary middle-aged women. *European Journal of Applied Physiology*, 115(12), 2671–2679.

Mohr, M., Lindenskov, A., Holm, P. M., Nielsen, H. P., Mortensen, J., Weihe, P., and Krustrup, P. (2014). Football training improves cardiovascular health profile in sedentary, premenopausal hypertensive women. *Scandinavian Journal of Medicine & Science in Sports*, 24(S1), 36–42.

Molmen-Hansen, H. E., Stolen, T., Tjonna, A. E., Aamot, I. L., Ekeberg, I. S., Tyldum, G. A., Wisloff, U., Ingul, C. B., and Stoylen, A. (2011). Aerobic interval training reduces blood pressure and improves myocardial function in hypertensive patients. *Eur J Cardiovasc Prev Rehabil*, 19(2), 151–160.

Nielsen, G., Wikman, J. M., Jensen, C. J., Schmidt, J. F., Gliemann, L., and Andersen, T. R. (2014). Health promotion: the impact of beliefs of health benefits, social relations and enjoyment on exercise continuation. *Scandinavian Journal of Medicine & Science in Sports*, 24 (Suppl. 1), 66–75. doi:10.1111/sms.12275

Nikander, R., Sievänen, H., Heinonen, A., Daly, R. M., Uusi-Rasi, K., and Kannus, P. (2010). Targeted exercise against osteoporosis: a systematic review and meta-analysis for optimising bone strength throughout life. *BMC Medicine*, 8(1), 47.

Nybo, L., Sundstrup, E., Jakobsen, M. D., Mohr, M., Hornstrup, T., Simonsen, L., Bülow, J., Randers, M. B., Nielsen, J. J., Aagaard, P., and Krustrup, P. (2010). High-intensity training versus traditional exercise interventions for promoting health. *Med Sci Sports Exerc*, 42, 1951–1958.

Oja, P., Titze, S., Kokko, S., Kujala, U. M., Heinonen, A., Kelly, P., Koski, P., and Foster, C. (2015). Health benefits of different sport disciplines for adults: systematic review of observational and intervention studies with meta-analysis. *British Journal of Sports Medicine*, 49, 434–440.

Ørntoft, C., Fuller, C. W., Larsen, M. N., Bangsbo, J., Dvorak, J., and Krustrup, P. (2016). 'FIFA 11 for Health' for Europe. II: effect on health markers and physical fitness in Danish schoolchildren aged 10–12 years. *British Journal of Sports Medicine*, 50(22), 1394–1399.

Ottesen, L., Jeppesen, R. S., and Krustrup, B. R. (2010). The development of social capital through football and running: studying an intervention program for inactive women. *Scandinavian Journal of Medicine & Science in Sports*, 20(S1), 118–131.

Pattyn, N., Coeckelberghs, E., Buys, R., Cornelissen, V. A., and Vanhees, L. (2014). Aerobic interval training vs. moderate continuous training in coronary artery disease patients: a systematic review and meta-analysis. *Sports Medicine*, 44(5), 687–700.

Pedersen, B. K. and Saltin, B. (2006). Evidence for prescribing exercise as therapy in chronic disease. *Scand J Med Sci Sports*, 16, 3–63.

Pedersen, B. K. and Saltin, B. (2015). Exercise as medicine–evidence for prescribing exercise as therapy in 26 different chronic diseases. *Scandinavian Journal of Medicine & Science in Sports*, 25(S3), 1–72.

Pedersen, M. T., Randers, M. B., Skotte, J. H., and Krustrup, P. (2009). Recreational soccer can improve the reflex response to sudden trunk loading among untrained women. *Journal of Strength and Conditioning Research*, 23(9), 2621–2626.

Pollock, M. L., Gaesser, G. A., Butcher, J. D., Després, J. P., Dishman, R. K., Franklin, B. A., and Garber, C. E. (1998). ACSM position stand: the recommended quantity and quality of exercise for developing and maintaining cardiorespiratory and muscular fitness, and flexibility in healthy adults. *Med Sci Sports Exerc*, 30(6), 975–991.

Pottie, P., Presle, N., Terlain, B., Netter, P., Mainard, D., & Berenbaum, F. (2006). Obesity and osteoarthritis: more complex than predicted! *Annals of the Rheumatic Diseases*. 65(11), 1403–1405.

Póvoas, S. A., Castagna, C., Resende, C., Coelho, E. F., Silva P., Santos, R., Seabra, A, Tamames, J., Lopes, M., Randers, M. B., Krustrup., P. (2017) Physical and physiological demands of recreational team handball for adult untrained men. *BioMed Res Int*. Article ID 6204603.

Randers, M. B., Nielsen, J. J., Bangsbo, J., and Krustrup, P. (2014) Physiological response and activity profile in recreational small-sided football: no effect of the number of players. *Scandinavian Journal of Medicine & Science in Sports*, 24(Suppl. 1), 130–137. doi:10.1111/sms.12232

Randers, M. B., Nielsen, J. J., Krustrup, B. R., Sundstrup, E., Jakobsen, M. D., Nybo, L., Dvorak, J., Bangsbo, J., and Krustrup, P. (2010b). Positive performance and health effects of a football training program over 12 weeks can be maintained over a 1-year period with reduced training frequency. *Scandinavian Journal of Medicine & Science in Sports*, 20, 80–89.

Randers, M. B., Nybo, L., Petersen, J., Nielsen, J. J., Christiansen, L., Bendiksen, M., Brito, J., Bangsbo, J., and Krustrup, P. (2010a). Activity profile and physiological response to football training for untrained males and females, elderly and youngsters: influence of the number of players. *Scandinavian Journal of Medicine & Science in Sports*, 20(Suppl. 1), 14–23.

Randers, M. B., Petersen, J., Andersen, L. J., Krustrup, B. R., Hornstrup, T., Nielsen, J. J., Nordentoft, M., and Krustrup, P. (2012). Short-term street soccer improves fitness and cardiovascular health status of homeless men. *Eur J Appl Physiol, 112*, 2097–2106.

Randers, M. B., Ørntoft, C., Hagman, M., Nielsen, J. J., Krustrup, P. (2017). Activity profile and physiological response during small-sided recreational football for untrained men – effect of number of players with a fixed pitch size. *J Sports Sci.*, to be published.

Schjerve, I. E., Tyldum, G. A., Tjonna, A. E., Stolen, T., Loennechen, J. P., Hansen, H. E., Haram, P. M., Heinrich, G., Bye, A., Najjar, S. M., Smith, G. L., Slordahl, S. A., Kemi, O. J., and Wisloff, U. (2008). Both aerobic endurance and strength training programmes improve cardiovascular health in obese adults. *Clin Sci (Lond), 115*, 283–293.

Schmidt, J. F., Andersen, T. R., Horton, J., Brix, J., Tarnow, L., Krustrup, P., Andersen, L. J., Bangsbo, J., and Hansen, P. R. (2013). Soccer training improves cardiac function in men with type 2 diabetes. *Med Sci Sports Exerc, 45*, 2223–2233.

Sheppard, J. M., Gabbett, T. J., & Stanganelli, L. C. R. (2009). An analysis of playing positions in elite men's volleyball: considerations for competition demands and physiologic characteristics. *The Journal of Strength & Conditioning Research*, 23(6), 1858–1866.

Smekal, G., Von Duvillard, S. P., Rihacek, C., Pokan, R., Hofmann, P., Baron, R., Tschan, H., and Bachl, N. (2001). A physiological profile of tennis match play. *Medicine and Science in Sports and Exercise*, 33(6), 999–1005.

Sui, X., LaMonte, M. J., Laditka, J. N., Hardin, J. W., Chase, N., Hooker, S. P., and Blair, S. N. (2007). Cardiorespiratory fitness and adiposity as mortality predictors in older adults. *JAMA*, 298(21), 2507–2516.

Sundstrup, E., Jakobsen, M. D., Andersen, J. L., Randers, M. B., Petersen, J., Suetta, C., Aagaard, P., and Krustrup, P. (2010). Muscle function and postural balance in lifelong trained male footballers compared with sedentary elderly men and youngsters. *Scand J Med Sci Sports*, 20(Suppl 1), 90–97.

Thayer, J. F. and Lane, R. D. (2007). The role of vagal function in the risk for cardiovascular disease and mortality. *Biol Psychol, 74*, 224–242.

Uth, J., Hornstrup, T., Christensen, J. F., Christensen, K. B., Jørgensen, N. R., Helge, E. W., Schmidt, J. F., Brasso, K., Helge, J. W., Jakobsen, M. D., and Krustrup, P. (2016). Football training in men with prostate cancer undergoing androgen deprivation therapy: activity profile and short-term skeletal and postural balance adaptations. *European Journal of Applied Physiology*, 116(3), 471–480.

Uth, J., Hornstrup, T., Christensen, J. F., Christensen, K. B., Jørgensen, N. R., Schmidt, J. F., . . . Helge, E. W. (2015b). Efficacy of recreational football on bone health, body composition, and physical functioning in men with prostate cancer undergoing androgen deprivation therapy: 32-week follow-up of the FC prostate randomised controlled trial. *Osteoporosis International*, 27(4), 1507–1518.

Uth, J., Hornstrup, T., Schmidt, J. F., Christensen, J. F., Frandsen, C., Christensen, K. B., Helge, E. W., Brasso, K., Rørth, M., Midtgaard, J., and Krustrup, P. (2014). Football training improves lean body mass in men with prostate cancer undergoing androgen deprivation therapy. *Scandinavian Journal of Medicine & Science in Sports*, 24(S1), 105–112.

Vicente-Rodriguez, G., Jimenez-Ramirez, J., Ara, I., Serrano-Sanchez, J. A., Dorado, C., and Calbet, J. A. L. (2003). Enhanced bone mass and physical fitness in prepubescent footballers. *Bone*, 33(5), 853–859.

Wei, M., Kampert, J. B., Barlow, C. E., Nichaman, M. Z., Gibbons, L. W., Paffenbarger, R. S., Jr., and Blair, S. N. (1999). Relationship between low cardiorespiratory fitness and mortality in normal-weight, overweight, and obese men. *JAMA*, 282, 1547–1553.

Weston, K.S., Wisløff, U., Coombes, J.S. (2014). High-intensity interval training in patients with lifestyle-induced cardiometabolic disease: a systematic review and meta-analysis. *British Journal of Sports Medicine*, 48(16), 1227–1234.

Whelton, S. P., Chin, A., Xin, X., and He, J. (2002). Effect of aerobic exercise on blood pressure: a meta-analysis of randomized, controlled trials. *Ann Intern Med*, 136, 493–503.

Wiklund, P., Toss, F., Weinehall, L., Hallmans, G., Franks, P. W., Nordstrom, A., and Nordstrom, P. (2008). Abdominal and gynoid fat mass are associated with cardiovascular risk factors in men and women. *J Clin Endocrinol Metab*, 93, 4360–4366.

Wu, C. H., Yao, W. J., Lu, F. H., Wu, J. S., and Chang, C. J. (1998). Relationship between glycosylated hemoglobin, blood pressure, serum lipid profiles and body fat distribution in healthy Chinese. *Atherosclerosis*, 137, 157–165.

Zribi, A., Zouch, M., Chaari, H., Bouajina, E., Zouali, M., Nebigh, A., and Tabka, Z. (2014). Enhanced bone mass and physical fitness in prepubescent basketball players. *Journal of Clinical Densitometry*, 17(1), 156–162.

Chapter 11

Healthy sport consumption

Moving away from pies and beer

*Keith D. Parry, David Rowe, Emma S. George
and Timothy J. Hall*

Introduction

Some Australian sports teams are struggling to encourage an increasingly sedentary population to attend live events, while the amount of sport available on television and via the Internet is rising. For example, in 2016 Australia's Channel 7 (a free-to-air broadcaster) aired 3,000 hours of Olympic content across three mainstream television stations and live-streams through the 7 Olympics app. In June 2016, Fox Sports (a subscription television service owned by News Corp Australia) delivered round-the-clock coverage of Wimbledon and offered 12 sport channels, providing 24/7 sports coverage – with one channel dedicated to rugby league. Fans in Australia (and elsewhere) can now watch sport on television at any time of the day or night, and stream sport endlessly on their mobile devices. The struggle to encourage spectators to attend sporting venues is also compounded by negative factors such as poor quality, high priced food and beverages at the stadium. The high prices at some Australian venues have resulted in concerns that watching sport at stadiums may no longer be affordable for 'the common person', particularly those with families (Sutton, 2017).

A sport stadium is a specific environment that, like airports and concert venues, is physically sealed off from the outside world. It is a space where there is contestation over the consumptive behaviour of sport fans. As an enclosed commercial domain, the economy of the sport stadium is designed around offering food and beverages in the context of a monopoly or oligopoly (depending on how many independent suppliers are contracted to service it). Within this environment, a small number of licensed suppliers rent the limited available space, and pass on the costs of supplying their necessarily limited offerings to sport fans. For those who wish to evade this control, as noted later they can either consume as much as possible before entering the stadium, or seek to smuggle in their own food and drink by evading the on-entry security measures involving searches not only for items that may endanger those attending (such as weapons), but also those that may 'injure' the profit margins of the suppliers of hospitality or the owners of intellectual property (in the case of so-called ambush marketing).

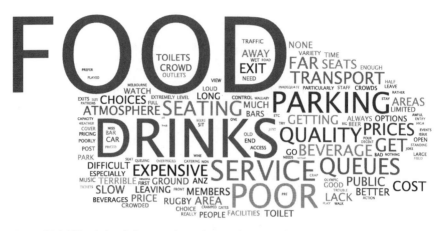

Figure 11.1 Word cloud showing Australian rugby union fans' responses to the questions: What aspects of the stadium do you consider to be particularly negative?

Keith Parry, created from survey responses of Australian Rugby Union fans

When attending a sports match, food and alcohol have been identified as the primary purchases of sports fans (Jones, 2002) but, as noted by Carter *et al.* (2012), there is little academic research into the actual offerings in stadiums and, therefore, discussions of food and drink within them remain largely anecdotal. Nevertheless, stadium food has a reputation for being of poor quality and is a point of frustration for many fans (see Figure 11.1). Although it is difficult to find a definition of healthy eating options, the World Health Organization highlights those foods that are low in fat, sugars and cholesterol (WHO, 2015). The food available in stadiums has been typically high in saturated fat, sugars, and sodium and would, therefore, be conventionally considered to be unhealthy. Although the European Healthy Stadia Network has called for healthier food options in stadiums (as part of a settings-based approach to health promotion (Martin *et al.*, 2016), there is yet to be a significant change in many European (and Australian) venues. This chapter explores the role of food and drink in the Australian sporting experience and highlights issues surrounding the quality and price of stadium food and drink. It begins with a brief contextualisation of the modern Australian sporting experience and recent shifts towards the mediated consumption of sport (Rowe, 2004).

Twenty-first century sport consumption

Humans have long engaged in physical activity or 'practices resembling the individual or recreational or theatrical activities we now call 'sport' (Mandell, 1999, p. xi). Sport is used by many nations to define themselves (Hallinan,

Hughson and Burke, 2007; Harris, 2008) and this is particularly the case in Australia, where sport is deeply embedded in the national culture (Rowe, 2013). It is a 'key cultural institution in Australia' (McKay *et al.*, 2001, p. 233) where matters of state are disrupted for one of two reasons – the first being issues of national or international importance, and the second updates on the top sporting events (Kell, 2000). Sport may be described as a 'national necessity', and it is certainly one of the principal amusements of Australians (Stewart, 1990). Stewart argues that playing and watching sport has been one of the key sources of meaning in the life of Australians for well over half a century, and many use it to escape the rigours and stresses of modern life (Booth, 2000).

Although over 17 million Australians are estimated to have participated in sport or physical activity between October 2015 and September 2016 (ASC, 2016), only 43 per cent of Australian adults met or exceeded the recommended levels of physical activity in 2011–2012 (ABS, 2013). It is important, however, to distinguish between sport and physical activity. While physical activity can be defined as 'any bodily movement produced by skeletal muscles that requires energy expenditure' (Caspersen, Powell and Christenson, 1985, p. 126), organised sport is structured physical exercise, a particular form of culture that offers a unique platform for social inter-action. Unfortunately, rates of sport participation are far lower than rates of sport spectatorship, both in terms of watching sport at a stadium or from home via the media. While the physical and mental health benefits of physical activity have been well-documented, participation in organised sport offers additional benefits, including improvements in health-related quality of life (Eime *et al.*, 2010) and social and mental wellbeing (Eime *et al.*, 2013). Yet, as Rowe (2017) notes:

> A national survey [conducted in 2015] of 1,200 people found that 61.2 per cent of respondents never play any kind of organised sport, 55.5 per cent had watched sport live at a venue in the last year, and 84.9 per cent had watched it live through the media.

Furthermore, the minority who participate in sport is not evenly spread across all social groups (Dollman and Lewis, 2010; Hardy *et al.*, 2010; Spaaij, 2012), and is predominantly the domain of young, well-off, and well-educated males (Bennett, Emmison and Frow, 2001). Australian sport participation decreases with age (ABS, 2015) and is essentially dominated by those who live in cities, with those based in the country or suburbs, migrants, and Indigenous Australians having lower levels of participation. But, as noted earlier, Australians do watch live sport in large numbers.

Australians are obviously not alone in their love of watching sport. Fans have existed for as long as athletes have competed against each other (Osborne and Coombs, 2013), and watching sport is one of the most popular leisure choices in many societies. This popularity is reflected in the high average attendance figures at games in sports leagues such as the National Football League (NFL) (68,278), German Bundesliga (43,331), English Premier League (36,464), and Major League Baseball (30,517) (Barrett, 2016). At an individual club level, German Association football team Borussia Dortmund averaged 80,451, NFL team the Dallas Cowboys 88,531, and NCAA American Football team Michigan 112,252 fans per match in 2012. Leading the way for Australian attendance is the Australian Football League (AFL) with an average of over 33,000 fans per game in 2012 (Sporting Intelligence, 2013), while the Big Bash League (cricket) is now the ninth most-watched sports league in the world, having an average crowd of 28,279 for the 2015-2016 season (Barrett, 2016). Attendances at other Australian sporting codes do not match these numbers and, for instance, the average figure in the National Rugby League (NRL) was only 16,423 in 2012 (Sporting Intelligence, 2013). Falling attendance numbers in some sports (Stensholt, 2014) have been attributed to various factors, such as ticket prices and the proliferation of sport on television, as will now be discussed.

Sport has popular, global appeal that has been recognised by media companies, who have exploited this capacity. The founder of one such multinational media corporation, Rupert Murdoch, stressed that his media conglomerate planned to 'use sport as a battering ram and a lead offering in all our pay television operations' (quoted in Cashmore, 2005, p. 365). People from countries around the world are now able to tune in via satellite broadcasts or the Internet to watch elite players performing in a small number of sports leagues (Maguire, 2001), creating a global market for both televised and live sporting events (Rookwood and Millward, 2011; Rowe, 2011). Mediated sport has now grown to such an extent that, while attending sporting events is a common practice among adults, consumers from Europe, North America, and Australia are now much more likely to watch it on television than to attend a sports event in person (Parry, Jones and Wann, 2014). For example, over two-fifths of the Australian population watched televised sports such as Australian football, horse racing, and cricket in 2009–2010 (ABS, 2010), while in North America 33 billion hours of sport were watched on television in 2013 (Nielsen, 2014). Sport dominates Australian television viewing habits, so much so that in 2015 the top five most watched programs on Australian television were live sport broadcasts (Rossi, 2016). As noted previously, it is more common for Australians to watch sport on television than to participate in sport or physical activity. The prolonged periods of sedentary behaviour, and screen time in particular, that are now associated with modern sport consumption can have a detrimental impact on the health of fans (Grøntved and Hu, 2011).

With physical activity levels falling and sedentary time increasing, almost two in three Australians (63 per cent) are now overweight or obese, a rise of 10 per cent from 1995 (AIHW, 2017). Australia is now in the 'worst' third of all Organisation for Economic Co-Operation and Development (OECD) countries for adult obesity (WHO, 2017). In response to the 'obesity epidemic' and increasing rates of chronic lifestyle-related diseases, such as Type 2 diabetes and cardiovascular disease, there is an increasing need to promote healthy lifestyle behaviour in innovative ways. To achieve health benefits, it is recommended that Australian adults accumulate at least 150 minutes of moderate-to-vigorous physical activity per week. In addition, adults are encouraged to limit the amount of time spent sitting (particularly in prolonged bouts), and to be aware of the time spent in front of screens (Department of Health, 2014).

Watching sport has the potential positively to influence people's motivation to be physically active; yet evidence from the *Sydney* 2000 Olympics, the *Vancouver* 2010 Winter Olympics, and the *London* 2012 Olympics has revealed that this is not the case. While major sporting events such as the Olympic Games can provide an increased awareness of sport, physical activity and sport participation levels remain largely unchanged and it seems that sporting organisations are failing to capitalise on the true potential of *sport* and the 'spirit' of the Olympics (Bauman, Bellew and Craig, 2014; Craig and Bauman, 2014; Mahtani *et al.*, 2013). This contradiction also opens up an important discussion around the social obligation of professional sporting bodies not only to use sport as a spectacle for television, but also to encourage fans to be more active as part of a healthier lifestyle (Anagnostopoulos, 2011; Inoue *et al.*, 2015; Parnell *et al.*, 2015). Such promotion should also be encouraged with regard to fans attending live sport, particularly through the provision of healthier eating options. The following section examines the food on offer to spectators when they attend professional sport matches.

Stadium food

Although Ko *et al.* (2011) claim that some North American sports teams use high-quality food and drinks as key promotional tools, the food in sports venues is widely perceived to be of poor quality (Lee, Parrish and Kim, 2015). As far back as the mid-1990s, Wakefield and Sloan (1995) identified stadium food prices as an area of dissatisfaction for many sports fans, and the results from a number of more recent studies suggest that many sport attendees are still not satisfied with the offerings of stadium concession stalls (Ireland and Watkins, 2010; Martin and O'Neill, 2010; Parry, Hall and Baxter, 2017; Sukalakamala, Sukalakamala and Young, 2013). In the United Kingdom, fans have described the food on offer at sporting stadiums as 'awful', 'abysmal' and 'atrocious' (Ireland and Watkins, 2010), while in Australia fans bemoan the 'terrible food choices' that are perceived to be of poor quality (Parry, Hall and Baxter, 2017). Indeed, some fans report going 'out of their way to not purchase food and beverage once inside the stadium . . .

[even] "loading up" on food and beverages before entering or sneaking such items into the stadium' (Martin and O'Neill, 2010, 14). Significantly, such 'loading up' practices are contrary to healthy eating guidelines that encourage smaller, balanced, and regular meals (National Health and Medical Research Council, 2013).

Another way in which fans avoid purchasing stadium food is by bringing pre-prepared meals with them. However, as mentioned previously, not all venues allow spectators to enter with their own food and drink (particularly if it is commercially prepared food), often prohibit opened drinks containers, or place restrictions on the size of food storage bags or coolers. While safety and licensing concerns may be behind some of these decisions, they serve to constrain the choices of fans. It should be noted that the issues discussed here are primarily pertinent for attendees in general admission, non-corporate seating. Spectators with access to hospitality facilities are more satisfied with stadium offerings than those in the 'cheap seats' (Lambrecht, Kaefer and Ramenofsky, 2009). Such 'corporate' fans are provided with better quality food, often without limits, and, as is particularly the case with corporate attendees at Japanese sumo wrestling tournaments, they are almost encouraged to eat excessive amounts (White, 2004). Such over indulgence is, again, contrary to healthy eating guidelines.

The standard food available in sporting stadiums has been compared to offerings found in fast food restaurants, which are traditionally high in carbohydrate, fat, sugar and calories. Indeed, it is not uncommon to see big-brand fast food outlets in sporting venues and, during the London 2012 Games, the Olympic Park boasted four McDonald's restaurants, including the world's biggest McDonald's for the duration of the Games (Ho, 2012). The healthiness of food offerings, or lack thereof, at many stadiums is a key factor in the decision of some fans not to eat at stadiums and, according to a YouGov report, attendees at UK sports events believe that the food is unhealthy (Tobin, 2013). In Australia, where very few teams own the stadium in which they play, fans have also highlighted the lack of healthy options at venues, with some claiming that they cannot find healthy or fresh food at stadiums, and so do not eat there for this reason (Parry, Hall and Baxter, 2017). Indeed, observations by the authors at Australian stadiums reveal few fresh/healthy choices, with those that are available often unappealing in appearance and higher in price than less healthy alternatives. It should also be noted that stadium menus rarely provide nutrition information to allow spectators to make informed choices on their food. In Europe, stadiums are often found in less affluent areas, surrounded by low-quality housing whose inhabitants are more familiar with fast food-style options, and so it has been argued that fans in such venues either have poorer health literacy and are consequently unaware of the health implications of their food choices, or are generally satisfied with lower quality, less healthy food offerings (Drygas et al., 2013). However, as mentioned previously, sport often constitutes a release from everyday life, and so is not bound by the same rules as other spheres of participants' lives. As a consequence, even when fans eat healthily at other times, some see attending sport as an excuse to eat unhealthily – it is a guilty treat, and so they get 'into the spirit of it, and have a pie' (Ireland and Watkins, 2010, p. 684). In Australia, the meat pie is much more than an occasional treat; it is the nation's most popular fast-food choice, with 270 million sold each year (Barr, 2015). It is also a traditional accompaniment to sporting events, on a par with the hotdog in North America (Kovaricek 2010). In 2013, an iconic Australian venue, the Melbourne Cricket Ground (MCG), sold over 300,000 pies (Veenhuyzen, 2014). Other popular fast food choices at the MCG include hot chips (600,000 servings in 2013), jam doughnuts (95,000), burgers (65,000) and pizzas (40,000) (Rolfe, 2014).

Contrastingly, in North America there is a longer history of healthy food choices in stadiums, with Roan (1997) reporting the availability of frozen yoghurt, teriyaki bowls and fresh fruit at Major League Baseball (MLB) stadiums in the 1990s. More recently, New York City's Icahn Stadium has offered wraps, grilled sandwiches, pizzas made on whole-wheat pitas, and low-fat organic parfaits (Fabricant, 2005). Again, North American venues appear to lead the way with food-based healthy stadium initiatives. It is estimated that approximately a dozen North American venues have installed either organic gardens or farms, growing food both to use in the catering outlets and for donation to the local community. For instance, Fenway Park (home of the Boston Red Sox baseball team) has a 5,000-square-foot rooftop farm and San Jose Earthquakes' Avaya Stadium has an 'edible garden' which includes fruit trees. Produce from these two initiatives are used by the stadiums' concession providers (Johnston, 2015). Meanwhile, the MLB's San Diego Padres combine healthy and competitively priced foods with in-game physical activity breaks for spectators (Yancey *et al.*, 2009). Australian and European venues have much to learn from such initiatives.

Martin *et al.* (2008) identify that it is not just the quality of food that is a concern for fans; along with the choices available, they list the price of food as a point of dissatisfaction. Indeed, studies in Europe and Australia have found that fans are more concerned about the price of food than the availability of healthy options (Ireland and Watkins, 2010; Miles and Rincs, 2004; Parry, Hall and Baxter, 2017; Sukalakamala, Sukalakamala and Young, 2013). As in many other countries, the food available in Australian stadiums has been criticised by fans and the media for being overpriced (Tarbert, 2015), with rugby union fans describing the prices as 'extreme' and 'exorbitant' (Parry, Hall and Baxter, 2017). Similarly, British fans believe that venues '"played on their loyalty" [to a club] to ensure their custom, whatever the price' (Ireland and Watkins, 2010, p. 685). Fans expect to pay more for food and drink at venues (Martin and O'Neill, 2010), but they now demand 'value for money' and an improved customer experience.

For the current prices, increasingly savvy fans want higher quality options. Because of the aforementioned globalisation and commercialisation of sport, fans are aware of overseas prices and make comparisons with local offerings. Australians baulk when they are asked to pay AU$5 for a bottle of water or AU$5 for a pie of poor quality when they are aware that other venues maintain much lower prices and offer a wider range of options. British fans similarly believe that they are now more sophisticated in their culinary tastes and are prepared to challenge the traditional fare offered in stadiums (Ireland and Watkins, 2010). If sporting organisations are to increase stadium attendances, they will need to provide a range of quality, healthy food options to meet the needs of twenty-first century consumers.

In a bid to reduce spectator dissatisfaction and to enhance the in-stadium fan experience, a number of venues have innovations such as in-seat food delivery (Jones, 2015; PRNewswire, 2009), pre-ordering of food and drink to eliminate the need for queuing (IRFU, 2014; SCG, 2014), and smartphone apps that show the length of queues at concession stands (Parry, Hall and Baxter, 2017). The Western Sydney Wanderers, an Australian association football team, have even partnered with a leading cinema chain to provide a 'Gold Class Experience' at matches, with private catering delivered to superior-quality seats for an additional fee (WSWanderers, 2017). Such moves add a degree of comfort and luxury to the fan experience, but they also increase the amount of time that stadium attendees are sedentary during games and the price of consumption. Significantly, evidence suggests that breaking up prolonged bouts of sedentary behaviour can be beneficial for metabolic health (Healy *et al.*, 2008). Therefore, if stadiums are to play a role in health promotion, they may also need to introduce activities that encourage spectators to reduce their sedentary behaviour and engage in regular physical activity breaks – following the lead of teams such as the aforementioned San Diego Padres. Yet, it is not merely stadium food that may play a role in promoting a healthy lifestyle during the fan experience; stadium beverage offerings should also be considered.

The price and quality of drinks

While many of the world's stadiums offer a range of beverages for fans, watching sport is frequently associated with the consumption of alcohol. Sports fans are more likely to drink alcohol, engage in binge drinking, and report alcohol-related problems than nonfans (Nelson and Wechsler, 2003). It is young, male fans (in the 20- to 35-year-old age group) that are typically the heaviest consumers of alcohol at sports matches (Wolfe, Martinez and Scott, 1998). As Wenner and Jackson (2009) have recorded in their collection about the relationship between sport and beer across the world, there is a historically powerful connection between gendered identities and practices and beer consumption in sporting contexts. In Australia, beer is especially important to sport as a major sponsor and advertiser consistently producing images of active men and passively admiring women made available for the male gaze (McKay, Emmison and Mikosza, 2009; Rowe and Gilmour, 2009). The predominantly male fan subcultures routinely and often excessively consume alcohol (Palmer, 2010).

Sociologists Jim McKay *et al.* (2001) argue that a strong masculine inflexion heavily influences Australian sport and that, through sport, hegemonic forms of masculinity are asserted, promoted, and defended against alternative versions of masculinity and/or femininity. The ability to drink large volumes of alcohol symbolically represents this masculinity, and can be evidenced through spectator boasts over the number of beers that they will be able to drink, tales of their drunken exploits at previous games, and drunken fights (Parry, 2014). It is not only spectators that have turned drinking large volumes of beer into a national 'sport'. In 1994, Australian cricketer David Boon set a 'world record' by consuming 52 cans of beer during a flight from Sydney to London. Boon overtook another former cricketer, Rodney Marsh, who was the former holder of this record (McKay, Emmison and Mikosza, 2009). Such feats have been celebrated by Australian newspapers and as part of television advertising campaigns, positioning them as signifying heroic masculine ideals to be copied by fans.

This excessive masculinisation of Australian sport, allied with the consumption of large amounts of alcohol at sports matches, may be partially to blame for the large number of violent incidents observed at some Australian sporting venues. One of the country's oldest and premier sporting institutions, the Sydney Cricket and Sports Ground Trust, which runs the Sydney Cricket Ground (SCG) and Allianz Stadium, reported 12 violent incidents in 2015, and as a result was classified as one of the most violent venues in New South Wales (NSW) – the first time that a sporting venue had been included on this list (Nicholls, 2015). This is not a new phenomenon – indeed, in *Crowd Violence in Australian Sport* (O'Hara, 1992), Cashman (1992, p. 1) notes that 'Violence was very much part and parcel of sport in Sydney prior to 1850', while Cashman (1984) and Lynch (1992) detail many disorderly incidents up to the late twentieth century at Australian cricket grounds. The causal role of alcohol in these events is, of course, in question, but the sport-masculinity-beer-violence nexus is powerful and enduring.

In NSW, the sale of alcohol in stadiums is permitted under liquor laws through an on-premises licence allowing alcohol to be sold on premises where the supply of alcohol is not the primary source of business. Repeated violent alcohol-related offences mean that venues face increasingly harsh penalties that impact on which types of alcohol can be served, when it can be served, and in what quantities. In the event that these incidents are not addressed by the venue, they can be closed or have their ability to sell alcohol withdrawn. To mitigate such measures, those serving alcohol in venues are required to complete a Responsible Service of Alcohol (RSA) training course, which teaches employees to recognise signs of insobriety and so to help prevent spectators from becoming intoxicated. In addition, the drinks served in general bar areas are often low-strength or non-alcoholic, and spectators may be limited to buying four alcoholic drinks at a time. Indeed, the SCG has addressed alcohol-related issues with the 1998 introduction of a 'low alcohol beer policy for public concourse areas at international cricket fixtures', and of dedicated non-alcohol seating areas (Sydney Cricket and Sports Ground Trust, 2017). It is instructive to note that many North American venues go further and allow no more than two alcoholic drinks per single sale, with Soldier Field in Chicago only selling one beer per purchase in their seating areas during NFL games (Lenk *et al.*, 2010). However, such measures are largely enforced to limit public disorder rather than strictly for health promotion purposes.

Fans will often look for ways to circumvent the rules, regulations, and laws around alcohol consumption, and in 2004 the SCG Trust was required to take additional steps to outlaw 'beer wenches'. These are usually attractive females employed by a group of male fans to accompany them to the sporting matches for the purpose of acting as personal waitresses. This sexist practice brings attention to the male group, and reinforces their sense of hegemonic masculinity and its association with drinking at sporting matches. Because the beer wench serves the fans, their level of intoxication is never assessed by trained staff hired by the stadium and their vendors, thus breaching the venue's liquor licence. Consequently, the practice was outlawed by the SCG Trust (and subsequently other venues), much to the frustration of some male fans.

As with stadium food, the price of drinks at venues has been criticised in the media (Murray, 2016; Sutton, 2017) and identified as a point of dissatisfaction for Australian fans (Parry, Hall and Baxter, 2017). Parry and Hughes (2016) compared stadium beer prices in various European, North American, and Australian leagues and revealed that fans typically pay more inside stadiums than in other venues (see Table 11.1). For example, the average price for a beer in Australian stadiums was found to be AU$6.90, compared to an average of AU$6.44 across the country. Again, the higher prices in stadiums are not designed to limit the consumption of alcohol as part of a strategy that encourages spectators towards healthier lifestyles, but are aiming to increase profit margins.

It is not just the price of drinks that is a point of frustration for spectators. In Australia, the beer served in general admission sections is largely limited to low-mid strength options, as detailed earlier. This issue is being addressed to a degree by stadiums that have incorporated the growing boutique market of craft beers into their beverage offering (Parry and Hughes, 2016). Traditionally, craft brew options are focused more on the taste and overall drinking experience as opposed to the masculinist display associated with

Table 11.1 Average prices of beer in global leagues in 2016

League/Nation	Local price	Price in AU$ correct on 02/12/16	Average serving size	Standardised price AU$/100 ml
Bundesliga Germany	€3.85	5.59	478 ml	1.17
Premier League England	£3.99	6.76	568 ml	1.19
Various Australia	AU$6.68	6.90	401 ml	1.73
MLB USA	US$5.90	7.91	15 oz = 443.603 ml	1.78
NBA USA	US$7.5	10.14	18.23 oz = 539.223 ml	1.88
NHL USA	US$7.07	9.55	16 oz = 473.176 ml	2.02
NFL USA	US$7.38	9.99	16 oz = 473.176 ml	2.11

the consumption of more mainstream beers. It may, therefore, be that spectators focus on the quality of such products, rather than the quantity that they are able to consume.

Although NSW venues that serve alcohol are required to provide free drinking water as part of their on-premises licence, fans are encouraged to purchase bottled water (which also involves negative environmental consequences – Hawkins, Potter and Race, 2015) or fizzy drinks, with limited or no healthy alternatives, despite the sustained popularity of freshly squeezed or cold-pressed juices and 'smoothies'. Consumption of sugar-sweetened beverages, including fizzy drinks and sports drinks, has gained attention in recent years, and in an attempt to combat the obesity epidemic there is a push for countries including Australia to introduce a tax on these types of beverage and on unhealthy food (Thow, Dans and Jan, 2014; Veerman et al., 2016). As mentioned previously, the social obligation of stadiums and sporting organisations to promote a healthy lifestyle should be emphasised. If they are to do so, a holistic approach would be required, incorporating a healthy eating policy and commitments to measures such as at least one healthier food option within the stadium (Drygas et al., 2013). Yet, in a European study, few stadiums (only 16 out of 88) had such a policy, and only one-quarter employed a specially designated person to deal with food/healthy food issues. Although some venues have developed their own catering brands (Pierpoint, 2000), stadium food and drink is frequently outsourced to external contractors (Lee, Heere and Chung, 2013; Parry, Hall and Baxter, 2017), thereby significantly relinquishing control over the options made available to spectators (Drygas et al., 2013) and the quality and value for money that they can receive (Pierpoint, 2000). These external contractors are often large organisations which can negotiate advantageous deals with food providers (Ackerman, 1994), typically aiming to minimise their costs. Food and beverages that are cheap to produce, such as low-quality pies and other fast food options, generally provide greater returns than more expensive or more time intensive, healthier alternatives. However, the venue must still take responsibility for the food and beverage contracts that it signs, and can make the provision of reasonably priced healthy offerings a key contractual condition.

As noted by Drygas et al. (2013), it is often fast food, fizzy drinks, alcohol, gambling, and (previously) tobacco companies that are the main sponsors of sport, particularly for mega events and venues, making sport stadiums a difficult setting for health promotion. Although several studies have investigated the negative impact of (less healthy) food and beverage companies sponsoring sporting events (Carter et al., 2012; Garde and Rigby, 2012; Sherriff, Griffiths and Daube, 2010), there may be little appetite from venues and sports organisations to sever or loosen ties with their most profitable sponsors. Consequently, health-promoting policies regarding stadium food are difficult to introduce, and require a series of interventions involving both voluntary measures and binding regulations.

The way forward for stadium food and drink in Australia (and elsewhere)

Parry, Hall and Baxter (2017) provide a list of principles that healthier stadium food options should follow for them to be considered realistic alternatives to the current stadium fare. Their list includes: being at a similar or better price than existing offerings; being quick to order/be served and easy to eat using one hand; portion controlled; and to be an existing popular choice in the city where the stadium is located. They cite the Australian version of the Japanese Nori or sushi roll as an example for Sydney-based stadiums to adopt. In addition, Parry and Hughes (2016) make a series of suggestions for Australian stadiums to improve their beverage (and, in particular, their beer) offerings. They identify innovations such as: making locally brewed craft beer available; measures to keep beer colder for longer (and presumably reduce the need to drink it quickly); and the introduction of designated driver programs which provide nominated drivers with free soft drinks. To these points, a further set of recommendations for venues are now added:

- Accessible nutrition information, particularly nutrient values for stadium food should be included at the point of sale (as is now common on much packaged food). Recent legislation in several Australian states requires the energy content of meals and menu items to be shown on menu boards in restaurants along with information on the average daily adult energy intake. While it has been found that energy menu labelling reduces the energy content of purchases, Wellard et al. (2015), in their study of nutrition information in fast food outlets, argue that more detailed information is required for customers to be able to make informed decisions on the nutritional value of food at stadiums.

- It is also recommended that stadiums publish menus online (with prices and nutrition information) to allow spectators to make reasonable decisions on their food and beverage options in advance of their arrival at venues.
- Venues should provide healthier beverage options, capitalising on the rising popularity of squeezed/pressed juices and smoothies.
- More venues should include activities that encourage spectators to be physically active at games.
- At a wider level, sporting organisations should also consider the ethical issues arising from partnering with companies associated with unhealthy lifestyle choices (such as fast food, fizzy drinks, alcohol, and gambling companies).
- Finally, stadiums in Australia and Europe should consider following the examples of North American venues and install organic gardens to supply healthy produce for their catering outlets.

Sporting stadiums offer a unique opportunity to promote healthy lifestyle choices. The above recommendations reflect public health messages, current research evidence, and fan perceptions. Sports organisations and venues need to take them into account if they are to invest in the health and wellbeing of their fans and wider community. After all, given that sporting activity is widely celebrated and often publicly subsidised as health affirming, attending a stadium to watch it being performed should not have an unduly unhealthy impact on the bodies and the bank accounts of co-present spectators.

References

ABS (2010). *Spectator Attendance at Sporting Events, 2009–10*. Australian Bureau of Statistics: Canberra.

ABS (2012). *Sport and Recreation: A Statistical Overview*. Australian Bureau of Statistics: Canberra.

ABS (2015). *4177.0 – Participation in Sport and Physical Recreation, Australia, 2013–14*. Australian Bureau of Statistics: Canberra.

Ackerman, M. A. (1994). Privatization of public-assembly-facility management. *The Cornell Hotel and Restaurant Administration Quarterly*, 35 (2), 72–83.

AIHW (2017). Overweight and obesity. *Australian Institute of Health and Wellness*, viewed 22 February 2017, http://aihw.gov.au/overweight-and-obesity/

Anagnostopoulos, C. (2011). From Corporate Social Responsibility (CSR) to . . . Club Stakeholder Relationship (CSR): the case of football. *The Social Responsibility Review*, 3, 4–7.

ASC (2016). AusPlay: participation data for the sport sector. *Australian Sports Commission*, www.ausport.gov.au/__data/assets/pdf_file/0007/653875/34648_AusPlay_summary_report_accessible_FINAL_updated_211216.pdf

Barr, E. (2015). Meat pies are Australia's national fast food choice, with Australians eating 270 million every year, viewed 5 July 2016, http://dailytelegraph.com.au/newslocal/inner-west/meat-pies-are-australias-national-fast-food-choice-with-australians-eating-270-million-every-year/news-story/3ab90bcb3467d1b57203cfbbc065fdbc

Barrett, C. (2016). Big Bash League jumps into top 10 of most attended sports leagues in the world, viewed 20 January 2016, http://smh.com.au/sport/cricket/big-bash-league-jumps-into-top-10-of-most-attended-sports-leagues-in-the-world-20160110-gm2w8z.html

Bauman, A., Bellew, B., and Craig, C. L. (2014). Did the 2000 Sydney Olympics increase physical activity among adult Australians? *British Journal of Sports Medicine*, 49(4), 243.

Bennett, T., Emmison, M., and Frow, J. (2001). Social class and cultural practice in contemporary Australia. In T. Bennett and D. Carter (eds), *Culture in Australia: Policies, Publics and Programs* (pp. 193–216). Cambridge: Cambridge University Press.

Booth, D. (2000). 'Surf lifesaving: the development of an Australasian "sport"'. *The International Journal of the History of Sport*, 17 (2–3), 166–87.

Carter, M.-A., Edwards, R., Signal, L., and Hoek, J. (2012). Availability and marketing of food and beverages to children through sports settings: a systematic review. *Public Health Nutr*, 15(8), 1373–9.

Cashman, R. (1984). *'Ave a Go Yer Mug! Australian Cricket Crowds from Larrikin to Ocker*. Collins: Sydney.

Cashman, R. (1992). Violence in sport in Sydney before 1850. In J. O'Hara (ed.), *Australian Society for Sports History Studies in Sports History Number 7* (pp. 1–9).

Cashmore, E. (2005), *Making Sense of Sports*, 4th edn. London: Routledge.

Caspersen, C. J., Powell, K. E., and Christenson, G. M. (1985). Physical activity, exercise, and physical fitness: definitions and distinctions for health-related research. *Public Health Reports (1974–)*, 100(2), 126–31.

Craig, C. L. and Bauman, A. E. (2014). The impact of the Vancouver Winter Olympics on population level physical activity and sport participation among Canadian children and adolescents: population based study. *International Journal of Behavioral Nutrition and Physical Activity*, 11(1), 107.

Department of Health (2014). *More Than Half of All Australian Adults Are Not Active Enough*. Canberra, Australia: Department of Health, Commonwealth of Australia.

Dollman, J. and Lewis, N. (2010). The impact of socioeconomic position on sport participation among South Australian youth. *Journal of Science and Medicine in Sport*, 13(3), 318–22.

Drygas, W., Ruszkowska, J., Philpott, M., Björkström, O., Parker, M., Ireland, R., Roncarolo, F., and Tenconi, M. (2013). Good practices and health policy analysis in European sports stadia: results from the 'Healthy Stadia' project. *Health Promotion International*, 28(2), 157–65.

Eime, R. M., Harvey, J., Brown, W., and Payne, W. (2010). Does sports club participation contribute to health-related quality of life? *Med Sci Sports Exerc*, 42.

Eime, R. M., Young, J. A., Harvey, J. T., Charity, M. J., and Payne, W. R. (2013) A systematic review of the psychological and social benefits of participation in sport for adults: informing development of a conceptual model of health through sport. *International Journal of Behavioral Nutrition and Physical Activity*, 10, 135.

Fabricant, F. (2005). Healthier food lineup at new stadium. *New York Times*, 27 April 2005, p. 10.

Garde, A. and Rigby, N. (2012). Going for gold – should responsible governments raise the bar on sponsorship of the Olympic Games and other sporting events by food and beverage companies? *Communications Law*, 17(2), 42–9.

Grøntved, A. and Hu, F. (2011). Television viewing and risk of type 2 diabetes, cardiovascular disease, and all-cause mortality: a meta-analysis. *JAMA*, 305(23), 2448–55.

Hallinan, C. J., Hughson, J. E., and Burke, M. (2007). Supporting the 'world game' in Australia: a case study of fandom at national and club level. *Soccer & Society*, 8(2–3), 283–97.

Hardy, L. L., Kelly, B., Chapman, K., King, L., and Farrell, L. (2010). Parental perceptions of barriers to children's participation in organised sport in Australia. *Journal of Paediatrics and Child Health*, 46(4), 197–203.

Harris, J. (2008). Match day in Cardiff: (re)imaging and (re)imagining the nation. *Journal of Sport & Tourism*, 13(4), 297–313.

Hawkins, G, Potter, E., and Race, K. (2015). *Plastic Water: The Social and Material Life of Bottled Water Opens*. Cambridge, MA: The MIT Press.

Healy, G., Dunstan, D., Salmon, J., Cerin, E., Shaw, J., Zimmet, P., and Owen, N. (2008). Breaks in sedentary time: beneficial associations with metabolic risk. *Diabetes Care*, 31(4), 661–6.

Ho, E. (2012). World's biggest McDonald's restaurant is coming to the London Olympics. *Time*, viewed 1 March 2017, http://olympics.time.com/2012/05/02/worlds-biggest-mcdonalds-restaurant-is-coming-to-the-london-olympics/

Inoue, Y., Yli-Piipari, S., Layne, T., Chambliss, H., and Irwin, C. (2015). A preliminary study of a professional sport organization's family-centered health promotion initiative. *International Review on Public and Nonprofit Marketing*, 12(2), 189–205.

Ireland, R. and Watkins, F. (2010). Football fans and food: a case study of a football club in the English Premier League. *Public Health Nutrition*, 13(5), 682–7.

IRFU (2014). Beat the queue at Aviva Stadium with 'My order app', viewed 19 April 2015. http://irishrugby.ie/news/30247.php

Johnston, M. W. (2015). Sports teams build food recovery awareness. *BioCycle*, 56(5), 34–8.

Jones, C. (2002). The stadium and economic development: Cardiff and the Millennium Stadium. *European Planning Studies*, 10(7), 819–29.

Jones, G. (2015). New app will allow football lovers to have food ordered and delivered to their stadium seats, viewed 19 April 2015. http://dailytelegraph.com.au/lifestyle/food/new-app-will-allow-football-lovers-to-have-food-ordered-and-delivered-to-their-stadium-seats/story-fnov1g0j-1227238025816

Kell, P. (2000). *Good Sports: Australian Sport and the Myth of the Fair Go*. Pluto Press, Annandale.

Ko, Y. J., Zhang, J., Cattani, K., and Pastore, D. (2011). Assessment of event quality in major spectator sports. *Managing Service Quality*, 21(3), 304–22.

Kovaricek, E. (2010). The glorious meat pie and humble pie floater, *ABC Adelaide*, viewed 20 July 2015. http://blogs.abc.net.au/sa/2010/05/the-glorious-meat-pie-and-humble-pie-floater.html?site=adelaide&program=adelaide_afternoons

Lambrecht, K. W., Kaefer, F., and Ramenofsky, S. D. (2009). Sportscape factors influencing spectator attendance and satisfaction at a professional golf association tournament. *Sports Marketing Quarterly*, 18(3), 165–72.

Lee, S., Heere, B., and Chung, K.-S. (2013). Which senses matter more? The impact of our senses on team identity and team loyalty. *Sport Marketing Quarterly*, 22(4), 203–13.

Lee, S. S., Parrish, C., and Kim, J.-H. (2015). Sports stadiums as meeting and corporate/social event venues: a perspective from meeting/event planners and sport facility administrators. *Journal of Quality Assurance in Hospitality & Tourism*, 16(2), 164–80.

Lenk, K. M., Toomey, T. L., Erickson, D. J., Kilian, G. R., Nelson, T. F., and Fabian, L. E. A. (2010). Alcohol control policies and practices at professional sports stadiums. *Public Health Reports (1974–)*, 125(5), 665–73.

Lynch, R. (1992). A symbolic patch of grass: crowd disorder and regulation on the Sydney Cricket Ground hill. In J. O'Hara (ed.) *Australian Society for Sports History Studies in Sports History Number* (pp. 7, 10–48).

Maguire, J. A. (2001). *Global Sport: Identities, Societies, Civilizations*. Cambridge: Polity.

Mahtani, K. R., Protheroe, J., Slight, S. P., Demarzo, M. M. P., Blakeman, T., Barton, C. A., Brijnath, B., and Roberts, N. (2013). Can the London 2012 Olympics 'inspire a generation' to do more physical or sporting activities? An overview of systematic reviews. *BMJ Open*, 3(1).

Mandell, R. D. (1999). *Sport: A Cultural History*. New York: Columbia University Press.

Martin, A., Morgan, S., Parnell, D., Philpott, M., Pringle, A., Rigby, M., Taylor, A., and Topham, J. (2016). A perspective from key stakeholders on football and health improvement. *Soccer & Society*, 17(2), 175–82.

Martin, D., O'Neill, M., Hubbard, S., and Palmer, A. (2008). The role of emotion in explaining consumer satisfaction and future behavioural intention. *Journal of Services Marketing*, 22(3), 224–36.

Martin, D. S. and O'Neill, M. (2010). Scale development and testing: a new measure of cognitive satisfaction in sports tourism. *Event Management*, 14 (1), 1–15.

McKay, J., Lawrence, G., Miller, T., and Rowe, D. (2001). Gender equity, hegemonic masculinity and the governmentalisation of Australian amateur sport. In T. Bennett and D. Carter (eds), *Culture in Australia: Policies, Publics and Programs* (pp. 233–52). Cambridge: Cambridge University Press.

McKay, J., Emmison, M., and Mikosza, J. (2009). Lads, larrikins and mates: hegemonic masculinities in Australian beer advertisements. In L. Wenner and S. Jackson (eds), *Sport, Beer, & Gender: Promotional Culture and Contemporary Social Life* (pp. 163–179). New York: Peter Lang.

Miles, L. and Rines, S. (2004). *Football Sponsorship & Commerce: An Analysis of Sponsorship and Commercial Opportunities in Football*. Buckfastleigh, UK: International Marketing Reports.

Murray, O. (2016). How the cost of beer at Australian sporting events compares to rest of the world, *news.com.au*, viewed 19 December 2016. http://news.com.au/sport/sports-life/how-the-cost-of-beer-at-australian-sporting-events-compares-to-rest-of-the-world/news-story/78ffd150a2e2bacdcfc8dd2d4ad537a3

National Health and Medical Research Council (2013). *Australian Dietary Guidelines: Summary*, viewed 23 February 2017. https://nhmrc.gov.au/guidelines-publications/n55

Nelson, T. F. and Wechsler, H. (2003). School spirits: alcohol and collegiate sports fans. *Addictive Behaviors*, 28(1), 1–11.

Nicholls, S. (2015). Sydney Cricket Ground Trust on most violent venues list, *Sydney Morning Herald*, viewed 28 February 2016. http://smh.com.au/nsw/sydney-cricket-ground-trust-on-most-violent-venues-list-20151127-gl9mh2.html

Nielsen (2014). *Year in the Sports Media Report: 2013*, viewed 4 April 2014. http://nielsen.com/us/en/insights/reports/2014/year-in-the-sports-media-report-2013.html

Osborne, A. C. and Coombs, D. S. (2013). Performative Sport Fandom: an approach to retheorizing sport fans. *Sport in Society*, 16(5), 672–81.

Palmer, C. (2010). Everyday risks and professional dilemmas: fieldwork with alcohol-based (sporting) subcultures. *Qualitative Research*, 10(4), 421–40.

Parnell, D., Pringle, A., McKenna, J., Zwolinsky, S., Rutherford, Z., Hargreaves, J., Trotter, L., Rigby, M., and Richardson, D. (2015). Reaching older people with PA delivered in football clubs: the reach, adoption and implementation characteristics of the Extra Time Programme. *BMC Public Health*, 15(1), 220.

Parry, K. D. (2014). Boxing Day Test: sunny spectacle on a stadium-sized stage, *The Conversation*, viewed 26 December 2014. https://theconversation.com/boxing-day-test-sunny-spectacle-on-a-stadium-sized-stage-34300

Parry, K. D., Hall, T., and Baxter, A. (2017). Who ate all the pies? The importance of food in the Australian sporting experience. *Sport in Society*, 20(2), 202–18.

Parry, K. D. and Hughes, B. (2016). The price is not right: how much is too much for a beer at sporting events?, *The Conversation*. https://theconversation.com/the-price-is-not-right-how-much-is-too-much-for-a-beer-at-sporting-events-69708

Parry, K. D., Jones, I., and Wann, D. L. (2014). An examination of sport fandom in the United Kingdom: a comparative analysis of fan behaviors, socialization processes, and team identification. *Journal of Sport Behavior*, 37(3), 251–67.

Pierpoint, B. (2000). 'Heads above water': business strategies for a new football economy. *Soccer & Society*, 1(1), 29–38.

PRNewswire (2009). In-seat food delivery available stadium-wide at Rio Tinto. *PR Newswire*, 23 July 2009.

Roan, S. (1997). Buy me some peanuts and yogurt? Food: survey finds healthy choices have become available at all major league stadiums. *Los Angeles Times*, 11 June 1997, pp. 3–4.

Rolfe, P. (2014). Price rises for food and drink at MCG and Etihad Stadium hit footy fans, *Herald Sun*, viewed 10 August 2014. www.heraldsun.com.au/news/victoria/price-rises-for-food-and-drink-at-mcg-and-etihad-stadium-hit-footy-fans/news-story/98f16a4aeb80c146764058f9aba481df

Rookwood, J. and Millward, P. (2011). 'We all dream of a team of Carraghers': comparing 'local' and Texan Liverpool fans' talk. *Sport in Society*, 14(1), 37–52.

Rossi, M. (2016). Game on! Live sport dominates Aussie TV viewing over the past 15 years, *Nielsen*, viewed 16 August 2016. http://nielsen.com/au/en/insights/news/2016/game-on-live-sport-dominates-aussie-tv-viewing-over-the-past-15-years.html

Rowe, D. (2017). Australia needs to make sport a more equal playing field: here's why. *The Conversation*, 17 January. https://theconversation.com/australia-needs-to-make-sport-a-more-equal-playing-field-heres-why-71144

Rowe, D. (2013). Sport: scandal, gender and the nation. *Institute for Culture and Society Occasional Paper Series*, 4(3), 1–17.

Rowe, D. (2011). *Global Media Sport: Flows, Forms and Futures*. London and New York: Bloomsbury Academic.

Rowe, D. (2004). *Sport, Culture and the Media: The Unruly Trinity*, 2nd edn. Maidenhead, UK and New York: Open University Press/McGraw-Hill Education.

Rowe, D. and Gilmour, C. (2009). Lubrication and domination: beer, sport, masculinity and the Australian gender order. In L. Wenner and S. Jackson (eds), *Sport, Beer, & Gender: Promotional Culture and Contemporary Social Life* (pp. 203–21). New York: Peter Lang.

SCG (2014). Fact sheet on new grandstands, viewed 19 April 2015. http://sydney cricketground.com.au/news/2014-ashes-media-kit/new-grandstands/fact-sheet-on-new-grandstands/

Sherriff, J., Griffiths, D., and Daube, M. (2010). Cricket: notching up runs for food and alcohol companies? *Australian and New Zealand Journal of Public Health*, 34(1), 19–23.

Spaaij, R. (2012). Beyond the playing field: experiences of sport, social capital, and integration among Somalis in Australia. *Ethnic and Racial Studies*, 35(9), 1519–38.

Stensholt, J. (2014). NRL, AFL aim to get fans back in seats, *Australian Financial Review*, viewed 1 October 2015. http://afr.com/business/nrl-afl-aim-to-get-fans-back-in-seats-20140810-j76iq

Stewart, B. (1990). Leisure and the changing patterns of sport and exercise. In D. Rowe and G. Lawrence (eds), *Sport and Leisure: Trends in Australian Popular Culture* (pp. 174–88). Sydney: Harcourt Brace Jovanovich.

Sukalakamala, P., Sukalakamala, S., and Young, P. (2013). An exploratory study of the concession preferences of generation Y consumers. *Journal of Foodservice Business Research*, 16(4), 378–90.

Sutton, M. (2017). Adelaide Oval's 'ridiculous' food prices and ticket costs making it 'untenable' for families: punters, *ABC*, viewed 22 February 2017. http://abc.net.au/news/2017-02-22/prices-at-adelaide-oval-becoming-untenable-for-families/8289382

Sydney Cricket & Sports Ground Trust (2017). Alcohol policy, viewed 8 March 2017. http://sydneycricketground.com.au/news/2014-ashes-media-kit/faq-crowd-policies/alcohol-policy/

Tarbert, K. (2015). High cost of hydration: sports stadiums facing pressure to reduce food and drink prices, *The Daily Telegraph*, viewed 20 July 2015. http://daily telegraph.com.au/newslocal/west/high-cost-of-hydration-sports-stadiums-facing-pressure-to-reduce-food-and-drink-prices/story-fngr8i5s-1227245839561

Thow, A. M., Downs, S., and Jan, S. (2014). A systematic review of the effectiveness of food taxes and subsidies to improve diets: understanding the recent evidence. *Nutrition Reviews*, 72(9), 551–65.

Tobin, B. (2013). Stadium food is bottom of the league for sports fans, viewed 20 January 2016. https://yougov.co.uk/news/2013/12/19/stadium-food-bottom-league-sports-fans/

Veenhuyzen, M. (2014). Meat pie: a great Australian dish, *The Guardian*, viewed 20 July 2015. http://theguardian.com/lifeandstyle/australia-food-blog/2014/may/07/meat-pie-a-great-australian-dish

Veerman, J. L., Sacks, G., Antonopoulos, N., and Martin, J. (2016). The impact of a tax on sugar-sweetened beverages on health and health care costs: a modelling study. *Plos One*, 11(4), p. e0151460.

Wakefield, K. L. and Sloan, H. J. (1995). The effects of team loyalty and selected stadium factors on spectator attendance. *Journal of Sport Management*, 9(2), 153–72.

Wellard, L., Havill, M., Hughes, C., Watson, W. L., and Chapman, K. (2015). The availability and accessibility of nutrition information in fast food outlets in five states post-menu labelling legislation in New South Wales. *Australian and New Zealand Journal of Public Health*, 39(6), 546–9.

Wenner, L. and Jackson, S. (eds). (2009). *Sport, Beer, & Gender: Promotional Culture and Contemporary Social Life*. New York: Peter Lang.

White, M. (2004). Feeding your face: fan fare and status at a Sumo tournament. *Gastronomica*, 4(1), 54.

WHO (2015). *Healthy Diet*, World Health Organisation, viewed 28 January 2016. http://who.int/mediacentre/factsheets/fs394/en/

WHO (2017). *Australia: Health Profile*, World Health Organisation, viewed 27 February 2017. http://wpro.who.int/countries/aus/2AUSpro2011_finaldraft.pdf?ua=1

Wolfe, J., Martinez, R., and Scott, W. A. (1998). Baseball and beer: an analysis of alcohol consumption patterns among male spectators at major-league sporting events. *Annals of Emergency Medicine*, 31(5), 629–32.

WSWanderers (2017). Experience gold class at Wanderland, viewed 23 February 2017. http://wswanderersfc.com.au/article/gold-class-at-wanderland/ufuc5nxwlicb1h80envh0oah6

Yancey, A., Winfield, D., Larsen, J., Anderson, M., Jackson, P., Overton, J., Wilson, S., Rossum, A. and Kumanyika, S. (2009) 'Live, Learn and Play': building strategic alliances between professional sports and public health. *Preventive Medicine*, 49(4), 322–5.

Chapter 12

Healthy Stadia

A settings-based approach to health promotion

Daniel Parnell, Kathryn Curran and Matthew Philpott

Introduction

Public health is a major concern of our time, with healthy lives and wellbeing listed as one of the United Nations key Sustainable Development Goals (Goal 3: Ensure healthy lives and promote wellbeing for all at all ages). Public health focuses on the entire spectrum of health and wellbeing, not only the eradication of particular diseases, and has been defined as 'the art and science of preventing disease, prolonging life and promoting health through the organised efforts of society' (Acheson, 1988). Importantly, public health considers health and wellbeing through the preventative lens of population groups as opposed to individual illnesses. At the same time, research suggests that there are growing health inequalities in the Western world (Marmot *et al.*, 2010), which may already have been exacerbated as a result of the economic downturn and subsequent austerity policy measures in many countries (Rukert and Ronald, 2017). In response to ongoing public health concerns such as the development of non-communicable diseases (i.e., cardiovascular disease, Type 2 diabetes, a range of cancers, and the debilitating effects of mental health issues across the life-course), a number of public health strategies and programmes of work at both global and national level have been implemented.

One increasingly successful health promotion strategy is the concept of a 'settings-based approach' to promote health and reduce health inequalities. The World Health Organization's (WHO) Ottawa Charter began the momentum towards this new way of bringing to bear public health resources on everyday sites of mass interaction (WHO, 1986). This helped shift the emphasis away from the individual and towards the living environment and organisational structures where people lived, worked, socialised and gathered (WHO, 1986). The settings-based approach has been implemented successfully in a number of locations where populations interact and gather, including hospitals (i.e., Healthy Hospitals (Johnson, 2000; Pelikan *et al.*, 2001)), schools (i.e., Healthy Schools (Clift and Jensen, 2005), prisons (i.e., Healthy Prison Programmes (Whitehead, 2006; Møller *et al.*, 2007), and workplaces (i.e., Healthy Cities (De Leeuw and Skovgaard, 2005).

Given the recognition afforded to the settings-based approach to health promotion, reflected in policies and statements by international stakeholders, there has been a recognised increase in sports-based health initiatives (Parnell and Richardson, 2014; Parnell and Pringle, 2016; Parnell, Curran and Philpott, 2017). Furthermore, the hyper commodification of sport has seen increasing interest, expectation and pressure from stakeholders, to deliver a social return on their operations, whether with fans, within their stadia or local community (Anagnostopoulos and Shilbury, 2013; Parnell *et al.*, 2013). In particular there has been a rise in interest from governments, club owners and researchers in how sports venues can provide a setting to both deliver on corporate objectives *and* public health outcomes (Drygas, *et al.*, 2013).

The Healthy Stadia movement

It was during the mid-2000s that a group of sports clubs and venue operators pioneered the way for a nascent healthy stadia movement. The club and venues, located in the North West region of the United Kingdom, catered for rugby league, horseracing and football, with many additional sports such as cycling, rugby union, cricket and multipurpose venues joining this initial network in the years following. Their initial endeavour was coordinated by the cardiovascular disease prevention charity, Heart of Mersey. The primary aim of this work was to trial new healthy stadia initiatives across a variety of different sports using the following definition of a healthy stadia setting:

> *Healthy Stadia are . . . those which promote the health of visitors, fans, players, employees and the surrounding community . . . places where people can go to have a positive healthy experience playing or watching sport.*
>
> (see Crabb and Ratinckx, 2005)

Such initiatives at participating venues included policies and interventions to promote healthy lifestyles incorporating three cross-cutting themes: (i) healthier stadium environments for fans and non-match day visitors (e.g. smoke-free environments); (ii) healthier club workforces (e.g. active transport options for staff commuting to work); and (iii) delivering against the health needs of local communities (e.g. childhood obesity interventions). Examples of this early work included:

- Declaring stadiums completely smoke-free for all users at least 18 months ahead of national smoke-free legislation which came into effect in the United Kingdom in 2007
- Displaying and promoting the fruit and vegetable 5-a-day message to supporters and visitors. For one stadium this included a fruit delivery

scheme in the main reception area, with a range of healthier food choice options made available in staff canteens.

- Players' diets and healthy eating messages were included on club websites in a 'Healthy Stadia' section.
- Local health walks were developed to and from stadia for both fans and staff with encouragement to progress to more advanced exercise, with pedometers provided.

Following this initial work and interest from venues in the United Kingdom, Heart of Mersey was successful in securing funding from the EU's Public Health Programme in 2007 to run a 30-month project entitled 'Sports Stadia and Community Health – European Healthy Stadia Programme'. Working in partnership with public health, sports and research agencies in Finland, Greece, Italy, Latvia, Ireland, Poland, Spain and the United Kingdom, the project was tasked with piloting the healthy stadia concept with clubs and stadia in a cross-section of European countries.

Building on an initial evidence base garnered through a current practice survey among sports venues in Europe, the key deliverable from this European project was a Healthy Stadia guidance 'Toolkit'. This document was aimed at stadium management and intermediary partner agencies, and drew heavily on pilot projects that were run with sports stadia in Finland, Ireland, Spain and Latvia. The toolkit provides users with a walk-through of the basic steps needed to roll out Healthy Stadia initiatives, such as putting an action plan together, finding partners, evaluating interventions and embedding healthy initiatives. The guidance is supported by a host of case studies drawn together from stadia participating in the programme, which are grouped under the broad public health themes of lifestyle, social and environmental.

This EU-funded project set the foundations for the initiation of a 'European Healthy Stadia Network', to act as a facility for sharing good practice and emerging research among clubs, stadium operators, governing bodies of sport, public health practitioners and academic institutions. Healthy Stadia is now an established and successful social enterprise based in the United Kingdom with over 300 members from a cross-section of European countries, and long-term partnerships established with the World Heart Federation and the Union of European Football Associations (UEFA) (http://healthystadia.eu/).

The EU 'Sport Stadia and Community Health' project, is one of five EU-funded health and sport programme Healthy Stadia has participated in as either coordinating of partners agency since 2010. This has included work with young people not in education, employment or training – NEETs (Health 25), a programme enhancing the health and well-being education of young performance level athletes (Fit 4 Health), a new programme on health enhancing physical activity advocacy (Active Voice) and a ground-breaking 5-year clinical research project entitled EuroFIT, improving levels of physical activity and reducing sedentary time in male football fans.

Healthy Stadia is considered a spearhead in advocating for sports stadia, clubs and governing bodies of sport to develop health-promoting sports settings. Healthy stadia practices, policies and research have grown over the last decade across a wide number of different sports and European settings. It is apparent that clubs, governing bodies of sport, league operators and – perhaps most importantly outside of sport – agencies commissioning public health interventions, are beginning to recognise that sports settings offer a unique opportunity for health promotion. Such growth includes population-level approaches to improving public health (e.g. smoke-free stadia at sports mega events such as UEFA EURO, Olympic Games and FIFA World Cup), and targeted interventions attempting to change the individual behaviours of target groups (e.g. addressing low levels of physical activity and sedentary behaviour in male football fans).

Healthy Stadia toolkits and guidance documents

Healthy Stadia also play an important role capturing and sharing examples of good practice across its network of members and decision makers within clubs, governing bodies of sport, league operators and agencies commissioning health interventions. In order to encourage further uptake of good practices, Healthy Stadia has developed a number of themed toolkits and guidance documents to advocate and assist clubs and stadium operators in adopting population level public health policies. In addition to Healthy Stadia assessments of competition venues (e.g. UEFA club competition host venues), and the development of healthy lifestyle intervention toolkits for events and campaigns such as EURO 2012 and the annual World Heart Day, Healthy Stadia has worked with a range of partners to develop step-by-step guidelines and training modules concerning:

- Active travel to sports stadia (2014)
- Development and enforcement of tobacco-free sports venues (2016)
- Online healthier catering benchmarking and guidance (2017)

(To view guidance see: http://healthystadia.eu)

There have been some considerable successes in the area of tobacco control and sports stadia over the last 5 years, both in terms of advocacy and policy change. Healthy Stadia has worked closely with UEFA over the last 6 years to ensure tobacco-free environments at club competition finals, and the European football championships (EURO) in 2012 and 2016. Further, in 2016 Healthy Stadia launched its tobacco-free guidance and training documents through a programme of work with governing bodies of sport and other key stakeholders in European sport and health, advocating for all European sport venues to be completely smoke-free by the year 2020 (Parnell, Curran and Philpott, 2017). Already, this work is starting to pay dividends, with a number of clubs and league operators in countries such as Netherlands and Belgium pledging their support for tobacco-free stadium environments that exceed national tobacco control legislation.

The rise of research and evaluation

In recent years there has been a rise in the interest, volume of academic papers and wide range of academic research and evaluation on the role of sports stadia and related public health interventions (see Parnell, Curran and Philpott, 2017). Examples of this work include; using a club's badge (or brand) to engage fans and communicate positive messages on health-related behaviours on match days and non-match days including engaging match going fans in health screening, contact with health services, and disseminating positive health related messages through the sport clubs' official channels (Witty and White, 2011; Curran, Drust and Richardson, 2014; Trivedy et al., 2017). Other examples include; the introduction of healthier catering options in sports stadia (Ireland and Watkins, 2010), the exposure of fans to unhealthy sponsorship logos and advertising (Sherriff, Griffiths, and Daube, 2009), the development of smoke-free and tobacco-free sports venues (Philpott and Sagar, 2014), and the development of sport-club and foundation-led community physical activity and health programmes targeting a range of at-risk and hard-to-reach populations (Hunt et al., 2014; Parnell and Richardson, 2014; Curran et al., 2014; Hulton et al., 2015; Parnell et al., 2015; Curran et al., 2016; Parnell and Pringle, 2016). Research is a key strand in substantiating and further developing the Healthy Stadia agenda, and it is incumbent upon Healthy Stadia and a range of wider stakeholders to ensure that research findings are widely disseminated to policy holders and relevant practitioners.

An important and significant moment for the healthy stadia movement, was the publication of a special issue on the 20th Anniversary of the Routledge journal Sport in Society, titled *Healthy Stadia: An Insight From Policy to Practice* (Parnell, Curran and Philpott, 2017). The volume examines the relationship between professional and amateur sport clubs, stadia and health promotion, through a collection of papers aligned to philosophical, political, environmental and practical health-related interventions enabled through sport stadia settings. Notably, the collection of articles, commentaries and research notes offer an insight into sport stadia as a setting for public health promotion and sport-based physical activity and health-promotion programmes delivered by amateur and professional sport clubs.

Insights and considerations: case study examples

In order to provide industry and research insights into considerations for promoting public health within sport stadia settings, the following are three case study examples drawn from this collection of papers (Parnell, Curran and Philpott, 2017). First, we offer an insight into the process and results of delivering health checks to fans at professional cricket venues on match days (Trivedy et al., 2017). Next, we explore the impact of a community-based physical activity intervention delivered by a professional football club which engaged hard-to-reach men (Lewis, Reeves and Roberts, 2017). Finally, we consider the community impact of artificial grass football pitches: a case study of Maidstone United FC (May and Parnell, 2017).

Health checks at professional cricket matches

In the United Kingdom, a population level health screening programme was established for people over the age of 40 years, which has been delivered by the National Health Service since 2009. The focus of this service was to identify and treat the leading causes of preventable disease and death, including cardiovascular disease and diabetes. Data showed that in 2013 there were over 3.2 million diabetics living in the United Kingdom and this figure was projected to increase to 5 million by 2025 (Diabetes UK, 2013). The costs associated with treating these conditions are extremely high, with diabetes alone costing £10 billion pounds a year in the United Kingdom (or 10 per cent of the annual NHS budget. Checks are offered every 5 years through scheduled appointments at primary care settings, and uptake of such checks has been relatively low to date with 12.7 per cent of those eligible to have a NHS health check receiving one between 2009 and 2013 (Robson et al., 2016).

Non-clinical settings such as sports stadia have previously been used to offer health interventions and opportunistic health checks. The efficacy of such projects to date has been mixed, with lower than anticipated levels of engagement from fans in health-related behaviours, and time pressures being cited as a main barrier to participation (Witty and White, 2011; Curran, Drust, and Richardson, 2014). Despite these relatively modest results in football and rugby settings, professional cricket fixtures may offer high footfall and higher levels of uptake and participant satisfaction, and provide a novel setting for engaging BME communities. This research concerned the process and results from the Boundaries For Life initiative that delivered health checks at professional cricket matches over the 2014 and 2015 seasons (Trivedy et al., 2017).

The Boundaries for Life health check service was delivered at professional cricket venues by a team of clinicians, including doctors, dentists, nurses and medical students. There was no cost to either fans or staff to undertake a health check. While anyone over the age of 18 could access the service, it was promoted primarily to people over the age of 40. Overall, 513 participants undertook the checks. Of the 499 where data were available, 338 (67.7 per cent) were fans attending the match, and another 161 (32.3 per cent) were staff employed at the cricket ground as either club staff or event specific staff (e.g. security or catering staff). A total of 84 per cent gave their ethnicity as white (British), 14 per cent were of Asian origin, 1 per cent Chinese and another 1 per cent falling into the 'other' category. Uptake of the checks was significantly high in comparison to other sports settings, with very strong feedback from participants on the convenience of service. These findings provide positive support for cricket as a setting for health promotion in comparison to professional rugby or football matches which have cited problems with recruitment (Whitty and White, 2011; Curran, Drust and Richardson, 2014).

The findings of this pilot study suggests that cricket stadia may be a feasible setting for providing health promotion interventions in populations that may not otherwise engage with primary care. While these checks are not intended to replace NHS health checks, it is clear that such work may play a role in supporting the uptake of statutory checks. In this case, the brand of sport is being capitalised upon to modify health perceptions and ultimately health behaviour. Further research is required to examine the scalability and cost-effectiveness of rolling out similar initiatives on a larger scale.

Improving physical and mental wellbeing: Active Rovers

There is a growing number of studies that health interventions conducted in partnership with professional sport organisations can recruit, retain and improve aspects of physical and mental health (Parnell et al., 2015; Curran et al., 2017). An example of this is the Premier League Health football 12-week intervention programme for men. Despite drawing solely on self-report measures, the study demonstrated how men from diverse backgrounds, with less than optimal lifestyles, improved their health behaviour (Zwolinsky et al., 2013). Professional sport clubs, in particular football, have targeted men with health promotion interventions (Bingham et al., 2014).

Active Rovers is an intervention that targets hard-to-reach men to deliver a programme of physical activity. The intervention aimed to trial a physical activity lifestyle knowledge programme, with respect to changes in mental well-being, health perceptions, and lifestyle knowledge in older hard to reach men living in Wirral, North West England. This intervention was delivered in by Tranmere Rovers Football Club 'Football in the Community' programme. Active Rovers was designed through a partnership between

Tranmere Rovers FC and NHS England, from initial funding received by The Football Foundation, whom are the United Kingdom's largest sports charity and funder of sport-based social projects (Parnell *et al.*, 2015) and was later fully funded by NHS England. Active Rovers comprised a series of mixed exercise programmes delivered on a weekly basis at Prenton Park, the home of Tranmere Rovers FC. The activities include football, walking football, yoga and Tai Chi. The associated football activities were delivered by the (1st4Sport Level 2 Certificate in Coaching Football to the UEFA B Certificate qualified) community coaches. Healthcare professionals, who worked for NHS Wirral, were responsible for delivering the remaining activities (i.e. yoga and Tai chi) health checks (i.e. blood pressure, cholesterol levels and body mass index).

Since the Active Rovers programme commenced in 2010, over 15,000 participants have registered and taken part in the designated activities. The participants were initially recruited via advertisements in Tranmere Rovers FC match-day programmes, social media outlets, and from NHS referral schemes for hard-to-reach (HTR) men. In addition, adverts were placed in the two local newspapers (i.e. The Wirral Globe and The Wirral News). The participants reported improvements in the shortened seven-item Likert scale Warwick-Edinburgh Mental Well-Being Scale (SWEMWBS), alongside positive changes in perceptions of the danger of excessive alcohol. Less successful outcomes were the participants' casual (or other) physical activity outside of the Active Rovers intervention. Despite this, it was suggested that the football club brand and location, Prenton Park may have helped recruit and motivate participants in physical activity, as found elsewhere (Parnell *et al.*, 2015). The practitioner-researcher responsible for the planning and the delivery of the Active Rovers intervention highlighted common problems with rigorous data collection on such stadia-based interventions.

Artificial grass pitches: club and community use

Football in the United Kingdom has seen a sweeping growth in the development of AGPs across the various structures of the games based on the need for a quality assured surface and increased access and use. The development of AGPs has seen significant growth in Western Europe and Scandinavia, where natural pitches can be adversely affected by weather conditions and regular use. While, grassroots football has received significant investment, football clubs have also chosen to install AGPs at their training facilities (Andersson, Ekblom, and Krustrup, 2008; Bjorneboe, Bahr, and Andersen, 2010; Almutawa *et al.*, 2014). The impact of investment in an AGP at a football club is largely unexplored. This research explored the impact of AGP facilities within a semi-professional football club setting for both the football club benefit and the health of the local community.

Maidstone United Football Club were pioneers in the development of AGPs in England, only second to Sutton Coldfield Town in terms of installing an AGP. It is worthwhile noting that no full-time professional clubs in the English league system have installed an AGP. This is because they are currently banned for use in the Football League and Premier League. This means that clubs in the National League (i.e., semi-professional) with ambitions to get promoted into the Football League have not installed AGPs either. English football represents an anomaly in its ban on artificial surfaces in full-time professional football, even within the UK. Scottish Premier League teams Kilmarnock and Hamilton Academical have installed an artificial surface, as have Scottish Championship clubs Queen of the South and Alloa Athletic. Welsh Premier League champions The New Saints also play on an AGP. The uses of AGPs are an ongoing discussion for football stakeholders in England.

Having introduced the AGP, the football club has seen an automatic return in that the pitch was now available and useable, which was impossible previously with a natural pitch. The club now realised that stadium use was dramatically increased through the AGP being accessed for up to 80 hours per week. All 45 of the football clubs teams, from first team, academy and community, we are able to train at the stadium on the AGP. This in turn facilitated increased communication and improved talent identification and development. The AGP allowed for increased community access, allowing increase sports and physical activity participation supporting the public health agenda, while raising the clubs profile in the local community. Finally, the AGP delivered increased income generation supporting the financial sustainability of the club (May and Parnell, 2017).

Summary

This chapter has provided an insight into a settings-based approach to health promotion and an overview of the work of the European Healthy Stadia Network. Industry and research insights into considerations for promoting health within sport stadia settings have been offered, alongside some reflections for future interventions and research. The three case study examples offer an insight into the value and effectiveness of stadia-based health interventions, whether during match days, non-match days, within the stadium and through a novel innovation in the stadia playing surface. It is evident that the Healthy Stadia is, and has been, a key player and significant leader in the development of good practices and helping to establish policy change. Arguably, the growing body of evidence that relates to how amateur and professional sports clubs and their stadia can attend to public health outcomes for fans, visitors, workforces and local communities has also enhanced the movement of setting-based approaches in public health.

One overriding reflection is that we would like to continue the endorsement of commissioning agencies in local and national government in supporting a rigorous evidence base in understanding sport stadia as a setting for health promotion. Further research is needed to understand the impact of population level and individual behaviour change interventions. With this, such research skills need to be shared and developed within operational organisations, in many cases organisation analysts or sports coaches. This capacity building must equip those working in these frontline positions with the understanding of, and ability to, collect reliable and relevant data (for example, physical activity measures: accelerometer data; physical measures: heart rate; and psychosocial measures: interviews and surveys). At present, evidence is limited in some cases, to monitoring, which lacks rigour, depth and independence. We believe it is vital for clubs, national governing bodies of sport and league operators to establish academic partners to assist with programme design and the evaluation of projects.

Statement on intellectual property

The Healthy Stadia word mark and logo mark are registered as official trademarks to the European Healthy Stadia Network CIC Ltd at EU level. Healthy Stadia CIC has granted permission for the word mark 'healthy stadia' to be used by contributing authors, editors and the journal's publication house for this special edition only.

Acknowledgements

The authors would like to acknowledge all of the contributors to Special Issue, Healthy Stadia: An Insight From Policy to Practice. In particularly, authors of the research that we have featured in this chapter, Anthony May, Chet Trivedy, Ivo Vlaev, Russell Seymour, Colin J. Lewis, Matthew J. Reeves and Simon J. Roberts.

Disclosure statement

No potential conflict of interest was reported by the authors.

References

Acheson, D. (1998). *Independent Inquiry into Inequalities in Health: Report*. London: The Stationery Office.

Andersson, H., Ekblom, B., and Krustrup, P. (2008). Elite football on artificial turf versus natural grass: movement patterns, technical standards, and player impressions. *Journal of Sports Sciences*, 26(2), 113–122.

Almutawa, M., Scott, M., George, K. P., and Drust, B. (2014). The incidence and nature of injuries sustained on grass and 3rd generation artificial turf: a pilot study in elite Saudi national team footballers. *Physical Therapy in Sport*, 15, 47–52.

Anagnostopoulos, C. and Shilbury, D. (2013). Implementing corporate social responsibility in English Football: towards multi-theoretical integration. *Sport, Business and Management: An International Journal*, 3(4), 268–284.

Bjorneboe, J., Bahr, R., and Andersen, T. E. (2010). Risk of injury on third-generation artificial turf in Norwegian professional football. *British Journal of Sports Medicine*, 44, 794–798.

Clift, S. and Jensen, B. B. (eds). (2005). *The Health Promoting School: International Advances in Theory, Evaluation and Practice*. Copenhagen, Denmark: Danish University of Education Press.

Curran, K., Bingham, D., Richardson, D., and Parnell, D. (2014). Ethnographic engagement from within a football in the community programme at an English premier league football club. *Soccer and Society*, 15(6), 934–950.

Curran, K., Drust, B., Murphy, R., Pringle, A., and Richardson, D. (2016). The challenge and impact of engaging hard-to-reach populations in regular physical activity and health behaviours: an examination of an English Premier League 'Football in the Community' men's health programme. *Public Health, 135*, 14–22.

Curran, K., Drust, B., and Richardson, D. (2014). 'I just want to watch the match': a practitioner's reflective account of men's health themed match day events at an English premier league football club. *Soccer and Society*, 15(6), 919–933.

Crabb, J. and Ratinckx, L. (2005) *The Healthy Stadia Initiative: A Report for North West Public Health Team*. Preston, UK: Department of Health.

De Leeuw, E. and Skovgaard, T. (2005) Utility-driven evidence for healthy cities: problems with evidence generation and application. *Social Science and Medicine*, 61, 1331–1341.

Diabetes UK (2013). Diabetes in the UK 2013: key statistics on diabetes. *Diabetes UK*, 1 March, https://diabetes.org.uk/About-us/What-we-say/Statistics/Diabetes-in-the-UK-2013-Key-statistics-on-diabetes/ (accessed 30 January 2016).

Drygas, W., Ruszkowska, J., Philpott, M., Bjorkstrom, O., Parker, M., Ireland, R., and Roncarolo, F. (2013). Good practices and health policy analysis in European sports stadia: results from the 'Healthy Stadia' project. *Health Promotion International*, 28(2), 157–165.

Hulton, A., Drust, B., Flower, D., Richardson, D., and Curran, K. (2015). Effectiveness of a community football programme on improving physiological markers of health in a HTR male population. *Soccer and Society*, 17(2), 196–208.

Hunt, K., Wyke, S., Gray, C. M., Anderson, A. S., Brady, A., Bunn, C., and Donnan, P. T. (2014). A gender-sensitised weight loss and healthy living programme for overweight and obese men delivered by Scottish Premier League football clubs (FFIT): a pragmatic randomised controlled trial. *The Lancet*, 383(9924), 1211–1221. doi:http://dx.doi.org/10.1016/S0140-6736(13)62420-4

Ireland, R. and Watkins, F. (2010). Football fans and food: a case study of a football club in the English Premier League. *Public Health Nutrition*, 13(5), 682–687.

Johnson, J. L. (2000) The health care institutions as a setting for health promotion. In B. Poland, L. Green, and I. Rootman (eds), *Settings for Health Promotion: Linking Theory and Practice* (pp. 175–216). Thousand Oaks, CA: Sage Publications.

Lewis, C. J., Reeves, M., and Roberts, S. J. (2017). Improving the physical and mental well-being of typically hard-to-reach men: an investigation of the impact of the Active Rovers project. *Sport in Society*, 20(2), 258–268.

Marmot, M., Allen, J., Goldblatt, P., Boyce, T., McNeish, D., Grady, M., and Geddes, I. (2010). The Marmot review: fair society, healthy lives. *The Strategic Review of Health Inequalities in England Post-2010.*

May, D. and Parnell, D. (2017). The community impact of football pitches: a case study of Maidstone United FC. *Sport in Society*, 20(2), 244–257.

Møller, L., Stover, H., Jurgens, R., Gatherer, A., and Nikogosian, H. (2007) *Health in Prison. A WHO Guide to the Essentials in Prison Health.* WHO Regional Office for Europe, Copenhagen, Denmark.

Parnell, D. and Pringle, A. (2016). Football and health improvement: an emerging field. *Soccer and Society*, 17(2), 171–174.

Parnell, D. and Richardson, D. (2014). Introduction. *Soccer and Society*, 15(6), 823–827.

Parnell, D., Curran, K., and Philpott, M. (2017). Healthy stadia: an insight from policy to practice. *Sport in Society*, 20(2), 181–186.

Parnell, D., Stratton, G., Drust, B., and Richardson, D. (2013). Football in the community schemes: exploring the effectiveness of an intervention in promoting healthful behaviour change. *Soccer and Society*, 14, 35–51.

Parnell, D., Pringle, A., McKenna, J., Zwolinsky, S., Rutherford, Z., Hargreaves, J., Trotter, L., Rigby, M., and Richardson, D. (2015). Reaching older people with PA delivered in football clubs: the reach, adoption and implementation characteristics of the extra time programme. *BMC Public Health*, 15. doi:http://dx.doi.org/10.1186/s12889-015-1560-5. http://biomedcentral.com/1471-2458/15/220

Pelikan, J. M., Krajic, K., and Dietscher, C. (2001). The health promoting hospital (HPH): concept and development. *Patient Education and Counselling*, 45, 239–243.

Philpott, M. and Sagar, D. (2014). Survey of smoke-free policies at football stadia in Europe. *European Health Stadia Network*, 1 June. http://healthystadia.eu/resource-library/alcohol-and-substance-misuse/itemlist/user/63-matthew-philpott.html (accessed 20 December 2015).

Robson, J., Dostal, I., Sheikh, A., Eldridge, S., Madurasinghe, V., Griffiths, C., Coupland, C., and Hippisley-Cox, J. (2016). The NHS health check in England: an evaluation of the first four years. *BMJ Open*, 6(1).

Ruckert, A. and Ronald, L. (2017). Health inequities in the age of austerity: the need for social protection policies. *Social Science and Medicine*, http://dx.doi.org/10.1016/j.socscimed.2017.03.029

Sherriff, J., Griffiths, D., and Daube, M. (2009). Cricket: notching up runs for food and alcohol companies? *Australian and New Zealand Journal of Public Health*, 34, 19–23.

Trivedy, C., Vlaev, I., Seymour, R., and Philpott, M. (2017). An evaluation of opportunistic health checks at cricket matches: the Boundaries for Life initiative. *Sport in Society*, 20(2), 226–234.

Witty, K. and White, A. (2011). Tackling men's health: implementation of a male health service in a rugby stadium setting. *Community Practitioner*, 84(4), 29–33.

Whitehead, D. (2006). The health promoting prison (HPP) and its imperative for nursing. *International Journal of Nursing Studies*, 43, 123–131.

WHO (World Health Organization). (1986). Ottawa Charter for Health Promotion. *Canadian Journal of Public Health*, 77, 425–426.

Zwolinsky, S., McKenna, J., Pringle, A., Daly-Smith, A., Robertson, S., and White, A. (2013). Optimizing lifestyles for men regarded as 'hard-to-reach' through top-flight football/soccer clubs. *Health Education Research*, 28, 405–413.

Index